T0257578

Drug Carrier Systems Handbook

Drug Carrier Systems Handbook

Edited by **Erica Helmer**

FOSTER
A C A D E M I C S

New Jersey

Published by Foster Academics,
61 Van Reypen Street,
Jersey City, NJ 07306, USA
www.fosteracademics.com

Drug Carrier Systems Handbook
Edited by Erica Helmer

International Standard Book Number: 978-1-63242-119-7 (Hardback)

Contents

Preface

In my initial years as a student, I used to run to the library at every possible instance to grab a book and learn something new. Books were my primary source of knowledge and I would not have come such a long way without all that I learnt from them. Thus, when I was approached to edit this book; I became understandably nostalgic. It was an absolute honor to be considered worthy of guiding the current generation as well as those to come. I put all my knowledge and hard work into making this book most beneficial for its readers.

This book compiles contributions of prominent experts and researchers in the multidisciplinary arena of novel drug delivery systems. It gives insights into the ongoing and recent potentialities of various drug delivery systems. Emergence of analytical approaches and capabilities to determine particle sizes in nanometer ranges has focused interest towards nanoparticles for more effective methods of drug delivery. The book assesses and reviews procedures involved in the drug carrier systems to prepare and apply, along with the methodologies necessary to design, develop and characterize them. Some of the important topics are oral delivery of insulin, novel mucoadhesive polymers for nasal drug delivery, amphiphilic cyclodextrins, synthesis, utilities and application of molecular modeling.

I wish to thank my publisher for supporting me at every step. I would also like to thank all the authors who have contributed their researches in this book. I hope this book will be a valuable contribution to the progress of the field.

Editor

Miscellaneous

Amphiphilic Cyclodextrins, Synthesis, Utilities and Application of Molecular Modeling in Their Design

Atena Jabbari and Hamid Sadeghian

Additional information is available at the end of the chapter

1. Introduction

Drug delivery systems that traditionally are used by the patient do not respond the drug delivery's needs of the world. According to the large number of the hydrophilic and hydrophobic drugs, design and synthesis of new drug delivery system seems to be necessary. With the traditional drug delivery systems practically there is no control over the time, location and rate of drug release, in addition to the drug concentration was fluctuated in the blood frequently and may even go beyond the therapeutic dose and less effective and cause more side effects. With the new drug delivery systems that called controlled released drug delivery system, we will be able to control and determine the rate, time and location of drug release. CDs are potential candidate for such a role, because of their ability to change physicochemical and biological properties of guest molecules through the formation of inclusion complexes (Uekama et al,1998). The most common pharmaceutical application of cyclodextrins is to increase the stability, solubility and bioavailibity of drug molecules and other pharmacological benefits,such as the reduction of unwanted side effect (Hedges, 1998).

Cyclodextrins (CD) are macrocyclic oligosaccharides composed of D-(+)-glycopyranosyl units linked α (1→4). CDs are classified as α-,β- and γ-CD according to the number of glucose units: six, seven and eight, respectively. Cyclodextrins have a truncated cone shape with a hydrophilic exterior and a hydrophobic cavity. A guest molecule of appropriaty size and shape is incorporated into hydrophpbic cavity in aqueous media (Szejtli, 1998).

However, the potential use of CDs in biological system needs amphiphilic properties because natural CDs have relatively low solubility both in water and organic solvents, thus limits their uses in pharmaceutical formulations. Amphiphilic or ionizable cyclodextrins can modify the rate or time of drug release and bind to the surface membrane of cells, that may be used for the enhancement of drug absorption across biological barriers.

Amphiphilic cyclodextrins can be obtained by the introduction of lipophilic groups at primary and or secondary face of the CD. Amphiphilic CDs have been shown to form monolayers at the air-water interface (Parot-Lopez, 1992; Greenhall et al, 1995) and micelles in water (Auze'ly-Velty et al, 2000). Different self-organized amphiphilic CDs, such as nanospheres (Skiba et al, 1996), solid-lipid nanoparticles (Dubes, 2003) , liquid crystals (Ling et al, 1993) and vesicles (Ravoo & Darcy, 2000) were prepared with varying length of hydrophobic chains for their promising properties for farmaceutical applications.

Hydrophilic-hydrpphobic balance, molecular shape and solvation have all been enunciated as important criteria for formation of distinct lyotropic assemblies (Israelachvilli, 1985; Fuhrhop & Koning, 1994).

A particulary interesting example of self-assembly of amphiphilic CDs in water is bilayer vesicles. CDs vesicles consist of bilayers of CDs, in which the hydrophobic "tails" are directed inward and the hydrophilic macrocycle"head groups" are facing water, thereby enclosing an aqueous interior. Recently, vesicles composed entirely of nonionic, anionic, and cationic amphiphilic CDs was described (Falvey et al, 2005).

Nano capsules and nanospheres were prepared using amphiphilic β-and γ-CDs modified on the secondary face by nanoprecipitation and emulsion/solvent evaporated techniques avoiding the use of additional surfactant (Woussidjewe et al, 1996).

The first amphiphilic cyclodextrin were synthesized in 1986 by Kwabata et al. The primary OH-groups of β-CD were made lipophilic with alkyl sulfunyl groups with various length. This amphiphilic CD could form monolayer at the air-water interface (Kawabata et al, 1986).

2. Synthesis of amphiphilic cyclodextrins

β-CDs in synthesis of amphiphilic cyclodextrins was used more than α- and γ CDs. Common synthetic path to amphiphilic cyclodextrins was shown in Fig. 1.

2.1. Alkylated, arylated and lipid –Conjugated CDs

Synthesis of alkylated α- and β-CDs and their treatment at air –water interface, have been described by Jurczak et al (Wazynska et al, 2000). Silyl-protected α- or β-CDs was alkylated then desilated to achievement amphiphilic per-(2,3-di-O-alkyl)-CDs (5) (Fig. 2).

Compound (10) which contain amphiphilic chains, was synthesized from per-amino-β-CD using peptide chemistry (Imamura et al, 2002) (Fig. 3). Reason of suitable complexation of anilinonaphthalene sulfonic acid can ralativ to presence of Adipic-glucamine chains that enhance extension of the cavity in this structure. γ-CDs derivatives of this family, can complex with two molecules of anthraquinone-2-sulfonate (Ling & Darcy, 1993) (Fig. 4).

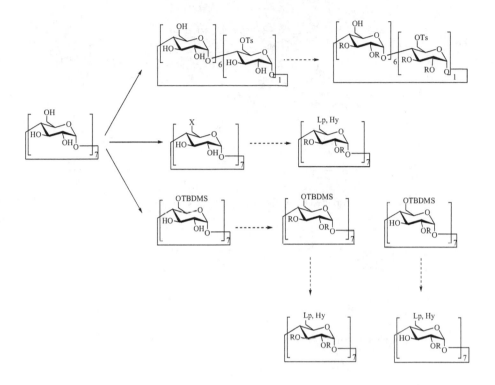

Lp=lipophile, Hy=hydrophile; for Lp,R, is hydrophilic; for Hy ,R ,is lipophilic

Figure 1. Common synthetic path to amphiphilic cyclodextrins

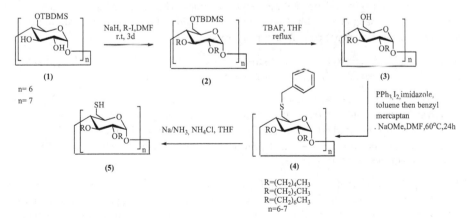

Figure 2. Synthesis of alkylated cyclodextrins

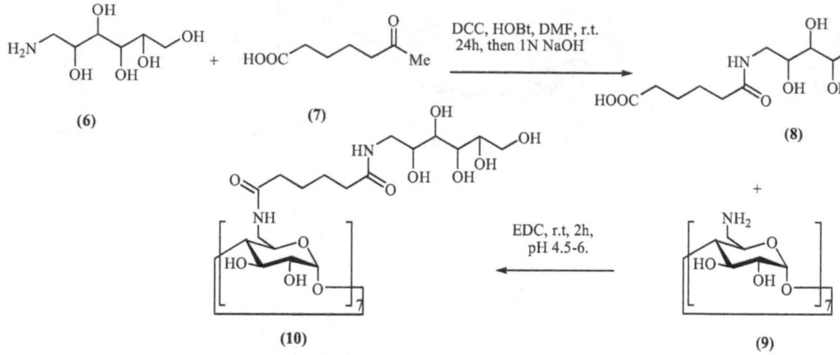

Figure 3. Peptide chemistry was used for synthesis of amphiphilic cyclodextrins

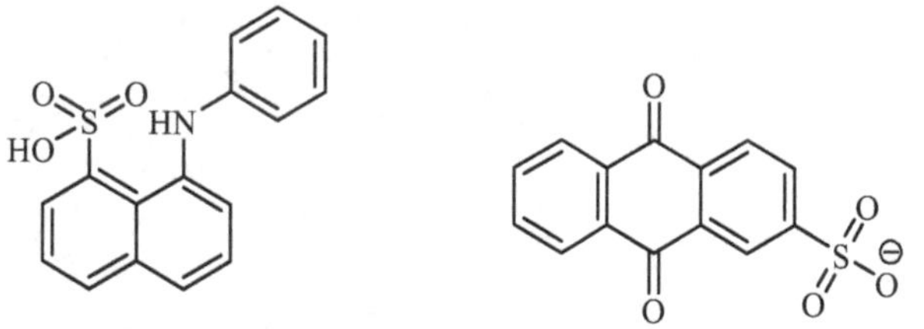

8-Anilino-1-naphtalenesulfonic acid   Anthraquinone-2-sulfonate

(11)   **(12)**

Figure 4. Structures of two guest molecules for complxation with compound (10)

Wu and coworkers in 2010 reported the synthesis of new amphiphilic biodegradable β-cyclodextrin/poly (L-leucine)(β-CD-PLLA) copolymer by ring-opening polymerization of N-carboxy-L-alanine anhydride in N,N-dimethylformamide(DMF) initiated by mono-6-amino-β-cyclodextrin (Zhang et al, 2010). These compound could self- assemble into nano-micelles in water and could be expected to find application in drug delivery systems (Fig. 5).

A novel thiolated carboxymethyl chitosan-g-β-cyclodextrin (CMC-g- β-CD) drug delivery carrier was synthesized by Gong et al (Prabaharan & Gong, 2008).

Thiolated CMC-g- β-CD was prepared using two steps. First ,carboxymethyl- β-CD (CM β-CD) was grafted onto carboxymethyl chitosan (CMC) using water-soluble 1-ethyl-3-(3-dimethylaminopropyl)carbodiimide (EDC) and N-hydroxysuccinimide (NHS) as the condensing agents. Next, the resultant product was further grafted with cycteine methyl ester hydrochloride (CMEH) (Fig. 6).

The drug release showed that thiolated CMC-g- β-CD tablets provided a slower release of the entrapped hydrophobic model drug, ketoprofen, than the chitosan control, and the release behavior was influenced by the amounts of thiol groups present on the polymer chains. These results suggest that thiolated CMC-g- β-CD with improved mucoadhesive

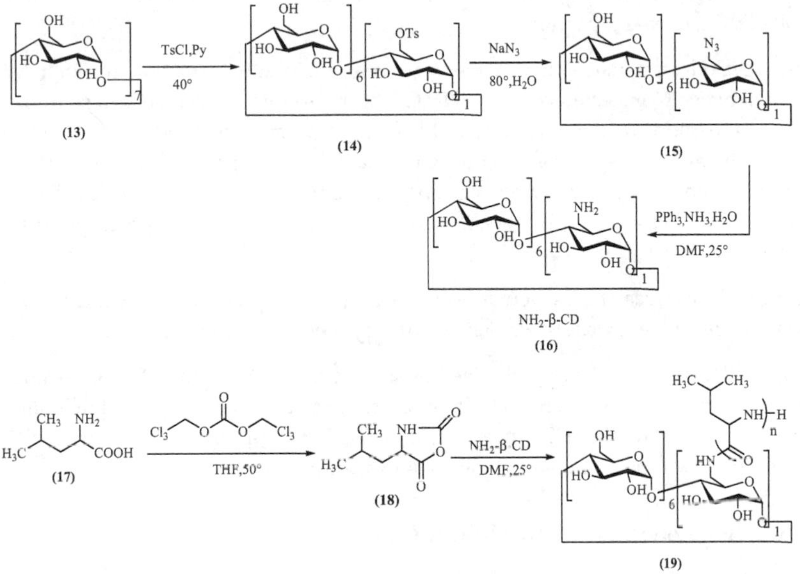

Figure 5. Synthetic pathway to amphiphilic biodegradable β-cyclodextrin/poly (L-leucine)(β-CD-PLLA) copolymer

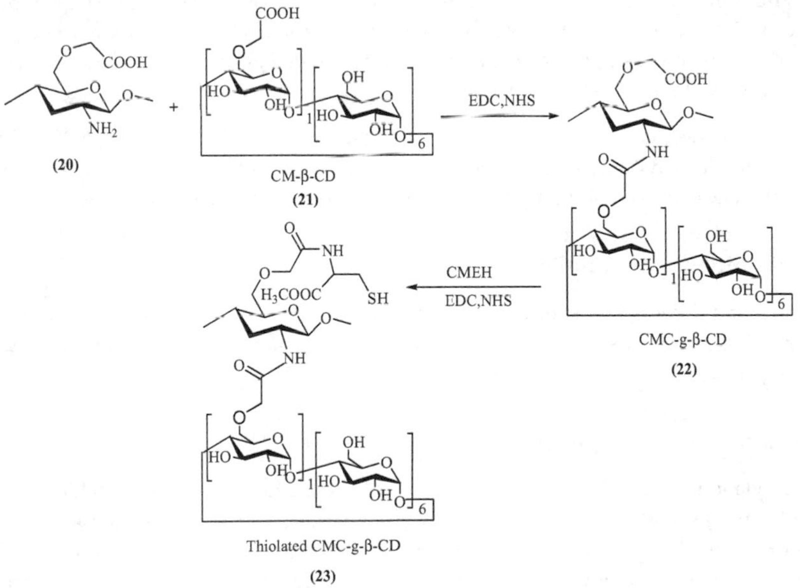

Figure 6. Preparation of thiolated CMC-g- β-CD

properties may potentially become an effective hydrophobic drug delivery system with controlled drug release capability.

Chitosan-cyclodextrin nanosphere were prepared by in situ formation through Michael addition between N-maleated chitosan (NMC) and per-6-thio- β-cyclodextrin sodium salt in an aqueous medium (Wang et al, 2011). This facil preparation method did not involve any organic solvent and surfactant. Through adjusting the preparation conditions, the nanosphere with a relatively narrow size analyzer. Doxorubicin hydrochloride (DOX-HCl), a water soluble anticancer drug, was loaded in the nanosphere with a high encapsulation efficiency (Fig. 7).

Chloesteryl derivatives of CDs were mostly investigated by Pilard and coworkers. Synthetic pathway of one of them was shown below (Auze'ly-Velty et al, 1999) (Fig. 8).

In 2007, Mallet and coworkers synthesized new derivatives of amphiphilic CDs (Collat et al, 2007). These compound were obtained from reaction between carboxylic acid that derivative of chlosterol with di-amino CDs in presence of DCC and 1-hydroxy benzo tri azol(HoBt). These compounds can act similar to biological membrans (Fig. 9).

2.2. Oligo(ethylene oxide) amphiphilic CDs

The first Amphiphilic CD to form bilayer vesicles were reported by Ravoo and Darcy in 2000 (Ravoo & Darcy, 2000; Mazzaglia et al, 2001; Falvey et al, 2005). Synthesis of them initiated from per-6-bromo and at the result of nucleophilic substituation with the sodium or potassium salt of alkyl thiols, per-alkyl thio CDs were prepared then hydroxyl groups that bind to C-2 of these compounds reacted with an excess of ethylene carbonat and finally average of two units of ethylene glycol were located in this position (C-2 of the CD) (Ravoo & Darcy, 2000; Mazzaglia et al, 2001) (Fig. 10).

This reaction was performed with α- and γ-CD subsequently (Falvey et al, 2005). In these derivatives, the cavity size and hydrophilic of the cyclodextrin headgroup increase. Oligo(ethylene oxide) amphiphiles can form bilayer, vesicoles, and nanoparticles.

2.3. Cationic CD amphiphiles

Donohue and coworkers reported the synthesis of CDs in which hydroxyl groups of oligo(ethylene oxide) were substitude with amine groups and their hydrochloride salts were used in gene delivery studies (Donohue et al, 2002) (Fig. 11).

2.4. Anionic CD amphiphiles

With alkylation of CDs by Declercq and coworkers (Leydet et al, 1998), achievement to versatile groups and so new structures were possible. For example Kraus et al with oxidation by osmium tetroxide in presence of 4-methyl morpholine prepared novel alcoholic stractures of mentioned allylic derivatives (Kraus et al, 2001). They converted the resulting diastreoisomeric diols to carboxylated CDs with oxidation (Fig. 12).

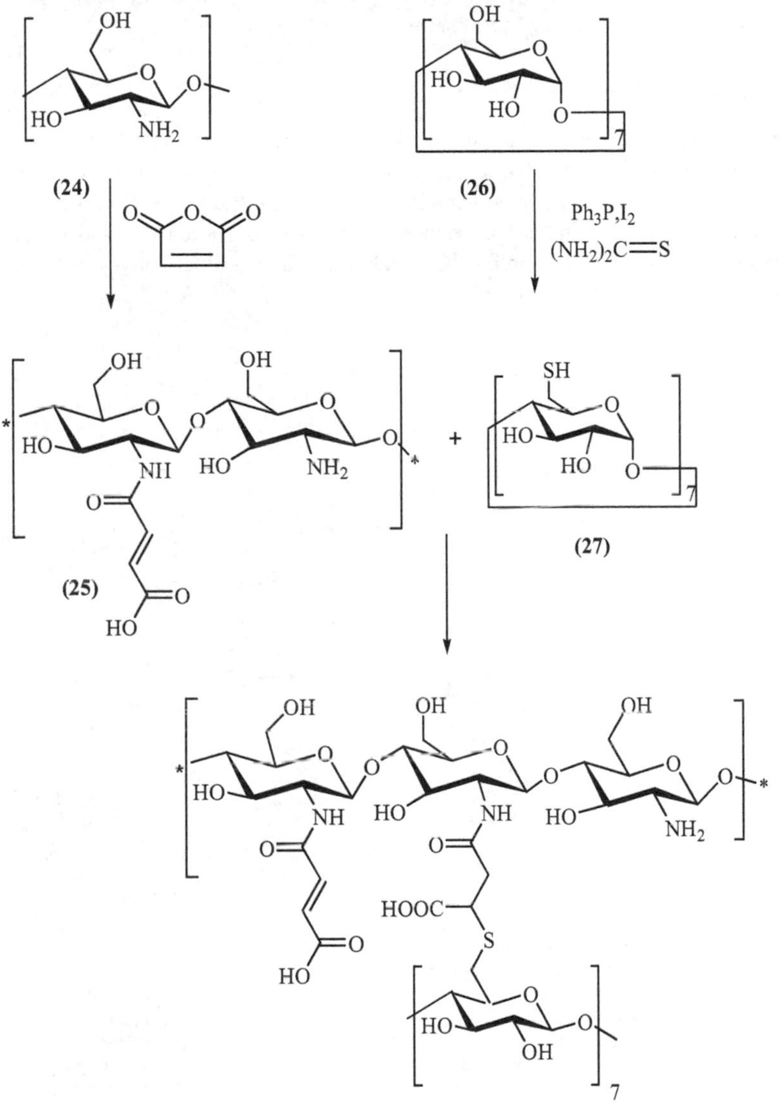

Figure 7. Synthetic path to Chitosan-cyclodextrin nanosphere

The first sulfated amphiphilic CD synthesized by Dubes (Dubes et al, 2001, 2003). They produced compound (48) via esterification of silyl-protected CDs (45) with hexanoic anhydride at position 2 and 3. After removal of the silyl groups, the primary hydroxyl groups were sulfated by SO₃.pyridine complex (Fig. 13).

2.5. Flurinated CD amphiphiles

Granjger and coworkers prepared the per tri fluromethyl thio-β-CD derivative (Granger et al, 2000), which formed monolayer at the air-water interface despite the short hydrophobic chains that applicable in oxygen delivery. Mono- di and per fluoro alkyl thio-CDs (Péroche et al, 2003, 2005) were made subsequently and demonstrated to self-organise into nanosphere in aqueous media, unlike their analogous alkylated derivatives that formed flat particle under same condition (Fig. 14).

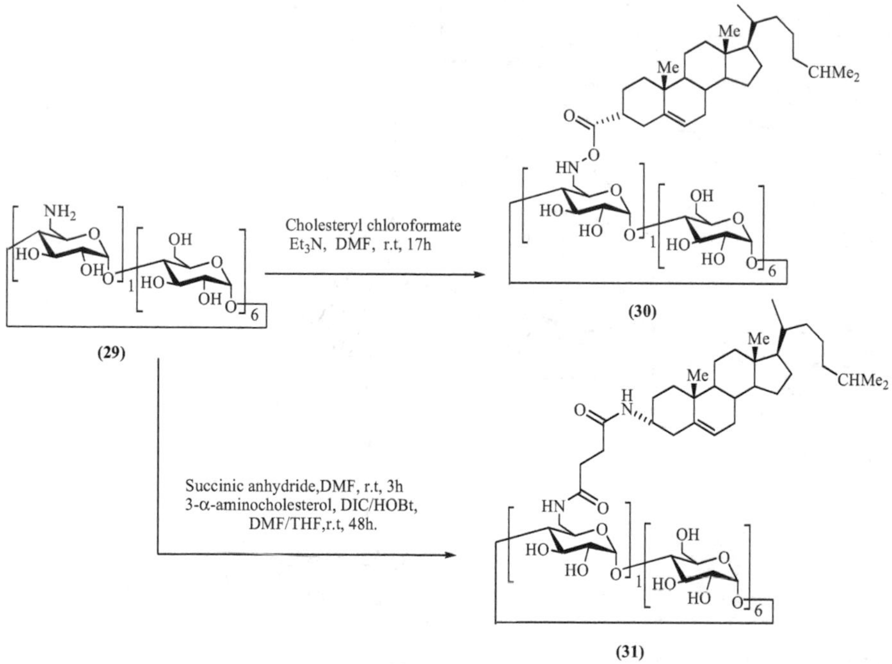

Figure 8. Synthesis of one of chlosteryl derivatives

The synthesis of a γ-CD 6-per fluroalkyl ester was reported by Lim et al (Lim et al, 2006). CD was easily reacted with an excess heptafluoro butanoic acid and finally, compounds were formed that complexes with many substances for example surfactants.

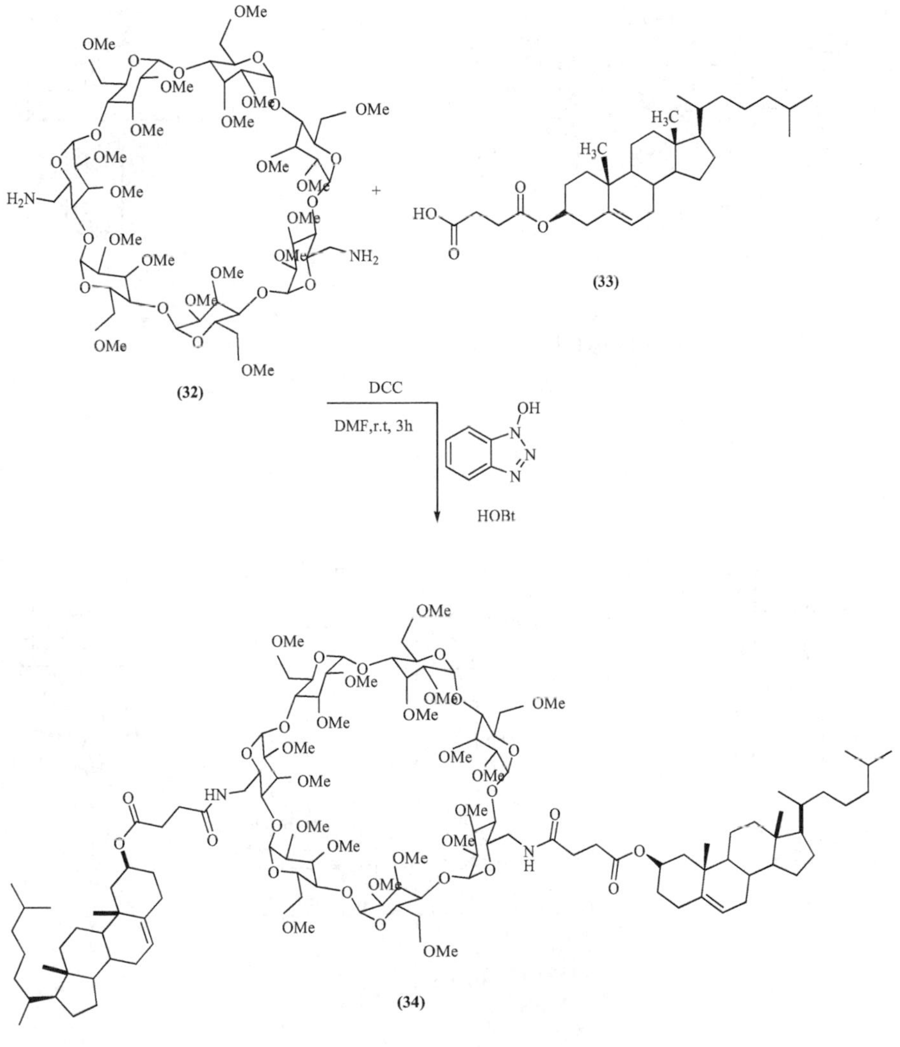

Figure 9. Synthesis of amphiphilic cyclodextrin that can act as similar to biological membrans

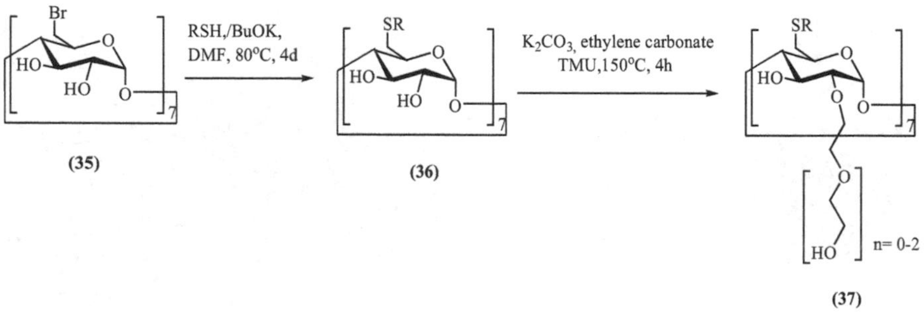

Figure 10. Synthesis of the first oligo(ethylene oxide) amphiphilic cyclodextrin

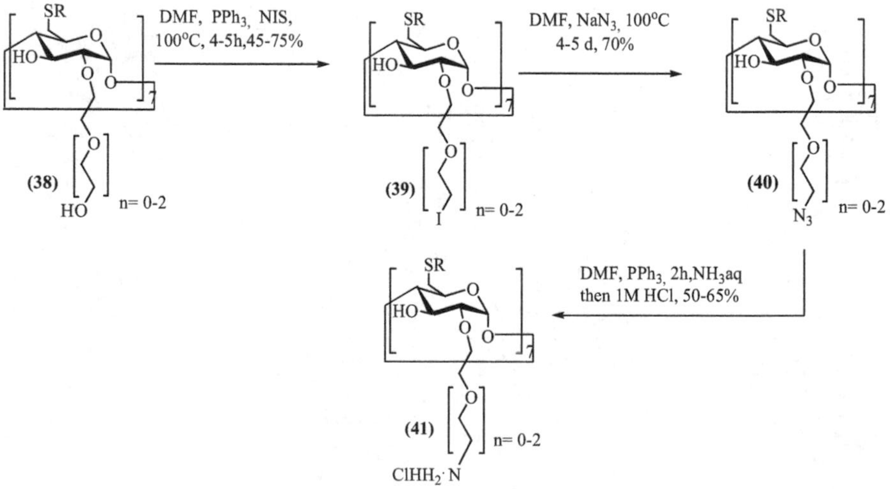

Figure 11. One of synthetic path to cationic cyclodextrin amphiphiles

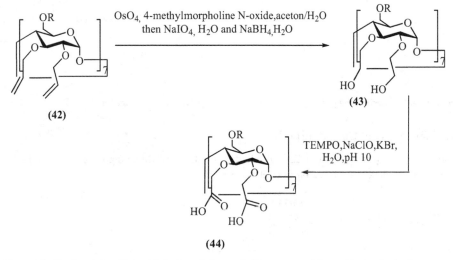

Figure 12. Osmium tetroxide beside to 4-methyl morpholine were used for synthesis of anionic cyclodextrin amphiphiles

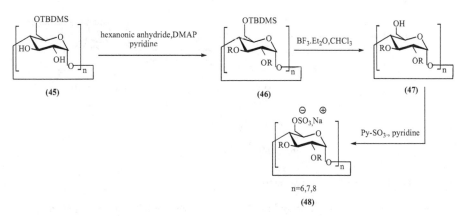

Figure 13. Synthesis of the first sulfated amphiphilic cyclodextrin

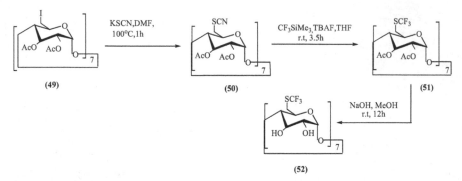

Figure 14. Synthesis of the per tri fluromethyl thio-β-CD derivative by Granger et al

2.6. Glycosylated CD amphiphilic

Sallas and coworkers prepared CDs esterified on the C-2 and C-3 and glycosylated on the C-6 position of glucose units (Sallas et al, 2004) (Fig. 15).

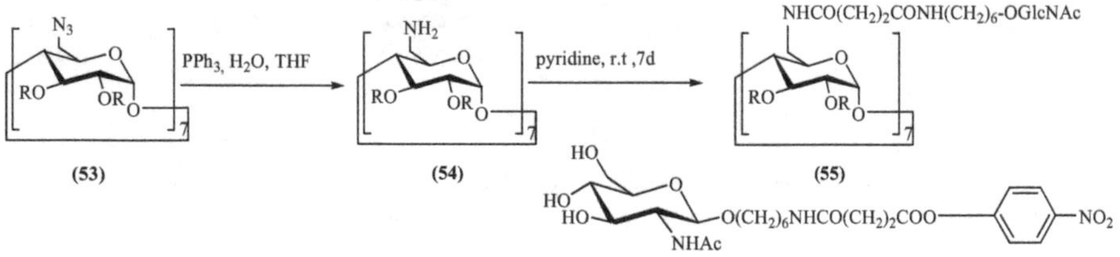

Figure 15. Preparation of glycosylated cyclodextrin amphiphilic

Glycosylation was occurred when a glucosamine having either a terminal amino group or an active ester group was reacted with amino CDs (Fig. 16).

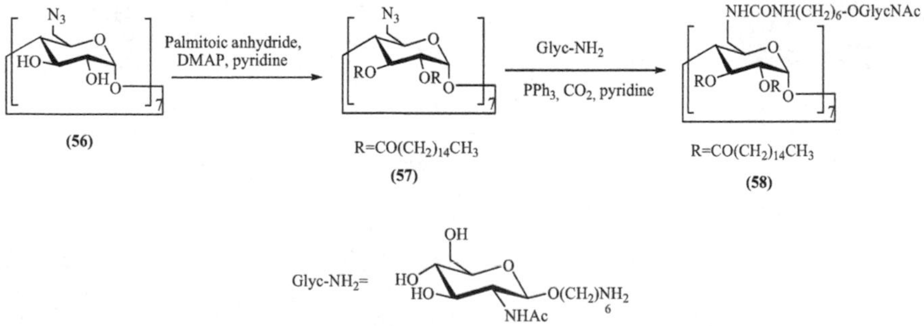

Figure 16. Glycosylation of amino cyclodextrins

A Staudinger reaction in pyridine and in presence of carbon dioxide led to the glycosylated CDs that having a urea function.

Other type of glycosylated amphiphilic CDs have been prepared from oligo(ethylene oxide) CD amphiphile by Mazzaglia et al (Mazzaglia et al, 2004). Despite the existence of seven glycosyl groups, these compound aggregrated in water into vesicles (Fig. 17).

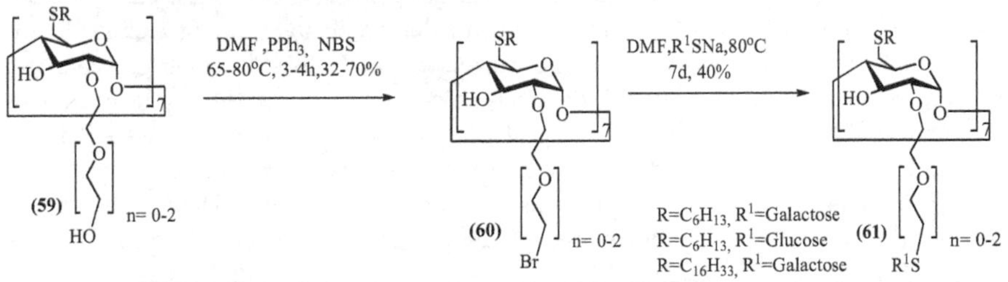

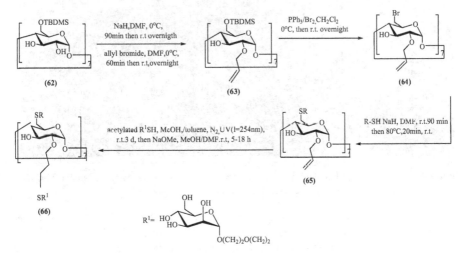

Figure 17. Glycosylation of oligo(ethylene oxide) cyclodextrin

Photochemical addition of sugar thiol to allylic groups on the CDs was another pathway for glycosylated CDs (Fulton & Stoddart, 2001). The hydroxyl groups can be protected with silyl groups, then allylated the hydroxyl groups (on the position 2). This pathway has been further developed to create a variety of glycosylated amphiphilic CD such as (66) (Nicholas, 2005) (Fig. 18).

Figure 18. Photochemical addition, another path for synthesis of glycosylated cyclodextrin

3. Molecular modeling in designing of host molecules

Prediction of host-geust binding affinity could be made by calculating the binding energy. It could be down in molecular modeling software such as HyperChem (http://www.hyper.com/). In such software we can design and optimize the geometry of host and gust molecule separately and then by introducing the guest molecule in the cavity of host molecule, the geometry of the combined structure is optimized. Then the total energy of the host, guest and host-guest structures are separately calculated by single point command under one of the molecular calculation methods: molecular mechanics, semi-empirical, *ab-initio* or DFT. By subtracting the single point energy of host-guest complex from sum of the host and guest energy, we can determine the binding energy. In this procedure there is some incompetency: Construction of the best geometry depends on oreintention loaded into the cavity of the host molecule. For example in fig.18 we can see two opposite and acceptable oreientaions of the dopamine in the cavity of the Heptakis [6-O-(N-acetyl-L-Valyl)]-α-cyclodextrin in the screen of the hyperchem software (Fig. 19). For this case, binding energy of both models must be separately calculated. The orientation with less energy is the preferable binding model for analyzing.

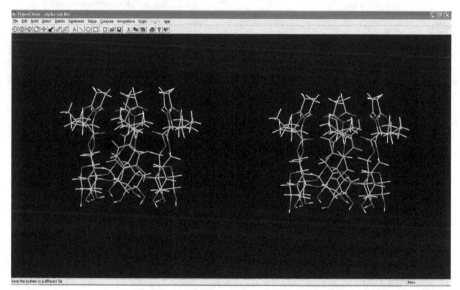

Figure 19. Stick view of the two binding model of dopamine loaded in the cavity of Heptakis [6-O-(N-acetyl-L-Valyl)]-α-cyclodextrin in the screen of the hyperchem software.

In docking software, there is not such a mentioned limitation. In this software we can search all of the possible oreientation and rise to further acceptable binding conformers. This kind of molecular modeling operates based on the two combined calculation methods: local search and genetic algorithm known as Lamarckian Genetic Algorithm (LGA) (Morris et al, 1998). In this procedure the best binding conformation of the gust molecule based on the intermolecular interactions such as hydrogen binding, electrostatic force and ... is achieved.

AutoDockTools, also known as ADT, is an easy-to-use graphical front-end to the automated docking software packages AutoDock and AutoGrid (Phyton, 1999). ADT provides menus to:

- set up a ligand (the 'moving' molecule to be docked) and write out a PDBQ file;
- set up a macromolecule (the 'fixed' molecule being docked to) and output a PDBQS file with solvation parameters;
- assign Kollman United Atom charged to a protein or peptide, or DNA or RNA;
- compute Gasteiger PEOE partial charges for small molecules or cofactors;
- add polar hydrogens, or 'merge' non-polar hydrogens;
- set up a grid box for atomic affinity grid maps and electrostatic potential maps around the target macromolecule (the box is a cubic space with definable center and dimension length);
- set various docking parameters;
- write GPF and DPF files (grid parameter and docking parameter files);
- launch AutoDock and AutoGrid calculations;
- read in DLG files (docking log files) and visualize AutoDock results;
- cluster and re-cluster docking results in various ways.

The ADT software is programmed for modeling of ligand-protein interactions. For small part of a protein (active site pocket) we set a restricted region as grid box, where docking operation performs in it. For host molecules with less than 4-5 KD, it could be defined so that all of the molecular structures located there (Fig. 20).

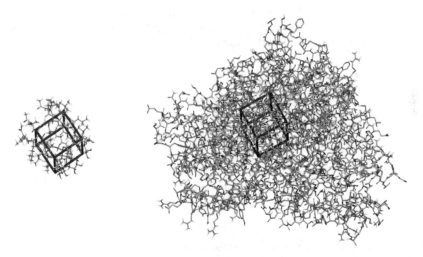

Figure 20. Comparison between the two host molecule grid boxes with the same size in ADT software: soybean 15-lipoxygenase enzyme (right) and a suggested host molecule with 2.6 KD molecular weight.

For reducing the formation of unfavorable binding conformer of gust molecules it is better to limit the size of the grid box around the internal space of the host molecule cavity. By doing the mentioned work, the external binding conformers will not originated by software and population of suitable conformers is increased.

In modeling project, for a series of homolog guest molecules, it ought to be the docking results compare with the experimental data (extraction content, binding affinity, phase transferring ability with considering of lipophilic factors such as logD, and ...). This comparison help us to reach the best binding conformation and it able us to predict the new structure of host molecule for better scavenging results. It lead us about how structure modifications, such as grafting of electronegative atoms, increase or decrease of lipophilic properties by introducing of hydrophobic substituents, could be made. Recently we have shown the ability of the mentioned calculating methods for a new series of peptide - βcyclodextrins as suitable host molecules for phase transferring of glucosamine (Seyedi et al, 2010).

3.1. Amphiphilic peptide-cyclodextrins: Synthesis, designing and their utility as drug carrier: A novel experience

Among the amphiphilic cyclodextrin, amphiphilic peptide-cyclodextrins (APCs) is one of the new and interesting case for studying in drug delivery field. In the aforementioned molecules, hydrophobic residues are aligned above the CD ring *via* amid or ester bonds and the cylindrical structure shape is observed in which the outer part is hydrophobic (duo to hydrophobic amino acids) while the head (CD ring) possess the hydrophilic nature. The structure was stabilized by cross intermolecular hydrogen bonds of amide groups. This molecular structure has ability for introducing the polar molecules into its cavity and transfer of them across the lipophil phases (Fig. 21).

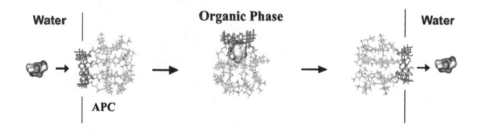

Figure 21. Transport of drug molecules across the organic phase by APC. The cyclodextrin ring and peptide moieties are distinguished by blue and green color respectively.

Our interested in design and synthesis of β-CD peptide derivatives emerges from the work of Imamura and co-workers in which preparation of amphiphilic compounds from per-amino-β-CD using peptide chemistry was reported. The desired amphiphilic structures have been produced from ester linkage between all the C-6 of β-CD and the carboxyl group of N-acetylated resides: H₂N-Leu-COOH, H₂N-Leu-Gly-COOH, H₂N-Leu-Gly-Leu-COOH and H₂N-Leu-Gly-Leu-Gly-COOH (Fig. 22).

In this molecular designing, L-leucine (Leu), the most lipophilic amino acid, was selected for extension of the cavity of β-CD and organizing an external lipophilic structure. Due to the inhibiting effect of pH on the amphiphilic property of the compounds, the *N*-acetyl form of the aforementioned residues was used. To prevent steric hindrance adjust to leucine, Gly was selected as the preferred connector of the two residues.

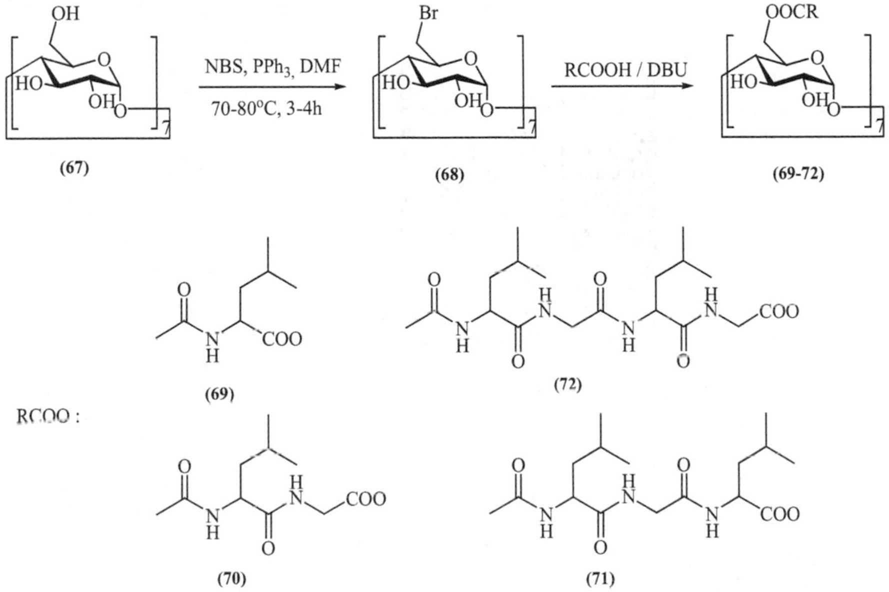

Figure 22. General procedure for the synthesis of amphiphilic peptide β-CDs (69-72).

Binding behavior was studied using glucosamine as a guest molecule. The relative binding affinity of 69-72 toward glucosamine was measured using a phase extraction method. the decrease in concentration of aqueous glucosamine (pH 7.4) after shaking for 12 h with a lipid phase (octanol) containing 69-72 and β-CD was determined and reported as extraction content (%E).

the equilibrium constant of extraction could be defined as the binding constant (K_b):

$$K_b = ([\text{host-Glu}])/([\text{Glu}][\text{host}] \tag{1}$$

$$\text{host} + \text{Glu} \rightleftarrows \text{host-Glu}$$

The observed glucosamine binding constants (K_b) of 69-72 are outlined in Table 2.

In the other experiment, phase transfer of glucosamine by 69-72 and β-CD was determined. In this work the tendency of each compound for glucosamine transferring between two aqueous phases, separated by octanol, was measured (Fig. 23). Two stirred aqueous phases (pH 7.4), in which one of them (primary phase) contained glucosamine (25 mM), were connected through octanol, containing test compound (69-72 and β-CD; 5 mM), without any solvent diffusion. After 24 h the glucosamine concentration of the intact aqueous phase (secondary phase), was determined. The ratio of glucosamine concentration of the primary and secondary phases was recorded as phase transferring extent (%T).

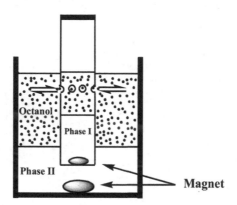

Figure 23. Schematic presentation of the apparatus used for phase transfer experiment

Case	%E	%T
69	24.4 ± 0.9	1.62 ± 0.3
70	23.8 ± 2.2	1.50 ± 0.2
71	28.6 ± 1.8	3.49 ± 0.3
72	26.3 ± 1.2	1.63 ± 0.4
CD	0.40 ± 0.2	0.74 ± 0.1
Ctr.	0.21 ± 0.1	0.43 ± 0.1

Table 1. Extraction and phase transferring percentage of glucosamine (%E and %T respectively) by compounds 69-72.

Among the tested compounds, a modest phase transfer was observed for 71, while the experiments with 69-70 and 72 showed worse results (Table 1). Phase transfer of glucosamine by β-CD was significantly lower.

To explore the origin of these effects, the octanol-water disturbtion coefficient (logD) of 69-72 was measured using shake flask method (Griffin et al, 1999). On the other hand by considering the logD values, the phase transfer results of 69-72 could be rationalized. It was concluded that more lipophilic host molecule (71: logD 1.57) has a higher capability for transferring glucosamine in determined period time.

To complete the study, the binding affinity of glucosamine toward 69-72 was calculated and reported as estimated binding free energy (ΔG_b). In this section, the 3D structures of 69-72 were modeled *via* grafting the desired residues on all primary hydroxyls of β-CD crystal structure followed by geometry optimization (PM3 methods). In the modeled molecules, residues are aligned above the β-CD ring and the cylindrical structure shape is observed in which the outer part is hydrophobic while the head (β-CD ring) possess the hydrophilic nature. The structure was stabilized by cross intermolecular hydrogen bonds of amide groups. The binding affinity was estimated in AuoDockTools software using autodock4.0 program (Python, 1999). 100 docked conformers of glucosamine were generated in ADT software for each of 69-72. The detailed assessment of all 100 docked models revealed as followings: 100% of docking results had nearly identical orientations in the β-CD ring with average ΔG_b of -5.81 kcal/mol for **69**; while for **70**, 68% of docking results had nearly identical orientations in the β-CD ring and 32% in the pocket formed by the residues with average ΔG_b of -6.13 and -6.25 kcal/mol respectively; for 71, 58% of docking results had nearly identical orientations in β-CD ring and 42% in the mentioned pocket with average ΔG_b of -5.62 and -5.45 kcal/mol respectively and finally for 72, 69% of docking results had nearly identical orientations in β-CD ring and 31% in the mentioned pocket with average ΔG_b of -6.14 and -6.08 kcal/mol respectively (table 2). Due to the orientation mentioned above, the docked conformers displayed hydrogen bonds with hydroxyl and amides of the sugars and residues in 69-72. Considering ΔG^o_b = -RTlnK$_b$ and equation (1), the high similarity between experimental and theoretical results (ΔG^o_b and ΔG_b respectively) was anticipated.

Compd.	ΔG_b	ΔG^o_b	K_b	logD
69	-5.81 ± 0.13	-2.62	84.2	1.17 ± 0.07
70	-6.17 ± 0.22	-2.60	80.8	1.05 ± 0.04
71	-5.55 ± 0.26	-2.79	110.8	1.57 ± 0.05
72	-6.11 ± 0.29	-2.70	95.6	1.11 ± 0.09

Table 2. Octanol-water disturbtion coefficient (logD), experimental free energy of binding (ΔG^o_b), binding constant (K$_b$) and average of estimated free energy of binding (ΔG_b) for compounds 69-72.

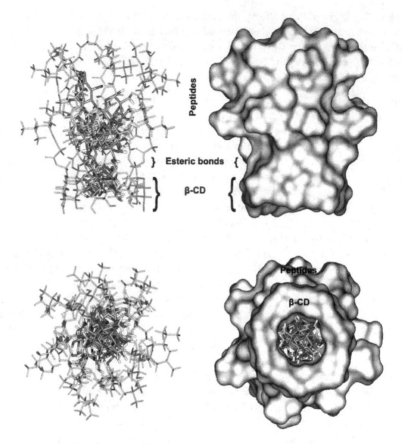

Figure 24. All of the Docked models of glucosamine in the cavity of 72. The below figure represents the cross view of docked models in 3d cavity.

Docking results of 69-72, showed that the binding free energy of glucosamine for all of the host molecules are almost equal and the docked models are mainly located in β-CD cavity. This could explain why the extraction contents and K$_b$ of 69-72 are similar.

Phase transfer properties of 69-72 is mainly depend on the external lipophilic character of their cavity while the host molecules have similar binding affinity toward glucosamine, the more lipophilic one (71), would transfer higher quantities of the guest molecule.

This kind of molecular modeling method operated based on the two calculation methods: local search and genetic algorithm. In this It could be useful for further design of host molecules. Recently we have show the ability of the menthioned calculating methods for a new series of peptide-α-cyclodextrins as a suitable host molecules for extracting of dopamine (Seyedi et al, 2011).

4. Conclusion

In summary, we have designed and synthesized a new series of hydrophobic peptide β-cyclodextrins as a phase transfer carrier for glucosamine. These types of cage-molecules could be a precursor for designing and synthesis of other similar molecules as carriers for desired biological compounds in the future. Considering the external hydrophobicity and terminal hydrophilicity of these molecular structures, it would be hypothesized, that the natural capacity of these compounds to locate in the bilayer membrane of the cells, act as a channel for transferring special compounds.

By using of the molecular modeling techniques, down by the molecular interaction stimulator softwares, we can design a suitable host APC for recognition and scavenging a desired guest molecule. The mentioned method helps us for predicting which of the cyclodextrin types (α, β or γ type), how long of the peptide chains and what kinds of the amino acids could be suitable for the synthesis of an efficient host APC. In this chapter we discussed about the principles of the APCs modeling, host-guest interactions, synthetic methods and the application of them in drug delivery systems.

Author details

Hamid Sadeghian
Department of Laboratory Sciences, School of Paramedical Sciences, Mashhad University of Medical Sciences, Mashhad, Iran

Atena Jabbari
Department of Chemistry, School of Sciences, Ferdowsi University, Mashhad, Iran

5. References

Auto Dock Tools (ADT), the Scripps Research Institute, 10550 North Torrey Pines Road, La Jolla, CA 92037-1000, USA Python, M. F. S. (1999). Python: A Programming Language for Software Integration and Development. *J. Mol. Graphics Mod.*, Vol.17,No.1, pp. 57-61, ISSN 1093-3263 http://www.scripps.edu/pub/olson-web/doc/autodock

Auze´ly-Velty, R.; Djedaı¨ni-Pilard, F.; De´sert, S; Perly, B. & Zemb T. (2000).Micellization of hydrophilic modified cyclodextrins.1. micellar structure. *Langmuir*, Vol.16, No.8, pp. 3727–3734, ISSN 0743-7463

Auzély-Velty, R.; Perly, B.; Taché, O.; Zemb, T.; Jéhan, P.; Guenot, J.-P. Dalbiez, P. & Djedaïni-Pilard, F. (1999). *Carbohydr. Res.* Vol. 318, No.1-4, pp. 82–90, ISSN 0008-6215

Collat, M.; Garcia-Moreno, M. I.; Fajolles, C.; Roux, M.; Mauclaire, L. & Mallet, J. M. (2007). Bis antenna amphiphilic cyclodextrins: the first examples. *Tetrahedron. Lett*, Vol.48, No.48, pp. 8566-8569, ISSN 0040-4039

Donohue, R.; Mazzaglia, A.; Ravoo, B. J. & Darcy, R. (2002). Cationic –β-cyclodextrin bilayer vesicles. *Chem.Commn.* Vol.2002, No.23, pp. 2864-2865, 0022-9936

Dubes, A.; Degobert, G.; Fessi, H. & Parrot-Lopez , H. (2003). Synthesis and characterization of sulfated amphiphilic α- β-and γ- cyclodextrins: application to the complexation of acyclovir. *Carbohydr. Res.*Vol.338, No.21, pp. 2185– 2193, ISSN 0008-6215

Dubes, A.; Parrot-Lopez, H.; Abdelwahed, W.; Degobert, G.; Fessi, H.; Shahgaldian , P. & Coleman, A.W. (2003). Scanning electron microscopy and atomic force microscopy imaging of solid lipid nanoparticles derived from amphiphilic cyclodextrins. *Eur. J. Pharm. Biopharm,* Vol.55, No.3, pp. 279–282, ISSN 0939-6411

Dubes, A.; Bouchu, D.; Lamartine, R. & Parrot-Lopez, H. (2001). An efficient region-specific synthesis route to the multiply substituted acyl-sulphated β-cyclodextrins. *Tetrahedron Lett,* Vol.42, No.11, pp. 9147–9151, ISSN 0040-4039

Falvey, P.; Lim, C. W.; Darcy, R.; Revermann, T.; Karst, U. M.; Giesbers, A.; Marcelis, M.; Lazar, A.; Coleman, A. W. D.; Reinhoudt, N. B. & Ravoo , J. (2005). Bilayer vesicles of amphiphilic cyclodextrins: host membranes that recognize guest molecules. *Chem. Eur. J,* Vol.11, No.6, pp. 1171–1180, ISSN 0947-6539

Fulton, D. A. & Stoddart, J. F. (2001). Synthesis of cyclodextrin-based carbohydrate clusters by photoaddition reactions. *J. Org. Chem,* Vol.66, No.25, pp. 8309– 8319, ISSN 0022-3263

Granger, C. E.; Félix, C. P.; Parrot-Lopez, H. P.& Langlois B. R. (2000). Flurine containing β-cyclodextrin: a new class of amphiphilic carriers. *Tetrahedron Lett,* Vol.41, No.48, pp. 9257–9260, ISSN 0040-4039

Greenhall, M.H.; Lukes, P.; Kataky, R.; Agbor, N.E.; Badyal, J.P.S;. Yarwood, J.; Parker, D. & Petty, M.C. (1995). Monolayer and multilayer flims of cyclodextrins substituted with two and three alkyl chains. *Langmuir,*Vol.11, No.10, pp. 3997–4000, ISSN 0743-7463

Griffin, S.; Wyllie, S. G. & Markham, J. (1999). Determination of octanol-water partition coefficient for terpenoids using reverswd-phase high-performance liquid chromatography. *J. Chromatogr.* Vol.846, No.2, pp.221-228.

Hedges, A.R. (1998). Industrial applications of cyclodextrins. *Chem. Rev,* Vol.98, No.5, pp. 2035-2044, ISSN 0009-2541

Imamura, K.; Ikeda, H. & Ueno, A. (2002). Enhanced binding ability of β-cyclodextrin bearing seven hydrophobic chains each with a hydrophilic end group. *Chem. Lett,* Vol.31, No.5, pp. 516–517, ISSN 0336-7022

Israelachvilli, J. N. (1985). Intermolecular and Surface Forces: With Application to Colloidal and Biological Systems, Academic Press, New York. (b) Fuhrhop, J.-H. & Koning, J. (1994). Membranes and Molecular Assemblies: The Synkinetic Approach, *Royal Society of Chemistry, Cambridge.*

Kawabata, Y. ; Matsumoto, M.; Tanaka, M.; Takahashi, H.; Irinatsu, Y.; Tamara, S.; Tagaki, W.; Nakahara , H. & Fukuda, K. (1986). Formation and deposition of monolayers of amphiphilic –β-cyclodextrin derivatives. *Chem. Lett.*Vol.11, No.12, pp. 1933–1934, ISSN 1157-1489

Kraus, T.; Budesinsky, M .& Zavada,J. (2001). General approach to the synthesis of persubstituted hydrophilic and amphiphilic cyclodextrin derivatives. *J. Org. Chem,* Vol.66, No.13, pp. 4595–4600, ISSN 0022-3263

Leydet, A.; Moullet, C.; Roque, J. P.; Witvrouw, M.; Pannecouque, C.; Andrei, G.; Snoeck, R. Neyts, J.; Schols, D. & De Clercq, E. (1998). Polycationic compound and polyzwitterionic compound derived from cyclodextrins as inhibitors of HIVtransmission. *J. Med. Chem*, Vol. *41, No*.25, pp. 4927–4932, 0022-2623

Lim, K. T.; Ganapathy, H. S., Lee, M. Y.; Yuvaraj, H.; Lee, W.-K. & Heo, H. (2006). Afacil one-pote synthesis of novel amphiphilic perfluoroalkyl ester functionalized γ-cyclodextrin and complex formation with anionic surfactants. *J. Fluorine Chem*, Vol.127, No.6, pp. 730–735, ISSN 0022-1839

Ling, C.-C. & Darcy, R. (1993). 6-S- hydroxyethylated 6- thiocyclodextrins: expandable host molecules. *J. Chem. Soc. Chem. Commun*, Vol.1993, No.1, pp. 203-205, ISSN 0022-4936

Ling, C.C.; Darcy, R. & Risse, W. (1993). Cyclodextrin liquid crystals: synthesis and self-organization of amphiphilic thio-β-cyclodextrins. *J. Chem. Soc. Chem. Commun*. Vol.1993, No.5, pp. 438–440, ISSN 0022-4936

Mazzaglia, A.; Donohue, R.; Ravoo, B. J. & Darcy, R. (2001). Novel amphiphilic cyclodextrins: graft- synthesis of heptakis (6-alkylthio-6-deoxy)-β-cyclodextrin 2-oligo(ethylene glycol) conjugate and their ω-halo derivatives. *Eur. J. Org. Chem*, Vol.2001, No.9, pp. 1715–1721, ISSN 1434-193X

Mazzaglia, A.; Forde, D.; Garozzo, D.; Malvagna, P.; Ravoo, B. J. & Darcy, R. (2004). Multivalent binding of galactosylated cyclodextrin vesicles to lectin. *Org. Biomol. Chem*, Vol.2, No.7, pp. 957–960.

Mc Nicholas, S .(2005). Ph. D. Thesis, University College Dublin, Dublin, Ireland.

Morris, GM.; Goodsell, DS.; Halliday, RS.; Huey, R.; Hart, WE.; Belew, RK. & Olson, JA. (1998). Automated docking using a lamarckian genetic algoritm and an empirical bonding free energy function. J Comput Chem, Vol.19, No.14, pp. 1639-1662, ISSN 1096-987X

Parrot-Lopez, H.; Ling, C.C.; Zhang, P.; Baszkin, A.; Albrecht, G.; De Rango, C. & Coleman, A.W. (1992). Self-assembling systems of the amphiphilic cationic per-6- amino-beta-cyclodextrin 2,3-Di-O-alkyl ethers. *J. Am. Chem. Soc*. Vol.114, No.13, pp. 5479–5480, ISSN 0002-7863

Péroche, S. & Parrot-Lopez, H. (2003). Novel fluorinated amphiphilic cyclodextrin derivatives: synthesis of mono-, di- and heptakis-(6-deoxy-6- per fluoroalkylthio)-β-cyclodextrin. *Tetrahedron Lett*. Vol.44, No.2, pp. 241–245, ISSN 0040-4039

Péroche, S.; Degobert, G.; Putaux, J.-L.; Blanchin, M.-G.; Fessi, H. & Parrot-Lopez, H. (2005). Synthesis and characterization of novel nanospheres made from amphiphilic perfluoroalkylthio-β cyclodextrins. *Eur. J. Pharm. Biopharm*, Vol.60, No.1, pp. 123–131, ISSN 1434-193X

Prabaharan, M. & Gong, S. (2007). Novel thiolated carboxymethyl chitosan-g-b-cyclodextrin as mucoadhesive hydrophobic drug delivery carriers. Carbohydrate Polymers , Vol.73, No.1, pp. 117–125, ISSN 0144-8617

Ravoo, B. J. & Darcy, R. (2000). Cyclodextrin bilayer vesicles. *Angew. Chem. Int. Ed*. Vol.39, No.23, pp. 4324–4326, ISSN 1433-7851

Ravoo, B.J. & Darcy, R. (2000). Cyclodextrin bilayer vesicles. *Angew. Chem. Int. Ed*. Vol.39, No.23, pp. 4324–4326, ISSN 1433-7851

Sallas, F.; Niikura, K. & Nishimura S.-I. (2004). Apractical synthesis of amphiphilic cyclodextrins fully substituted with sugar residue on the primary face. *Chem. Commun,* Vol.2004, No.5, pp. 596–597, ISSN 0022-9936

Seyedi, S. M.; Sadeghian, H.; Jabbari, A.; Assadieskandar, A. & Momeni, H. (2010). Design and synthesis of a new series of amphiphilic peptide-β-cyclodextrins as phase transfer carriers for glucosamine. *Tetrahedron,* Vol.66, No.34, pp. 6754-6760, ISSN 0040-4020

Seyedi, S. M.; Sadeghian, H.; Jabbari, A.; Assadieskandar, A. & Momeni, H. (2011). Synthesis of new series of α-cyclodextrin esters as dopamine carrier molecule. *Bioorg. Med. Chem,* Vol.19, No.14, pp. 4307-4311, ISSN 0968-0896

Skiba, M.; Duche`ne, D.; Puisieux, F. & Wouessidjewe D.(1996). Development of a new colloidal drug carrier from chemically modified cyclodextrins: nanospheres and influence of physicochemical and technological factores on particle size. *Int. J. Pharm,* Vol.129, No.2, pp. 113–121, ISSN 0975-1491

Szejtli, J. (1998). Introduction and general overview of cyclodextrin chemistry. *Chem. Rev,* Vol.98, No.5, pp. 1743–1754, ISSN 0009-2541

Uekama, K.; Hirayama, F. & Irie, T. (1998). Cyclodextrin drug carrier systems. *Chem. Rev,* vol.98, No.5, pp. 2045–2076, ISSN 0009-2541

Wang, J.; Zong, J.-Y.; Zhao, D.; Zhuo, R.-X. & Cheng, S.-X. (2011). In situ formation of chitosan-cyclodextrin nanospheres for drug delivery. *Colloids and Surfaces B: Biointerfaces,* Vol. 87, No.1, pp. 198– 202, ISSN 0927-7765

Wazynska, M.; Temeriusz, A.; Chmurski, K.; Jurczak. J. & Bilewicz, R. (2000). Synthesis and monolayer behavior of amphiphilic per (2,3-di-O-alkyl) - and β- cyclodextrins and hexakis (6-deoxy-6-thio-2,3-di-O-pentyl) –α- cyclodextrin at an air-water interface. *Tetrahedron Lett,* Vol.41, No.47, pp. 9119–9123, ISSN 0040-4039

Woussidjewe, D.; Skiba, M., Leroy-Lechat, F.; Lemos-Senna, E.; Puisieux, F. & Duchene D. (1996). A new concept in drug delivery based on skirt-shaped cyclodextrin aggregates, present state and future prospects. *STP Pharma Sci.* Vol.6, No.1, pp. 21–28.

Zhang, G.; Liang, F.; Song, X.; Liu, D.; Li, M. & Q.; Wu. (2011). New amphiphilic biodegradable-β- cyclodextrin/poly cyclodextrin/poly(L-leucine) copolymers, Synthesis, characterization, and micellization. *Carbohydrate Polymers ,* Vol.80, No.3, pp. 885–890, ISSN 0144-8617

Chapter 2

Oral Delivery of Insulin: Novel Approaches

Amani M. Elsayed

Additional information is available at the end of the chapter

1. Introduction

1.1. Insulin: physicochemical properties and function

Insulin is a hormone that is synthesized in the β-cells of the pancreas as a proinsulin precursor and is converted to insulin by enzymatic cleavage. The resulting insulin molecule is composed of 51 amino acids arranged into two polypeptide chains - the A and B chains - which are connected by two interchain disulphide bridges. In the A chain, there is an additional intrachain disulphide linkage [1]. The primary structure of human insulin is shown in **Figure 1 a**. In the secondary structure, chain A consists of two antiparallel α-helices (A_2 to A_8 and A_{13} to A_{20}), while chain B forms a single α-helix "B_9 to B_{19}" followed by a turn and a β strand "B_{21} and B_{30}" [2]. The folding of insulin into a tertiary structure is essential for its biological activity (Figure 1b). Insulin has an isoelectric point (pI) of 5.3 and a charge of -2 to -6 in the pH range 7-11. Another intrinsic property of insulin is its ability to readily associate into dimmers, hexamers and higher-order aggregates. At the low concentrations found in the blood stream (< 10^{-3} μM), insulin exists as a monomer, which is its biologically active form. Following biosynthesis, insulin is stored as crystalline zinc-bound hexamers in vesicles within the pancreatic β-cells from which secretion occurs in response to elevated blood glucose levels [3]. The biological actions of insulin are initiated when insulin binds to its cell surface receptor. Insulin is an anabolic hormone and when binding to its receptor begins, many protein activation cascades occur. These include: the translocation of the glucose transporter to the plasma membrane and the influx of glucose, glycogen synthesis, glycolysis and fatty acid synthesis. Insulin has been observed as promoting the transport of some amino acids and potassium ions. Insulin also inhibits the liberation of free fatty acids and glycerol from the adipose tissue [3].

Insulin is used for the treatment of diabetes, a disease which results from a defect in the secretion or action of insulin.

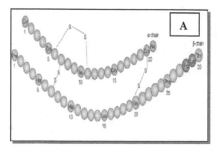 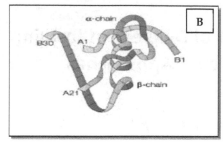

Figure 1. Insulin: a) Primary Structure b) Tertiary Structure

1.2. Oral delivery of insulin: Why?

Insulin is introduced by the parenteral route and two or three injections are needed for the better control of diabetes and in order to reduce the long term complications of hyperglycaemia (retinopathy, neuropathy and nephropathy). Patient non-compliance is common with the parenteral route. In addition, repeated injections will cause lipoatrophy or lipohypertrophy. Moreover, insulin injected into the subcutaneous tissues goes directly into general circulation and leads to peripheral hyperinsulinemia, which is associated with peripheral hypertension, the development of atherosclerosis, cancer, hypoglycaemia and other adverse metabolic effects [4]. Thus, the conventional subcutaneous injection of insulin is unphysiological because it deprives patients of the benefits of portal insulin since the liver is the major metabolic modulator of the glucose metabolism.

Oral insulin is a dream of patients and a challenge for scientists. For patients, not only are the pain and stress of injections relieved but it may also protect beta cells, avoid the weight gain associated with insulin injections and correct the blunting of the first-phase release of insulin [5]. All these effects are due to the fact that oral route provide insulin directly to the liver through portal circulation, resembling that which occurs in the non-diabetic individual [6]. The achievement of an adequate level of insulin in portal circulation has been associated with more a rapid and significant lowering of plasma glucose and haemoglobin A1c levels, the normalization of the plasma levels of three carbon precursors - such as lactate, pyruvate and alanine - and the hormones cortisol, growth hormone and glucagon [7].

Another advantage of oral insulin is that the gastrointestinal tract is immune tolerant compared to other routes of drug administration since immunogenicity has become a major issue for most biotechnology products. Immunogenicity decreases in the following order: (inhalation > subcutaneous > intramuscular > intravenous > oral).

For scientists, greater effort is needed to develop a nontoxic, stable, bioactive oral insulin delivery system. To develop such systems, many barriers must be explored.

1.3. Obstacles to oral delivery

The major barrier is that of absorption through the gastrointestinal membrane. Generally, the absorption of molecules can occur through the paracellular or the transcellular route.

The former is the preferred route for small hydrophilic molecules with a molecular weight below 500 Da [8]. Of course, molecules with a high molecular weight - such as insulin (about 6 KDa) - would not penetrate through this route. This large molecular size, its charge and its hydrophilicity all preclude insulin absorption by transcellular diffusion.

Another obstacle is those enzymes that are located throughout the GIT. In the stomach there is a family of aspartic proteases called pepsins. In the small intestine, pancreatic proteases consisting of the serine endopeptidase (trypsin, α-chymotrypsin, elastase and exopeptidases, carboxypeptidases A and B) are responsible for the degradation of proteins [9]. Other enzymes are located at the brush–border membrane (various peptidases) or within the enterocytes of the intestinal tract. It was demonstrated by Aoki et al. [10] that the enzymatic degradation activity for insulin in the mucous/glycocalyx layers tends to increase towards the upper small intestine in the following order: duodenum > jejunum > ileum.

Another challenge for the formulator is the stability of insulin. Insulin has a delicate structure, and both formulation and processing parameters could influence its stability [11]. The most common degradation reactions are deamidation and polymerization. Extensive deamidation at the residue Asn^{A21} of insulin occurs in acid solutions, while in neutral formulations deamidation takes place at Asn^{B3} at a substantially reduced rate [12]. High temperatures accelerate the formation of covalent insulin dimer and covalent insulin polymer [13].

The formulator could handle the enzyme and stability barriers. A well-formulated nanocarrier would protect insulin from enzymes. Also, and with the proper choice of excipients and a properly designed method of production, the stability of insulin could be preserved. Many investigated systems have overcome these two barriers. However, no system exhibits a reproducible and pronounced absorption.

1.4. Approaches explored to overcome the obstacles

To improve the bioavailability of insulin, different approaches have been explored, including chemical modification [14], co-administration with absorption enhancers and/or enzyme inhibitors [15] and incorporation into carriers, such as liposomes]16], mixed micelles, lipid-based systems, microspheres and nanoparticles [17-20].

1.4.1. Nanocarriers

These are carriers with a particle size of less than 1000 nm. Nanocarriers have received more attention recently due to their submicron size and their large specific surface area, both of which favour their absorption compared to larger carriers.

1.4.1.1. Types

Nanocarriers are categorized into: polymeric nanoparticles, nanovesicles and solid lipid nanoparticles **(Figure 2)**. There are two types of polymeric nanoparticles: the matrix particles termed 'nanospheres' and the reservoir-type named 'nanocapsules'. Vesicles have a hydrophilic core and hydrophobic bilayers. Conventionally, liposomal vesicles were developed by the self-assembly of phospholipid molecules in an aqueous environment. Recently, polymeric vesicles were prepared from amphiphilic polymers which form aggregates in aqueous solutions [21]. Solid lipid nanoparticles (SLN) are submicron colloidal carriers prepared from solid lipids (lipids being solid at room and body temperatures), such as triacylglycerols, complex acylglycerol mixtures or waxes, and dispersed either in water or in an aqueous surfactant solution [22]. The important features of different nanocarriers are illustrated in Table 1.

1.4.1.2. Applications

1.4.1.2.1 Liposomes

Insulin-loaded liposomes containing different kinds of bile salts (glycocholate, sodium taurocholate or sodium deoxycholate) were prepared by a reversed-phase evaporation method and their hypoglycaemic activity was assessed after oral administration to male Wistar rats. Liposomes containing sodium glycocholate elicited higher bioavailability - of approximately 8.5% and 11.0% - in non-diabetic and diabetic rats, respectively [23]. A hepatic-directed vesicle insulin system (HDV-I) was developed by Diasome Pharmaceuticals, Inc. The vesicles contain a specific proprietary hepatocyte-targeting molecule - biotin-phosphatidylethanolamine - in their phospholipid bilayer. Clinical trials in adult patients with type 1 diabetes mellitus demonstrated that the postprandial glycaemic control produced by 0.1 and 0.2 U/kg oral HDV-I was similar to that produced by 0.07 U/kg SC Humulin R [7].

1.4.1.2.2. Polymeric nanovesicles

Poly(lactic acid)-b-Pluronic-b-poly(lactic acid) block copolymers were synthesized [21]. This amphiphilic block copolymer aggregates in an aqueous solution to form vesicular nanoparticles. The oral administration of insulin-loaded vesicles to diabetic mice resulted in the reduction of blood glucose levels - 25% of the initial glucose level - which was maintained at this level for an additional 18.5 h [21].

1.4.1.2.3. Solid Lipid Nanoparticles (SLN)

Sarmento et al. [24] prepared insulin-loaded cetyl palmitate solid lipid nanoparticles and demonstrated their potential to deliver insulin orally. The drug loading capacity in solid lipid nanoparticles was improved by enhancing insulin liposolubility. Insulin was solubilized into mixed reverse micelles of sodium cholate and soybean phosphatidylcholine and transformed into SLN using a novel reverse micelle-double emulsion technique. Stearic acid and palmatic acid were used as a biocompatible lipid matrix [25]. The surface of the nanoparticles was modified by chitosan to enhance their penetration through GIT. In addition, chitosan was able to provide stealth properties to SLN, resulting in the absence of phagocytosis. Pharmacological availability values of 5.1–8.3% for SLN and 17.7% for chitosan-coated SLN were reported [26]. Lectins are proteins that bind sugar reversibly and are involved in many cell recognition and adhesion processes. They have been extensively adopted to target both absorptive enterocytes and M cells [27]. Wheat germ agglutinin binds (WGA) specifically to cell membranes and is taken up into cells by receptor-mediated endocytosis [28]. Zhang et al. [29] utilized the advantages of WGA and formulated SLN

Nanocarrier	Advantages	Shortcomings
Polymeric nanocarriers	Various polymeric materials (hydrophobic and hydrophilic) can be used to modulate the physicochemical properties of NPs (e.g., surface charge and mucoadhesivity), encapsulation efficiency, drug release profile and biological behaviour	Denaturation can occur during encapsulation in synthetic polymers, due largely to exposure to organic solvents, elevated temperatures and aqueous organic interfaces. Cytotoxicity of polymers after internalization into cells
Liposomes	Good permeation property since their bilayer structure is similar to that of the cell membrane	Poor entrapment efficiency Stability in biological fluids was relatively weak
Polymeric nanovesicles	More stable than liposomes The properties of polymeric vesicles, such as the size and the thickness of the bilayer, can be varied by changing the molecular weight and block composition of the polymer	Cytotoxicity of polymers after internalization into cells
Solid lipid nanoparticles	Tolerability, Biodegradability Composed of physiological lipids, which minimizes the risk of acute and chronic toxicity. Possibility of production on a large industrial scale	Poor encapsulation efficiency of water-soluble proteins and peptides into the lipid core The high temperatures required to melt the lipid may affect the stability of insulin Slow degradation

Table 1. Nanocarriers: general advantages and shortcomings

modified with WGA to enhance the oral delivery of insulin. Insulin-loaded SLNs or WGA-modified SLNs were administered orally to rats and elicited relative pharmacological bioavailability values of 4.46% and 6.08% and relative bioavailability values of 4.99% and 7.11%, respectively, in comparison with the subcutaneous injection of insulin.

Polymeric nanoparticles developed from biocompatible and biodegradable polymers are good candidates for insulin delivery

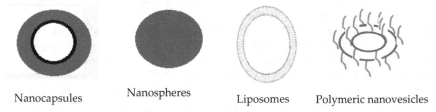

Nanocapsules   Nanospheres   Liposomes   Polymeric nanovesicles

Figure 2. Types of nanocarriers

1.4.1.3. Polymers used for the fabrication of polymeric nanoparticles

Both synthetic and natural polymers were investigated for the production of nanosystems. These polymers may be used alone or in combination to develop nanoparticles. Several fabrication techniques have been developed and can generally be subdivided into two categories, according to whether a preformed polymer is used or else whether nanoparticles are formed during the polymerization reaction. Methods from the first category include: emulsification/solvent evaporation, solvent displacement and interfacial deposition, emulsification/solvent diffusion, salting out with synthetic polymers, ionotropic gelation, coacervation and polyelectrolyte complexation. Meanwhile, the methods of the second category are: emulsion polymerization, interfacial polymerization and interfacial polycondensation. These methods were thoroughly discussed by Reis et al. [30].

1.4.1.3.1. Synthetic polymers

Usually, these are well-defined structures that can be modified to yield reasonable degradability and functionality. Synthetic biodegradable polymers such as poly ε-caprolactone (PCL) poly (lactic-co-glycolic acid) (PLGA) and polylactides (PLA) are widely used in drug delivery due to their good biocompatibility, biodegradability and novel drug release behaviour. The chemical structures of synthetic polymers were depicted in Table 2 and an example of insulin nanoparticles fabricated from these polymers is illustrated in Table 3.

1.4.1.3.1.1. PLGA

Poly (lactic-co-glycolic acid) (PLGA) is an aliphatic polyester synthetic biodegradable biopolymer which is successfully used for the development of nanomedicines. It was also investigated for the delivery of insulin. In the work of Yang et al. [31], insulin was encapsulated in PLGA nanoparticles. The administration of insulin-loaded PLGA nanoparticles for diabetes mellitus induced a rapid decrease in blood glucose levels for up to 24 h and increased insulin levels. The loading capacity was 78.35%. To facilitate loading efficiency, the lipophilicity of the insulin was increased by complexation with sodium lauryl sulphate or sodium oleate. Insulin encapsulation efficiency reached up to 90%. [32, 33]. Mucoadhesive PLGA nanoparticles were prepared to enhance the oral bioavailability of the negatively charged PLGA nanoparticles. The PLGA nanoparticles were coated with chitosan or Eudragit® RS (RS). The pharmacological availability of two kinds of nanoparticles - PLGA nanoparticles and chitosan-coated PLGA nanoparticles - relative to SC injection was calculated and found to be 7.6% and 10.5%, respectively, at an insulin dose of 15 IU/kg [34]. Meanwhile, the pharmacological availability of the 50 IU/kg Eudragit® RS (RS) coated PLGA nanoparticle was 9.2% [35]. The main shortcomings of PLGA are that the degradation products arising from degradation of PLGA (lactic and glycolic acid) result in the generation of acidic species which can provoke problems for long-term stability when encapsulating bioactive molecules. Antacid-insulin co-encapsulated PLGA were investigated with a view to increasing the microclimate pH and preventing structural losses and aggregation [36]. The antacids assessed were magnesium hydroxide and zinc carbonate. However, short-term stability was not reported.

1.4.1.3.1.2. PLA

Polylactides (PLAs) have similar properties to PLGAs but they are more hydrophobic than PLGAs and they degrade more slowly due to their crystallinity [37]. Cui et al. [38] reported enhanced insulin entrapment efficiency (up to 90%) in PLA and PLGA nanoparticles, where insulin was complexed with phosphatidylcholine (SPC) to improve its liposolubility. An oral bioavailability of 7.7% relative to subcutaneous injection was obtained.

1.4.1.3.1.3. PCL

Another interesting biodegradable polyester polymer is poly-ε caprolactone (PCL). Compared with PLGA and PLA, PCL is semi-crystalline, has superior viscoelastic properties and possesses easy formability. PCL has the advantage of generating a less acidic environment during degradation as compared with PLGA-based polymers [37]. Nevertheless, the hydrophobic nature of PCL affects the encapsulation of hydrophilic substances, such as peptides, enzymes and other proteins. Damgé et al. [39] prepared nanoparticles from a blend of a biodegradable polyester poly (ε-caprolactone) and a polycationic non-biodegradable acrylic polymer (Eudragit® RS). These nanoparticles were investigated as a carrier for the oral administration of insulin and demonstrated prolonged hypoglycaemic effect of insulin in both diabetic and normal rats. The same author loaded nanoparticles with regular insulin ((Actrapid, Novo Nordisk) or insulin-Aspart ((Novorapid). Regular insulin-loaded nanoparticles reduced glycaemia in a dose dependent manner with a maximal effect observed with 100 IU/kg. In contrast, insulin analogue did not elicit a dose-dependent hypoglycaemic effect. The maximal effect was observed with 50 IU/kg insulin while lower (25 IU/kg) and higher doses (100 IU/kg) did not show any significant reduction in glycaemia. The authors attributed these discrepancies to the saturation of the receptors when the dose of aspart-insulin increases to 100 IU/kg [40].

1.4.1.3.1.4. PACA

Poly (alkyl cyanoacrylate) is a biocompatible and biodegradable polymer. It is degraded by esterases in biological fluids and produces certain toxic products that will stimulate or damage the central nervous system. Thus, this polymer is not authorized for application in humans [41]. However, PACA polymers are used to encapsulate insulin using emulsion or interfacial polymerization. Damge et al. [42] prepared an insulin-loaded poly (alkyl cyanoacrylate) nanocapsule. The oral administration of nanocapsules dispersed in Miglyol 812 to diabetic rats resulted in a 50% reduction of initial glucose levels from the second hour for up to 10-13 days. This effect was shorter (2 days) or absent when the nanocapsules were dispersed in water, whether with surface active agents or not. Insulin-loaded poly (ethyl cyanoacrylate) nanoparticles were prepared from microemulsions with a different microstructure and were administered orally to diabetic rats. A consistent and significant hypoglycaemic effect over controls was found for up to 36 h depending upon the type of monomer (ethylcyanoacrylate or butyl cyanoacrylate). However, no significant serum insulin levels were detectable [43].

1.4.1.3.1.5. Poly (Acrylic acid)

These are non-degradable polymers with mucoadhesive properties based on acrylic or methacrylic acid. Anionic polymers, such as methyl acrylic acid (Eudragit L-100) and methyl methacrylate (S-100), have been used to formulate pH sensitive nanocarriers. Polymethacrylic acid–chitosan–polyethylene glycol nanoparticles were developed by Pawar et al. for the oral delivery of insulin. These nanoparticles displayed excellent binding efficiency on mucin from porcine stomach and elicited pH dependent release profiles in vitro [44]. The nanoparticles were formed by a complex coacervation method using EudragitL100-55 and chitosan of various molecular weights. Insulin release from these nanoparticles was pH-dependent [45]. The distribution, transition and bioadhesion of insulin-loaded pH-sensitive nanoparticles prepared from EudragitL100-55 and chitosan were investigated. The addition of the hydroxypropylmethylcellulose reduced the stomach- and intestine-emptying rates and enhanced the adhesion of the nanoparticles to the intestinal mucosa [46].

1.4.1.3.2. Natural polymers

The naturally-occurring polymers of particular interest in the oral delivery of insulin are either polysaccharides or else proteins. Polysaccharides include chitosan, hyaluronan, dextran, cellulose, pullulan, chondroitin sulphate and alginate. Meanwhile, the protencious polymers are casein and gelatin. They are nontoxic, biocompatible, biodegradable and hydrophilic. The structure of these natural polymers is illustrated in **Table 4**. Examples of the natural polymers used to prepare insulin-loaded nanoparticles and the methods used for their fabrication are shown in **Table 5.**

1.4.1.3.2.1. Dextran

Dextran sulphate is an exocellular bacterial polysaccharide consisting of linear 1,6-linked D-glucopyranose units and branches beginning from α-1,3-linkages with approximately 2.3 sulphate groups per glucosyl residue. It is a nontoxic, highly water-soluble, biodegradable and biocompatible branched negatively charged polyion. A nanoparticle insulin delivery system was prepared by the polyelectrolyte complexation of oppositely charged natural polymers - dextran sulphate and chitosan in an aqueous solution. These pH sensitive nanoparticles released insulin in the intestinal medium [47]. The natural uptake processes of the intestine were utilized for the oral delivery of peptides and proteins. Vitamin B12 is an example of such carriers and was investigated for delivering different peptides [48]. Due to the susceptibility of vitamin B12/peptide conjugate to gastrointestinal degradation, dextran nanoparticles were coated with vitamin B12 and used as a carrier for the oral delivery of insulin [49]. These nanoparticles were found to be targeted at the systemic circulation through vitamin B12-intrinsic factor receptor ligand-mediated endocytosis via ileocytes of the intestine [49]. The % pharmacological availability of nanoparticle conjugates containing 2, 3 and 4% w/w insulin was 1.1, 1.9 and 2.6 times higher, respectively, compared with nanoparticles without VB12.

Polymer	Chemical Structure
PLGA	 x = number of units of lactic acid y = number of units of glycolic acid
PLA	
Polycapolactone	
Ethyl cyanoacrylate monomer	
Poly (acrylic acid)	

Table 2. Chemical Structure of Synthetic Polymers

1.4.1.3.2.2. Alginate

Alginate is a naturally occurring polysaccharide obtained from marine brown algae. It is a linear copolymer composed of 1,4-linked-β-D-mannuronic acid and α-L-guluronic acid residues that gel in the presence of divalent cations. It is a nontoxic and biodegradable polyanion that forms polyelectrolyte complexes with polycations, such as chitosan. Insulin-loaded nanoparticles were prepared by the ionotropic pre-gelation of alginate with calcium chloride followed by complexation between alginate and chitosan [50]. The pharmacological effect of insulin-loaded nanoparticles was evaluated in diabetic rats. The pharmacological availability was 6.8% and 3.4% for the 50 and 100 IU/kg doses, respectively [51]. Alginate/chitosan nanoparticles form complexes with cationic β-cyclodextrin polymers. The nanoparticles protect insulin against degradation in simulated gastric fluid [52]. Reis et al. [53] evaluated nanoparticle systems composed of alginate/chitosan cores coated with chitosan-polyethylene glycol-albumin. Albumin was added to prevent protease attacks on the insulin and chitosan for its mucoadhesive properties, while PEG served as a nanosphere stabilizer to improve the half-live of the insulin and increase the residence time along the intestine. Chitosan-PEG-albumin coated nanospheres demonstrated a more than 70% blood glucose reduction, increased insulinemia by a factor of seven and significantly improved the response to the glucose oral tolerance test following oral administration to diabetic rats. In contrast, nanospheres lacking albumin and PEG in the coating material were ineffective. Multilayer nanoparticles consisting of calcium cross-linked alginate, dextran sulphate, poloxamer 188, chitosan and an outermost coating of albumin were developed. A 3-factor 3-level Box–Behnken statistical design was used to optimize the nanoparticle formulation. Solutions of 0.20% calcium chloride, 0.04% chitosan and 0.47% albumin constituted the optimum formulation of nanoparticles for orally-dosed insulin [54]. The relative pharmacological availability and bioavailability were calculated after oral administration of 50 IU/kg of insulin-loaded multilayered nanoparticles to diabetic rats and were found to be 11% and 13%, respectively [55].

Polymer	Method of preparation	Particle size (nm)	Pharmacological availability (PA)/ or relative bioavailability (RBA)	Ref.
PGLA	Double-emulsion/solvent evaporation technique	208	**Not calculated**	31
PLGA and chitosan	Water-in oil-in-water solvent evaporation technique	150	**PA: 10.5%**	34
PLGA, Eudragit® RS (RS) and Hydroxypropyl methylcellulose phthalate	Multiple emulsions solvent evaporation technique.	285	PA: 9.2%	35
PCL and Eudragit® RS	Double emulsion method	331	RBA: 13%	39

Table 3. Synthetic polymers used for the preparation of nanoparticles and the methods used for their fabrication

Polymer	Chemical Structure
Dextran	
Alginate	
Chitosan	

Table 4. Chemical Structure of Natural Polymers

As illustrated in Table 5, the most widely explored polymer is chitosan. This is because of its favourable biological properties, safety, low cost and easy modification. Compared to synthetic polymers, the degradation products of chitosan are amino sugars, which are easily metabolized by the body. Therefore, there is no concern of an acidic microclimate being generated by chitosan particles [56].

Polymer	Method of preparation	Particle size (nm)	Pharmacological Availability (PA)/ or Relative bioavailability (RBA)	Ref.
Chitosan and Poly (γ-glutamic acid)	Ionic-gelation method: the nanoparticles were freeze-dried and placed in enteric-coated capsules	232.9	RBA: approximately 20%.	70
Chitosan and Poly (γ-glutamic acid)	A penetration enhancer (DTPA) was covalently conjugated on poly (g-glutamicacid) followed by ionic-gelation with chitosan	246.6	RBA: approximately 20%	71
Chitosan, Alginate, Dextran, Poloxamer, and BSA	Ionotropic pre-gelation followed by polyelectrolyte complexation	396	RBA: 13.2±2.9	52
Dextran	Cross-linking of emulsion to prepare dextran nanoparticles. The surface was modified with succinic anhydride and conjugated with amino VB12 derivatives of the carbamate linkage.	160-250	PA: 26.5	49

Table 5. Natural polymers used for the preparation of nanoparticles and the methods used for their fabrication

What is Chitosan?

Chitosan is a linear copolymer consisting of ß (1-4)-linked 2-amino-2-deoxy–D-glucose (D-glucosamine) and 2-acetamido-2-deoxy-D-glucose (N-acetyl-D-glucosamine) units **(Table 4)**. It is obtained by the alkaline N-deacetylation of chitin, which is the primary structural component of the outer skeletons of crustaceans. Chitosan is a weak poly base due to the large quantities of amino groups on its chain [57]. Both high molecular weight (HMWC) and low molecular weight chitosans (LMWC) are available. The latter were obtained by the depolymerization of HMWC. This can be carried out by enzymatic [58,59], physical [60, 61] or chemical methods [62, 63]. Another important property of chitosan is the degree of deacetylation (DDA), defined in terms of the percentage of primary amino groups in the polymer backbone. The properties of chitosan and its biological role are dependent on the DDA and M.wt [64]. Chitosan dissolves easily at low pH due to the protonation of the amino groups, while it is insoluble at higher pH ranges since the amino groups become deprotonated, as the pH approach the pKa of chitosan (6-6.5). The solubility of chitosan depends upon the molecular weight and DDA.

Chitosan nanoparticles have been prepared using ionotropic gelation with tripolyphosphate or even simply polyelectrolyte complexation between insulin and chitosan. The interaction of chitosan and polyanions leads to the spontaneous formation of nanoparticles in an aqueous environment without the need for heating or the use of organic solvents [65]. In addition, to ease of preparation under mild conditions, a high level of drug entrapment can be achieved so that the protein secondary structure and biological activity is preserved [66]. Insulin-loaded chitosan nanoparticles were prepared by the ionotropic gelation of chitosan with tripolyphosphate anions [67]. These nanoparticles were effective at lowering the serum glucose level of streptozotocin-induced diabetic rats when administered orally at insulin doses of 50 U/kg and/or 100 U/kg. However, they dissociate easily in acidic gastric conditions. To protect insulin from harsh GIT conditions, chitosan nanoparticles were formulated with an enteric coating polymer - hydroxypropyl methylcellulose phthalate (HPMCP) - and evaluated for the oral delivery of insulin. HPMCP-chitosan nanoparticles showed a 2.8-fold increase in their hypoglycaemic effect when compared with chitosan nanoparticles without HPMCP [68]. Self-assembled nanoparticles were developed by mixing the anionic poly-γ-glutamic acid (γ-PGA) solution with the cationic chitosan solution in the presence of $MgSO_4$ and sodium tripolyphosphate (TPP). TPP and sulphate salts were physically added to crosslink chitosan by ionic gelation, while physical gelation may occur between Mg^+ and the carboxylate ions on γ-PGA via an electrostatic interaction. Chitosan-γ-PGA nanoparticles remained intact within the pH range of 2.0–7.2; however, at lower pH values they disintegrated. The pharmacodynamics and pharmacokinetics of insulin were evaluated in a diabetic rat model and the relative bioavailability was 15% [69]. For the further enhancement of bioavailability, two approaches were investigated: in the first, chitosan- γ-PGA nanoparticles were freeze-dried and placed in an enteric-coated capsule, while in the second, a penetration enhancer - diethylene triamine pentaacetic acid (DTPA) - was added. In both cases the bioavailability was approximately 20% [70,71].

The problem of the low solubility of chitosan in the neutral environment of the intestine was solved by synthesis of a partially quaternized derivative of chitosan - Trimethyl chitosan (TMC). TMC has good solubility and a permeation enhancing effect [72]. The targeting of trimethyl chitosan chloride to goblet cells was achieved through modification with a CSKSSDYQC (CSK) targeting peptide. The significant internalization of insulin via clathrin- and caveolae-mediated endocytosis on goblet cell-like HT29-MTX cells results in a better hypoglycaemic effect with a 1.5-fold higher relative bioavailability compared with unmodified TMC nanoparticles [73]. Trimethyl chitosan-cysteine conjugate and N-(2-hydroxyl) propyl-3-trimethyl ammonium chitosan were synthesized and demonstrated high mucoadhesion capability compared with TMC/insulin nanoparticles or native chitosan [74, 75]. Quaternized derivatives of chitosan have a high positive charge, which can easily interact with negatively-charged blood corpuscles, resulting in haemolysis and toxicity [76]. To overcome these problems, chitosan derivatives were modified with polyethylene glycol to reduce the interaction between the cationic polymers and cell membranes [77]. Chitosan was also modified with hydrophobic fatty acids, such as anacardic acid. Anacardoylated chitosan spontaneously formed nanoparticles in an aqueous insulin solution that sustained the release of insulin in the intestinal environment [78].

1.4.1.4. Mechanisms of the absorption of nanoparticles

The absorption of the nanoparticles was thoroughly reviewed by des Rieux [8]. A particle can traverse the intestinal epithelium by the paracellular (between cells) or transcellular route (through the cells). The transcellular route is the most common. With the transcellular transport of nanoparticles, the particles are taken up by cells through the endocytic process - which takes place at the cell apical membrane - transported through the cells and released at the basolateral pole. Two types of intestinal cells are important in nanoparticle transcytosis: the enterocytes lining the gastrointestinal tract and the M cells mainly located in Peyer's patches. The uptake of nanoparticles takes place by one of three endocytotic mechanisms: pinocytosis, macropinocytosis or clathrin-mediated endocytosis. Clathrin vesicles are for particles smaller than 150 nm while phagocytosis is for particulate matters of up to several µm. The uptake of particles, microorganisms and macromolecules by M cells occurs by fluid phase endocytosis, adsorptive endocytosis and phagocytosis [8].

1.4.2. Lipid-based systems

Lipid-based delivery systems (LDS) range from simple oil solutions to complex mixtures of oils, surfactants, cosurfactants and cosolvents [79]. The bioavailability of several peptides was improved when incorporated into LDS - e.g., cyclosporine (Neoral®). The enhancement in absorption was attributed to an increase in membrane permeability, the inhibition of efflux transporters, a reduction in cytochrome P450 enzymes, an increase in chylomicron production and lymphatic transport [80].

1.4.2.1. Types

The LDS investigated for the delivery of insulin are: multiple emulsions, microemulsions and solid in-oil-in water systems.

1.4.2.1.1. Water-in-oil-in-water

A water-in-oil-in-water (W/O/W) emulsion has been proposed to protect peptides against proteolysis and enhance their absorption. Multiple emulsions containing unsaturated fatty acids (oleic acid, linoleic acid and linolenic acid) have been reported to enhance the ileal and colonic absorption of insulin without tissue damage [81]. The transport enhancement of the W/O/W emulsion prepared with octanoic acid triacylglycerol was found to be affected by the size of oil droplets. When the oil-droplet median was 2.3 µm, an earlier hypoglycaemic response was observed compared with a multiple emulsion, having a diameter of 3.8 µm. In contrast, the emulsion with a diameter of 0.7 µm exhibited no effect [82].

1.4.2.1.2. Microemulsions

Microemulsions are clear, stable, isotropic mixtures of oil, water and surfactant, frequently in combination with a cosurfactant [83]. The average particle size of microemulsions falls in the range of 5-100 nm; they are polydispersed in nature and the polydispersity decreases with decreasing particle size [84]. Insulin-loaded microemulsions were developed using didodecyldimethylammonium bromide as the surfactant, propylene glycol as the co-surfactant, triacetin as the oil phase and insulin solution as the aqueous phase. These microemulsions displayed a 10-fold enhancement in bioavailability compared with a plain insulin solution administered orally to healthy rats [85]. The improved oral bioavailability of the w/o microemulsion system was also shown for a lecithin-based microemulsion of rh-insulin [86]. On the other hand, Kraeling and Ritschel [87] found that the oral pharmacological availability of insulin microemulsions as compared with intravenous insulin in beagle dogs was 2.1%, which further increased to 6.4% with the encapsulation of gelled microemulsions in hard gelatine capsules along with the protease inhibitor aprotinin and coating of the capsules for colonic release [87]. The improved oral delivery of insulin from a microemulsion system was also demonstrated by others [88]. A stable self-emulsifying formulation for the oral delivery of insulin was developed by Ma et al. [89]. It is composed of two non-ionic surfactants (polyethylene glycol-8-glycol octanoate/decanoate and polyglycerol-3 oleate). In diabetic beagle dogs, the bioavailability of this formulation was up to 15.2% at a dose of 2.5 IU/kg in comparison with the hypoglycaemic effect of native insulin (0.5 IU/kg) delivered by subcutaneous injection.

1.4.2.1.3. Solid-in-oil-in water (S/O/W) emulsions

S/O/W emulsions were also developed for the delivery of insulin whereby insulin was converted into a lipophilic complex by coating with surfactant molecules and dispersed in an oil phase of oil in a water emulsion to form the S/O/W emulsion [90]. The stability of this system was enhanced by lyophilization [91].

1.4.2.2. Mechanism of the absorption of lipid-based formulations

Suggested mechanisms of intestinal drug absorption, using lipid-based formulations include: an increase in membrane fluidity facilitating transcellular absorption, the opening of the tight junctions to allow paracellular transport (mainly relevant for ionized drugs or hydrophilic macromolecules), the inhibition of P-glycoprotein and/or cytochrome P450 to increase intracellular concentration and residence time, and the stimulation of lipoprotein/chylomicron production [92].

2. Chitosan-fatty acid systems

2.1. Rationale

Chitosan nanoparticles prepared by ionotropic gelation or polyelectrolyte complexation dissociate easily in an acidic medium. This might be related to the fact that both insulin and chitosan have net positive charges at pH 1.2, that the columbic repulsive forces lead to the dissociation of the complex and that the free insulin is subjected to degradation. For example, nanoparticles prepared from chitosan and poly (γ-glutamic acid) became unstable at pH 1.2 and broke apart [93] and nanoparticles composed of chitosan and tripolyphosphate rendered the protein more susceptible to acid and enzymatic hydrolysis [94]. In the present investigation, we benefited from the advantages of polyelectrolyte complexation between chitosan and insulin, its formulation in an aqueous environment without the need for heat or an organic solvent, and the solution of the shortcomings of burst release by the dispersion of nanoparticles in an oily phase. The oily vehicle was intended to reduce proteolytic degradation and improve absorption [95, 96]. In addition, the free chitosan amine groups may interact with any adjacent carboxylic acid groups of oleic acid, forming a protective hydrophobic coating layer at the surface of the dispersed phase, which may enhance stability in the GIT and promote lymphatic uptake. The particle size of the chitosan-oleic system is above 1 μm, due to the interaction. The reduction of the particle size of chitosan-oleic acid emulsion to nanosize was achieved by high pressure homogenization or else by the addition of surfactants. PEG-8 caprylic/capric glycerides (Labrasol) and polyglyceryl-6 dioleate were selected as surfactant and cosurfactant, respectively. Chitosan-insulin nanoparticles were solubilized in the inverted micelles. Chitosan plays an important role - as a matrix for nanoparticles and stabilizers of inverted micelles. In a previous work [97], we demonstrated the role of chitosan in the reduction of particle size of the w/o emulsion containing Labrasol, plurol oleique and oleic acid. This was attributed to the interaction of amine groups of chitosan with the surfactant-cosurfactant aggregates, resulting in the formation of a closer packing of surfactants at the interface, which leads to a reduction in particle size. This effect is more pronounced in 1:1 surfactant:cosurfactant rather than in 4:1 systems. Insulin is a water soluble protein that will be located inside the water droplets. Chitosan will be partly fixed near the surfactant head groups with the rest of it inside the water droplet. Interactions between chitosan, surfactants and insulin resulted in smaller microemulsion sizes [97]. Moreover, low molecular weight chitosans were chosen to prepare the nanoparticles, since their intestinal absorption is known to be significantly better than the high molecular weight candidates and showed a negligible cytotoxic effect on the Caco-2 cells [98].

The potential of chitosan-fatty acid or chitosan-fatty acid derivative nanoparticles as oral delivery carriers of insulin was investigated systematically.

2.2. Chitosan-fatty acid nanocarriers' development

Detailed descriptions of the compositions and preparation methods can be found in the relevant patents [99, 100]. Low molecular weight chitosans were obtained by the depolymerization of high molecular weight chitosan using 2 M hydrochloric acid. The resulting fractions were characterized by Fourier transformed infrared spectroscopy (FTIR), differential scanning calorimetry (DSC), X-ray powder diffraction (XRPD), nuclear magnetic resonance (NMR) and dynamic light scattering (DLS). The polyelectrolyte complexation method was utilized to prepare insulin-chitosan nanocomplexes. Chitosan was dissolved in deionized water and its pH was adjusted to 5.5 using 0.2 M NaOH. rh-insulin powder was dissolved in 0.1 M HCl, followed by the addition of 1M Tris (hydroxymethyl)-aminomethane buffer pH 7. Chitosan-insulin complexes were prepared by adding chitosan solution to an equal volume of insulin solution in a glass vial under gentle magnetic stirring, and incubating for a further 15 minutes at room temperature. The parameters affecting the encapsulation efficiency were investigated (final pH of the complex, molecular weight of chitosan, DDA of chitosan, initial concentration of chitosan and insulin, and chitosan: insulin ratio). A phase diagram was constructed and the results were used as guidance to select the suitable percentages of surfactants, oil and aqueous phases suitable for the nanoparticle dispersion system. The nanoparticle dispersion system was prepared by mixing two phases - the aqueous phase and the oily phase. The oily phase consists of Labrasol® and plurol oleique® at a fixed weight (1/1) ratio and oleic acid. The aqueous phase composed of a chitosan-insulin complex. To prepare the dispersion system, 50 µl of the aqueous phase was added to 2.5 g of the oily phase during mixing with a vortex mixer (VELP Scientifica, Europe) for 1 min. at room temperature (25 °C). The preparation was characterized: viscosity, particle size, morphology and encapsulation efficiency were all determined. The chemical and immunological stabilities of insulin after entrapment into nanoparticles were studied. The suitability of the preparation to preserve insulin activity, to withstand gut enzymes and to maintain the stability of insulin upon storage was investigated [101]. The hypoglycaemic effect of the preparation after oral administration to streptozotocin-diabetic rats was evaluated. The parameters that influence the pharmacological availability were characterized. The bioavailability of the preparation versus subcutaneous injection was calculated together with the pharmacokinetic parameters. Moreover, human studies were conducted where twenty-five healthy volunteers participated in five studies using a two-phase, two-sequence crossover design with a washout period of one day [102]. Other chitosan fatty acid systems were also formulated, for example chitosan sodium lauryl sulphate nanoparticles [103] and chitosan-oleic acid nanoemulsion (particle size reduced by a high pressure homogenizer) and their hypoglycaemic effects were evaluated and compared to the chitosan-oleic acid-surfactants system.

2.3. Results and discussion

2.3.1. Depolymerization and characterization of chitosan

Most commercially available chitosans possess quite large M.wts. LMWCs are better amenable for a wide variety of biomedical applications due to their solubility in water [104-106]. In addition, chitooligomers were found to be non-mutagenic and non-genotoxic when orally administered to mice [107]. To generate low molecular weight chitosans from high molecular weight candidates, hydrolysis by hydrochloric acid was adopted due to its practicability and reproducibility. IR spectrum spectroscopy demonstrated that there was no structure change during depolymerization. DDA was determined by NMR and it was about 99%. [101]. The solubility of chitosan increased with decreasing molecular weight. Chitosan has a positive zeta potential and its value is affected by the pH, molecular weight, DDA and concentration [108]. LMWCs with an average molecular weight of 13 KDa and DDA ~ 99% were used for further studies.

2.3.2. Chitosan-insulin polyelectrolyte complexes (PECs)

Insulin was first complexed with chitosan through the interaction of negatively charged insulin with positively charged chitosan to form PEC before incorporation into the oily vehicle. This is because chitosan has many beneficial effects, such as penetration enhancement. Chitosan was also found to stabilize insulin when incubated at 50 ± 1 °C while shaking at 100 strokes/min in a water bath [101]. As shown in **Figure 3**, the insulin solution was almost degraded while the chitosan-insulin complex protected the insulin from degradation for at least 24 h. In addition, chitosan has a role in protecting insulin from those enzymes present in the small intestine. This was reflected in the partial protection of insulin from pancreatin, as depicted in **Figure 4**, and the protection increases with the increase of the chitosan ratio. Moreover, chitosan may also protect insulin from destabilization at the oil/water interface when the PEC was dispersed in the oily vehicle. The PEC formation process is influenced by a variety of parameters, including the system pH, chitosan molecular weight and DDA. The most important factor appears to be the system pH [101].

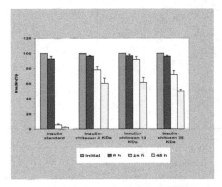

Figure 3. Effect of the temperature and shaking on the stability of the insulin

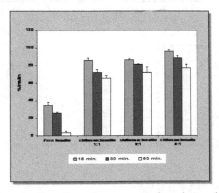

Figure 4. Effect of the chitosan:insulin ratio on the pancreatic degradation of insulin

2.3.3. Oily nanosystem preparation

Chitosan-insulin PECs were solubilized in an oily vehicle composed of a surfactant Labrasol, cosurfactant Plurol Oleique and an oily vehicle oleic acid. We attempted to formulate an oral insulin delivery system that combined the advantages of nanoencapsulation and the use of an oily vehicle. The nanoparticles were expected to translocate the intestinal epithelium, while the oily vehicle was intended to reduce proteolytic degradation and improve permeability [109, 110]. In addition, Labrasol and oleic acid are known penetration enhancers [111, 112]. Our expectation is that part of the chitosan will rest inside the water droplet of the inverted micelles where it forms PEC with insulin while the other part projecting near the surfactant head groups where it interacts with surfactants stabilizes the w/o microemulsion and resulted in smaller microemulsion sizes [97]. Chitosan at pH 6 will also interact with oleic acid to coat the particles with a hydrophobic layer. This interaction was studied by molecular mechanics, as illustrated in **Figure 5**. The structure of chitosan 13 KDa, oleic acid and chitosan-oleic acid

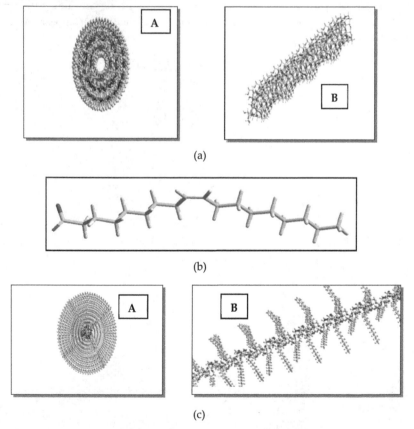

(a)

(b)

(c)

Figure 5. a. Top view (A) and side view of chitosan (B); b. The computed molecular geometries of oleic acid; c. Top view (A) and side view of the chitosan-oleic acid complex

complex, which were built up in Hyperchem®, was shown in **Figures 5.a, b** and **c**, respectively. The conformation of individual chitosan and oleic acid was the same as the complex.

It is obvious that the outer structure of the complex was hydrophobic due to presence of oleic acid while chitosan was embedded inside the structure. This is consistent with the immiscibility of the complex with water. The binding energy of the resulting chitosan oleic acid complex is calculated according to the following equation:

$$E \text{ binding} = E \text{ complex} - \left(E_{oleate} + E_{chitosan}\right)$$

$E_{complex} = -539.94$; $E_{oleic} = 2131.64$; $E_{chitosan} = 4526.58$; $E \text{ binding} = -7198.2 \text{ kcal / mol}$.

The value of the binding energy suggested a high degree of interaction between chitosan and oleic acid. The chitosan-oleic acid interaction was also studied using statistical design [108]. The effects of three formulation variables (the aqueous chitosan solution to oleic acid ratio, the chitosan molecular weight, and the degree of deacetylation of chitosan) on the viscosity of the system and the length of the emulsified layer (%) were studied in a conventional 2^3 factorial design. It was found that chitosan-oleic acid interaction is significantly influenced by pH. At a pH of around 6.5, chitosan is almost 50% ionized (pK_a NH$_3$/NH$_2$ ~ 6.5) and the ionized amine groups in chitosan will interact with the carboxylate ion of oleic acid. However, at pH 1.5, chitosan will be available as chitosan hydrochloride, and so no interaction was observed. 50% oleic acid and 50% chitosan aqueous solution (2%) at different pH were mixed and their viscosities were determined, as depicted in **Figure 6**. A sharp increase in viscosity was noticed when the pH of chitosan was ≥ 5.5. This indicates that the rheological properties of this dispersion were notably influenced by other factors - apart from the disperse phase volume fraction - such as the interaction between chitosan and oleic acid. These results were consistent with the surface tension measurements of the chitosan-oleic acid system [97].

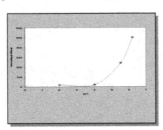

Figure 6. The effect of the pH of chitosan on the viscosity of oleic acid chitosan dispersions

2.3.4. Oily nanosystem characterization

The mean particle size was determined by dynamic light scattering - it was 111 ± 6.9 nm - and showed a unimodal particle size distribution. The particle size is affected by the molecular weight of chitosan, as shown in **Table 6**. An increase in the molecular weight of the chitosan polymer led to an increase in the dispersed phase particle size. The particles' shapes were assessed by a transmission electron microscope (TEM) and it was spherical, as depicted in **Figure 7**. The viscosity of the nanosystem was measured by a Vibro viscometer - it was 52.25 ± 2.6 mPa s. Neither the particle size nor the viscosity of the nanosystem changed upon storage at 4 or 25 ºC for one month, indicating the physical stability of the nanosystem. The preparation procedure is mild and the insulin is chemically and immunologically stable, as illustrated by RP-HPLC and ELISA, respectively. About 90% of the insulin was recovered from the preparation after incubation with pepsin, indicating the protective ability of the preparation for insulin under conditions simulating the gastric environment [97]. In addition, short term chemical stability demonstrates that the chemical stability of the insulin was maintained for at least 30 days of storage at 4 and 25 °C, according to the HPLC method. Moreover, the biological activity was reserved after one month at storage temperatures of 4 and 25 ºC.

Chitosan M.wt (KDa)	Mean diameter (nm) ± SD
3	79 ± 2.5
13	111 ± 6.9
30	205 ± 2.6

Table 6. The mean diameter of the oily nanosystem prepared from chitosans with different molecular weights

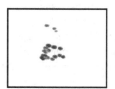

Figure 7. TEM image of the oily nanosystem

2.3.5. In vivo studies

The preliminary screening of the biological activity of nanoparticles prepared from different grades of chitosan (different molecular weights and DDA) and administered orally to STZ diabetic rats revealed a maximum effect with nanoparticles prepared from chitosan with a molecular weight of 13 KDa and DDA~ 99%. **Figure 8** illustrates changes in the plasma glucose levels after the oral administration of the nanoparticles prepared from chitosan with a molecular weight of 13 KDa and DDA 99%. As expected, the insulin oral solution showed no hypoglycaemic effect compared to the control group (P > 0.05). In contrast, the blood glucose levels of the rats decreased remarkably after the oral administration of insulin-loaded nanosystem, achieving a significant decrease at 3 h when compared with the control group (P< 0.05). More interestingly, the hypoglycaemic effect was maintained without recovery at the baseline for 12 h. A pharmacological availability value of 29% was obtained for the dose 5 IU/kg. An explanation of this positive behaviour of the oily nanosystem could be put forward in terms of the demonstrated ability of oily preparations to make the entrapped insulin more stable and protect it from degradation in the harsh conditions of the gastrointestinal tract as well as enhance its intestinal absorption.

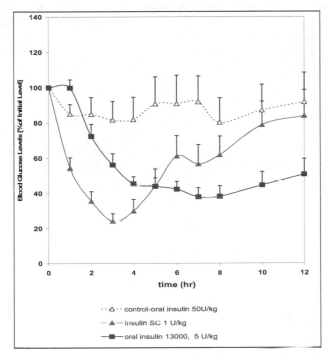

Figure 8. Changes in blood glucose level versus time profiles after a single oral administration of the oily dispersion of chitosan-insulin nanoparticles given at a dose level 5 IU/Kg (■ to STZ-diabetic rats compared to a free insulin solution given orally (50 IU/Kg) as a control group (Δ) and a subcutaneous injection of a free insulin solution (1IU/Kg) (▲ The results are expressed as the mean ± S.E.M (n = 12 per group)

A concomitant increase in plasma insulin levels was observed after the oral administration of the 5 IU/kg of insulin-loaded oily nanosystem to diabetic rats, as depicted in **Figure 9**. The pharmacokinetic parameters were determined based on the insulin concentration plasma profiles of **Figure 9**, as shown in **Table 7**. The subcutaneous injection group exhibited a rapid increase in serum rh-insulin concentration up to 279.2 µIU/ml over 30 min of administration. Meanwhile, the intragastric administration of 5 IU/kg of nanoparticles exhibited slower absorption and sustained elimination, reaching a maximum after 2 h (102.22 µIU/ml). Moreover, the serum rh-insulin levels of the nanoparticle group were significantly different from that of the control group (P < 0.001). The AUC$_{0-12}$ of orally administered nanoparticles was 664.99 µg hr/ml for the 5 IU/kg dose and 626.02 µg hr/ml for the 1 IU/kg subcutaneous rh-insulin dose. The corresponding relative bioavailability was calculated to be 21.24% [108].

These results clearly show that rh-insulin absorption was markedly enhanced by the nanoparticles dispersed in oily vehicle. As a proof of concept, early clinical trials have been performed by Badwan et al. [102]. The pharmacokinetic, pharmacodynamic and absorption kinetics of insulin-loaded oily nanosystem preparations of different particle sizes (57-220 nm) were compared with those of subcutaneous formulation in 25 healthy individuals using a euglycaemic clamp technique. The dose used was either 1, 2 or 3 IU/Kg. The effective permeability ratio (Peff*) was higher for preparations with a particle size of 57 nm than for those with a larger particle size. The preparation with the lowest particle size also exhibited the highest ratio in the dimensional analysis of the glucose infusion rate as a pharmacodynamic effect, while the other insulin formulations that were tested showed similar ratio profiles. The calculated intestinal permeability coefficients (×10–4) of the insulin best test and reference formulations were 0.084 and 0.179 cm/sec respectively. The total fraction of the insulin dose absorbed (Fa) for the test and reference products were 3.0% and 19% respectively. From these small studies, it was concluded that oral insulin bioavailability is promising for the development of oral insulin products.

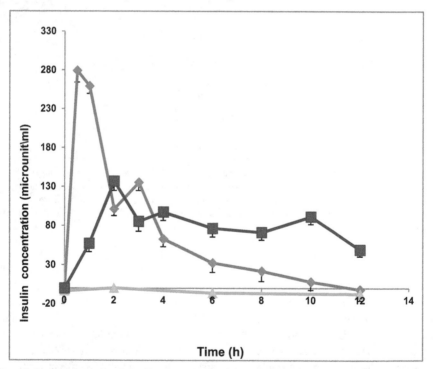

Figure 9. Insulin plasma levels profile after a single oral administration of the oily dispersion of chitosan-insulin nanoparticles (5 IU/Kg) (■ in fasted diabetic rats compared to the subcutaneous injection of free insulin (1 IU/Kg) (▲and an oral insulin solution (50 IU/kg) as a control (▲ The results are expressed as the average of the three independent experiments (n = 18)

Preparation	Cmax [μg/ml]	Tmax [hr]	MRT [hr]	AUC$_{0-12}$ [μg hr/ml]	F %
S.C injection (1 IU/kg)	279.19	0.5		626.02	
Oral formula (5 IU/kg)	102.22	2	6.72	664.99	21.24%.

Table 7. Pharmacokinetic parameters derived from the plasma level vs. the time profile for insulin

Other chitosan fatty-acid systems were also developed and compared to the above mentioned system. For example, chitosan-sodium lauryl sulphate nanoparticles dispersed in an aqueous vehicle elicited a pharmacological response after oral administration [103]. However, the pharmacological availability was poor - 1.1% versus 29% for nanoparticles dispersed in an oily vehicle. Another system was developed by dispersing PEC in oleic acid and the particle size was reduced using a high pressure homogenizer. The oral administration of this preparation resulted in a pronounced effect (P < 0.001) after 12 h of administration and the effect was sustained for 24 h (**Figure 10**). This indicates that chitosan-oleic acid nanoparticles were slowly absorbed in comparison with the preparation containing surfactants. This may be due to the permeation enhancing effect of surfactants [108]

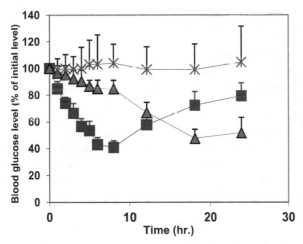

Figure 10. Changes in blood glucose level versus time profiles after a single oral administration of an oily dispersion of a chitosan-insulin oily nanosystem containing surfactant given at a dose level of 5 IU/Kg (■ to STZ-diabetic rats compared to a chitosan-insulin oily nanosystem without surfactant (▲ The control was given a placebo (a formula containing all excipient) (x). The results are expressed as the mean ± S.E.M (n = 12 per group)

In conclusion, the use of the combination strategy of nanoencapsulation and an oily vehicle has shown considerable improvement in insulin delivery along the following lines:

1) A significant hypoglycaemic action with a maximum pharmacological availability of 29.0% was obtained; 2) The relative bioavailability was 21.2%; 3) The antidiabetic activity was prolonged for many hours; 4) The insulin in the preparation was chemically and biologically stable for a period of one month at storage temperatures of 4 °C and 25 °C. 5). The system could be considered as a platform technology for the delivery of other peptides, such as calcitonin.

3. Oral insulin formulations in clinics

Oral systems in different clinical phases and the companies who have invested on them were listed in **Table 8.** The modification of proteins' structures by the attachment of proper moieties which alter their biopharmaceutical properties have been investigated by Biocon (Bangalore, India) and Nobex Corporation (Research Triangle Park, NC, USA). Nobex developed an orally active amphiphilic human insulin analogue, methoxy (polyethylene glycol) hexanoyl human recombinant insulin. Biological activity is retained and this compound is readily absorbed from the gastrointestinal tract. The effect of a single oral dose of hexyl-insulin monoconjugate 2 (HIM2) on the rate of whole-body glucose disposal (Rd) and endogenous glucose production (EGP) was investigated in healthy non-diabetic subjects using a euglycaemic clamp technique. Oral HIM2 suppresses EGP and increases tissue Rd in a dose-dependent manner. The effects of HIM2 on EGP and Rd persisted for 240 min. In patients with type 1 diabetes mellitus, a statistically significant effect of HIM2 on glucose excursion was observed [113]. The further development of the product was abandoned by the company. Biocon modified the hexyl insulin monoconjugate 2 (HIM2) developed by the Nobex Corporation. Conjugation with poly (ethylene glycol) improves the protein solubility, stability from enzymatic degradation and intestinal absorption [114]. The modified insulin (IN-105) was formulated as tablets and has a short duration of action (1.5-2 h). It was found that IN-105 reduced postprandial glucose excursion by 2 h in a dose-dependent manner and that it was readily tolerated by patients [115]. However, in Phase III studies, IN-105 did not meet the target of lowering the level of glycated haemoglobin by 0.7% compared to a placebo, as announced by the company. The level of glycated haemoglobin in the body is an indication of the effectiveness of a drug in controlling blood sugar levels. In contrast, the noncovalent interaction of macromolecules with small hydrophobic organic compounds, SNAC (n-(8-[2-hydroxybenzoyl]-amino) caprylic acid) and 5-CNAC (N-(5-chlorosalicyloyl)-8-aminocaprylic acid), was the technology developed by Emisphere's Eligen™. As a result of this interaction, the lipophilicity and absorption of the macromolecules increases and this is reflected in the rapid onset of action (about 10 minutes). Emisphere's oral insulin product was well tolerated and improved both glycaemic control and insulin sensitivity. However, a high dose (40 mg/day) is needed to decrease HbA1c significantly after 3 months of therapy [116]. ORMD 0801 is a capsule formulation of insulin developed by Oramed Pharmaceuticals (USA). An omega-3 fatty acid (carrier), a soya bean trypsin inhibitor (protease inhibitor) and sodium EDTA (absorption enhancer) were selected as adjuvants to protect the insulin from the harsh environment of the gastrointestinal tract and enhance its transport across the intestinal mucosa. ORMD is an intermediate insulin product with a duration of action of 5-6 h. This product demonstrated improved absorption, as indicated by a 28% increase in post-prandial serum insulin and it is well tolerated by patients [117]. However, the onset of action is delayed by 2 h, which may be due to the enteric coating of the capsules. Another capsule formulation (Capsulin) was developed by Diabetology (Jersey, UK). The capsule contains a mixture of penetration enhancers and solubilizers which are generally considered to be safe. The administration of the oral insulin Capsulin preparation to sixteen persons with type 2 diabetes demonstrated a significant hypoglycaemic action over a period of 6 h and was associated with only a small increase in circulating plasma insulin concentrations. Significant falls in HbA1c, weight and triglycerides were also observed [118].

Technology	Example	Company	Current status	Ref
Chemical modification	Hexyl-insulin monoconjugate-2 (HIM2)	Nobex corporation	Phase II	[113]
Chemical modification	IN-105	Biocon	Phase III	[115]
Delivery agent	Sodium N-[8-(2-hydroxybenzoyl) amino] carpylate (SNAC)	Emisphere	Phase II	[116]
Soft-gel capsule with enhancers	Oramed insulin capsule	Oramed Pharmaceuticals (USA).	Phase II	[117]
Absorption enhancers (Axcess™ delivery technology)	Capsulin™	Diabetology (Jersey, UK)	Phase II	[118]

Table 8. Systems currently being studied for the oral delivery of insulin

4. Conclusions and prospects for further investigations

Oral delivery is a physiological route for insulin administration. Improved disease management, the enhancement of patient compliance and the reduction of long-term complications of diabetes could be achieved by oral application. However, the challenges for developing oral insulin dosage forms are significant. A number of reports have appeared in the literature seeking to enhance insulin delivery via the oral route; however, the bioavailability in humans has not exceeded 10%. Most systems evaluated the pharmacodynamics and pharmacokinetics of oral insulin preparations on animal models. However, a few reports studied absorption mechanisms. The absorption of insulin is the major obstacle. Therefore, more focus should be directed on studying the very small details of absorption, especially with the development of many instrumental technologies that will help in this area. Nanotechnology will contribute largely to the success of oral insulin delivery. The investigators should plan to search for safer, simpler and scalable methods using biologically acceptable polymers. Nowadays, researchers from both academia and industrial fields work on oral insulin. With these efforts, the dream of oral insulin will become real in the near future.

Nomenclature

Da	Dalton
KDa	Kilodalton
HDV	Hepatic directed vesicles
PCL	poly ε -caprolactone
PLGA	Poly (lactic-co-glycolic acid)
PL	Polylactides
PACA	Poly (alkyl cyanoacrylate)
PEG	Polyethylene glycol
LMWC	Low molecular weight chitosan
HMWC	High molecular weight chitosan
DDA	Degree of deacetylation
M.wt	Molecular weight
HPMCP	Hydroxypropylmethylcellulose phthalate
γ-PGA	poly-γ-glutamic acid
TPP	Tripolyphosphate
TMC	Trimethyl chitosan
LDS	Lipid-based delivery systems
SLN	Solid lipid nanoparticles
GIT	Gastrointestinal tract
rh-insulin	Recombinant human insulin
WGA	Wheat germ agglutinin binds
FTIR	Fourier Transformed Infrared Spectroscopy
DSC	Differential Scanning Calorimetry
XRPD	X-Ray Powder Diffraction
NMR	Nuclear magnetic resonance
DLS	Dynamic light scattering
RP-HPLC	Reversed-phase high performance liquid chromatography
ELISA	Enzyme-linked immunosorbent assay
TEM	Transmission electron microscope
PECs	Protein Polyelectrolyte Complexes
AE	Association efficiency
SLS	Sodium lauryl sulphate
LDS	Lipid-based delivery systems
BSA	Bovine serum albumin
SGF	Simulated gastric fluid
SIF	Simulated intestinal fluid
W/O	Water in oil
O/W	Oil in water
W/O/W	Water-in-oil-in-water
S/O/W	Solid-in-oil-in water
RSD	Relative standard deviation

s.c.	Subcutaneous
PA	pharmacological availability
RBA	Relative bioavailability
STZ	Streptozotocin
Tmax	the time taken to reach the plasma peak level
Cmax	The plasma peak level
MRT	Mean residence time
AUMC	Area under the first moment curve
AUC	Area under the curve
F%	Relative bioavailability
AAC	Area above the curve
ANOVA	analysis of variance
MSE	Standard error of the mean
P	probability value
T_m	Melting temperature
GIT	Gastrointestinal tract
Rd	Rate of whole-body glucose disposal
EGP	endogenous glucose production

Author details

Amani M. Elsayed

Department of Pharmaceutics, Faculty of Pharmacy, Taif University, Taif, Saudi Arabia

Acknowledgement

The experimental work was carried out and financially supported by the Jordanian Pharmaceutical Manufacturing Company, Naor-Jordan. Dr. Adnan Badwan for his constructive comments and Dr. Mayyas El-Remawi for his revision of the manuscript.

5. References

[1] Beals J, Brader M, De Felippis M, Kovach P. Insulin. In: Crommelin D, Sindelar R. (2nd ed) Pharmaceutical biotechnology. London: Taylor and Francis group; 2002. 231-242.

[2] Whittingham J, Scott D, Chance K, Wilson A, Finch J, Brange J, Dodson G. Insulin at pH 2: structural analysis of the conditions promoting insulin fiber formation. J. Mol. Biol. 2002; 318: 479-490.

[3] Chien Y . Human insulin: Basic sciences to therapeutic uses. Drug Dev. Ind. Pharm. 1996; 22: 753-789.

[4] Nordestgard B, Agerholm-Larsen B, Stender S. Effect of exogenous hyperinsulinaemia on atherogenesis in cholesterol-fed rabbits. Diabetologia 1997; 40: 512-520.

[5] Iyer H, Khedkar A. Verm M. Oral insulin – a review of current status. Diabetes, Obesity and Metabolism. 2010; 12: 179–185.

[6] Arbit E. The physiological rationale for oral insulin administration. Diabetes Tech. & Therap. 2004; 6: 510-517.

[7] Geho W. Hepatic-directed vesicle insulin: A review of formulation development and preclinical evaluation. Journal of Diabetes Science and Technology. 2009; 3 (6): 1451-1459.

[8] des Rieux A, Fievez V, Garinot M, Schneider Y, Preat, V. Nanoparticles as potential oral delivery systems of proteins and vaccines: a mechanistic approach. J. Control Release. 2006; 116: 1-27.

[9] TenHoor C, Dressman J. Oral absorption of peptides and proteins. S T P Pharma Sci. 1992; 2: 301-312.

[10] Aoki Y, Morishita M, Takayama K. Role of the mucous/glycocalyx layers in insulin permeation across the rat ileal membrane. Int. J. Pharm. 2005; 297: 98-109.

[11] Bilati U, Allemann E, Doelker E. Strategic approaches for overcoming peptide and protein instability within biodegradable nano- and microparticles. Eur. J. Pharm. Biopharm. 2005; 59: 375-388.

[12] Brange J, Langkjaer L, Havelund S, Hougaard P. Chemical stability of insulin. 2. Formation of higher molecular weight transformation products during storage of pharmaceutical preparations. Pharm. Res.1992; 9: 727-734.

[13] Brange J, Hallund O, Sorensen E. Chemical stability of insulin. 5. Isolation, characterization and identification of insulin transformation products. Acta Pharm. Nord. 1992; 4: 223-232.

[14] Ashada H, Douen T, Mizokoshi Y, Fujita T, Murakami M, Yamamoto A, Muranishi S. Absorption characteristics of chemically modified insulin derivatives with various fatty acids in the small and large intestine . J. Pharm. Sci. 1995; 84: 682-687.

[15] Ziv E, Lior O, Kidron M. Absorption of protein via the intestinal wall. A quantitative model. Biochem. Pharmacol. 1987; 36: 1035-1039.

[16] Kisel M, Kulik L, Tsybovsky I, Vlasov A, Kholodova, Zabarovskaya Z. Liposomes with phosphatidylethanol as a carrier for oral delivery of insulin: studies in the rat. Int. J. Pharm. 2001; 216, 105-114.

[17] Scott-Moncrieff J, Shao Z, Mitra, K. Enhancement of intestinal insulin absorption by bile salt-fatty acid mixed micelles in dogs, J Pharm Sci. 1994; 83: 1465-1469.

[18] Silva-Cunha A, Chéron J, Puisieux F, Seiller M. W/O/W multiple emulsions of insulin containing a protease inhibitor and an absorption enhancer: preparation, characterization and determination of stability towards proteases in vitro. Int. J. Pharm. 1997; 158: 79-89.

[19] Kim B-Y, Jeonga J, Parkb K, Kim J-D. Bioadhesive interaction and hypoglycemic effect of insulin-loaded lectin–microparticle conjugates in oral insulin delivery system, J. Control. Release 2005; 102: 525–538.

[20] Sarmento B, Martins S, Rebeiro A, Veiga F, Neufeld R, Ferreira D. Development and comparison of different nanoparticulate polyelectrolyte complexes as insulin carriers, Int. J. Peptide Res. Therap. 2006; 12: 131-138.

[21] Xiong X, Li Y, Li Z, Zhou C, Tam K, Liu Z, Xie G. Vesicles from Pluronic/poly(lactic acid) block copolymers as new carriers for oral insulin delivery, J. Control Release 2007; 120: 11-17.

[22] Almeida A, Souto E. Solid lipid nanoparticles as a drug delivery system for peptides and proteins. Advanced Drug Delivery Reviews 2007; 59: 478–490.

[23] Niu M, Lua Y, Hovgaard L, Guan P, Tan Y, Lian R, Qi J, Wu W. Hypoglycemic activity and oral bioavailability of insulin-loaded liposomes containing bile salts in rats: The effect of cholate type, particle size and administered dose. European Journal of Pharmaceutics and Biopharmaceutics doi:10.1016/j.ejpb.2012.02.009

[24] Sarmento B, Martins S, Ferreira D, Souto E. Oral insulin delivery by means of solid lipid nanoparticles. International Journal of Nanomedicine 2007; 2(4): 743–749.

[25] Liu J, Gong T, Wang C, Zhong Z, Zhang Z. Solid lipid nanoparticles loaded with insulin by sodium cholate phosphatidylcholine-based mixed micelles: Preparation and characterization. International Journal of Pharmaceutics 2007; 340: 153–162.

[26] Fonte P, Andrade F, Arau´ jo F, Andrade C, Neves J, Sarmento B. Chitosan-Coated Solid Lipid Nanoparticles for Insulin Delivery. Methods Enzymol. 2012; 508: 295-314.

[27] Gabor F, Wirth M, Jurkovich B, Theyer G, Walcher G, Hamilton G. Lectin-mediated bioadhesion: proteolytic stability and binding characteristics of Wheat germ agglutinin and Solanum tuberosum lectin on Caco-2, HT-29 and human colonocytes. J. Control. Rel. 1997; 49: 27–37.

[28] Wirth M, Hamilton G, Gabor F. Lectin-mediated drug targeting: quantification of binding and internalization of wheat germ agglutinin and solanum tuberosum lectin using Caco-2 and HT-29 cells. J. Drug Targeting 1998; 6: 95–104.

[29] Zhang N, Ping Q, Huang, Wenfang X. Lectin-modified solid lipid nanoparticles as carriers for oral administration of insulin. International Journal of Pharmaceutics 2006; 327: 153–159.

[30] Reis C, Neufeld R, Ribeiro A, Veiga F. Nanoencapsulation I. Methods for preparation of drug-loaded polymeric nanoparticles. Nanomedicine 2006; 2: 8-21.

[31] Yang J, Sun H, Song C. Preparation, characterization and in vivo evaluation of pH-sensitive oral insulin-loaded poly(lactic-coglycolicacid) nanoparticles. Diabetes, Obesity and Metabolism 2012; 14: 358–364.

[32] Shi K, Cui F, Yamamoto H, Kawashima Y. Optimized formulation of high payload PLGA nanoparticles containing insulin-lauryl sulphate complex, Drug Dev. Ind. Pharm. 2009; 35: 177–184.

[33] Sun S, Liang N, Piao H, Yamamoto H, Kawashima Y, Cui F. Insulin-S.O (sodium oleate) complex-loaded PLGA nanoparticles: formulation, characterization an in vivo evaluation, J. Microencapsul. 2010; 27: 471–478.

[34] Zhang X, Sun M, Zheng A, Cao D, Bi Y, Sun J. Preparation and characterization of insulin-loaded bioadhesive PLGA. European Journal of Pharmaceutical Sciences 2012; 45: 632–638.

[35] Wu Z, Zhou L, Guo X, Jiang W, Ling L, Qian Y, Luo K, Zhang L. HP55-coated capsule containing PLGA/RS nanoparticles for oral delivery of insulin. International Journal of Pharmaceutics 2012; 425: 1– 8.

[36] Sharma G, van der Walle C, Kumar M. Antacid co-encapsulated polyester nanoparticles for peroral delivery of insulin: Development, pharmacokinetics, biodistribution and pharmacodynamics. International Journal of Pharmaceutics doi:10.1016/j.ijpharm.2011.12.038

[37] Bock N, Dargaville T, Woodruff M. Electrospraying of Polymers with Therapeutic Molecules: State of the Art. Progress in Polymer Science doi:10.1016/j.progpolymsci.2012.03.002.

[38] Cui F, Shi K, Zhang L, Tao A, Kawashima Y. Biodegradable nanoparticles loaded with insulin–phospholipid complex for oral delivery: Preparation, in vitro characterization and in vivo evaluation. Journal of Controlled Release 2006; 114 (2): 242–250.

[39] Damgé C, Maincent P, Ubrich N. Oral delivery of insulin associated to polymeric nanoparticles in diabetic rats. Journal of Controlled Release 2007; 117: 163–170.

[40] Damgé C, Socha M, Ubrich N, Maincent P. Poly(ε-caprolactone)/eudragit nanoparticles for oral delivery of aspart-insulin in the treatment of diabetes. Journal of pharmaceutical sciences 2010; 99 (2): 879–889.

[41] Davis S. Drug delivery systems. Interdisciplinary Sci. Rev. 2000; 25: 175-185.

[42] Damge´ C, Vranckx H, Balschmidt P, Couvreur P. Poly(alkylcyanoacrylate) nanospheres for oral administration of insulin. J. Pharm. Sci. 1997; 86: 1403–1409.

[43] Graf A, Rades T, Hook S. Oral insulin delivery using nanoparticles based on microemulsions with different structure-types: Optimisation and in vivo evaluation. European journal of pharmaceutical sciences 2009; 3 (7): 53–61.

[44] Pawar H, Douroumis D, Boateng J. Preparation and optimization of PMAA–chitosan–PEG nanoparticles for oral drug delivery. Colloids and Surfaces B: Biointerfaces 2012; 90: 102– 108.

[45] Jelvehgari M, Milani P, Siahi-Shadbad M, Loveymi B, Nokhodchi A, Azari Z, Valizadeh H. Development of pH-sensitive insulin nanoparticles using Eudragit L100-55 and chitosan with different molecular weights. AAPS PharmSciTech. 2010; 11 (3): 1237-1242.

[46] Li M, Lu W, Wang J, Zhang X, Wang X, Zheng A, Zhang Q. Distribution, transition, adhesion and release of insulin loaded nanoparticles in the gut of rats. International Journal of Pharmaceutics. 2007; 329: 182–191.

[47] Sarmento B, Ribeiro A, Francisco Veiga F, Ferreira D. Development and characterization of new insulin containing polysaccharide nanoparticles. Colloids and Surfaces B: Biointerfaces. 2006; 53: 193–202.

[48] Russell-Jones G, Westwood S, Farnworth P, Findlay J, Burger H. Synthesis of LHRH antagonists suitable for oral administration via vitamin B12 uptake system, Bioconjug. Chem. 1995; 12: 34–42.

[49] Chalasani K, Russell-Jones, G, Yandrapu, Diwan P, Jain S. A novel vitamin B12-nanosphere conjugate carrier system for peroral delivery of insulin. Journal of Controlled Release 2007; 117: 421–429.

[50] Sarmento B, Ferreira D, Veiga F, Ribeiro A. Characterization of insulin-loaded alginate nanoparticles produced by ionotropic pre-gelation through DSC and FTIR studies. Carbohydrate Polymers 2006; 66: 1–7.

[51] Sarmento B, Ribeiro A, Veiga F, Sampaio P, Neufeld R, and Ferreira D. Alginate/Chitosan Nanoparticles are Effective for Oral Insulin Delivery. Pharmaceutical Research, 2007; 24 (12): 724-733.

[52] Zhang N, Li, Jiang W, Ren C, Li J, Xin J, Li K. Effective protection and controlled release of insulin by cationic β-cyclodextrin polymers from alginate/chitosan nanoparticles. International Journal of Pharmaceutics 2010; 393, 212–218.

[53] Reis C, Veiga F, Ribeiro A, Neufeld R, Damage C. Nanoparticulate biopolymers deliver insulin orally eliciting pharmacological response. J. Pharm. Sci. 2008; 97 (12) 5290-5305.

[54] Woitiski C, Veiga F, Ribeiro A, Neufeld R. Design for optimization of nanoparticles integrating biomaterials for orally dosed insulin. European Journal of Pharmaceutics and Biopharmaceutics 2009; 73, 25–33.

[55] Woitiskia C, Neufeld R, Veiga F, Carvalhoc R, Figueiredo. Pharmacological effect of orally delivered insulin facilitated by multilayered stable nanoparticles. European Journal of Pharmaceutical Sciences 2010; 41, 556–563.

[56] Sonia T, Sharma C. An overview of natural polymers for oral insulin delivery. Drug Discov Today 2012; http://dx.doi.org/10.1016/j.drudis.2012.03.019.

[57] Muzzarelli R. Chemical and technological advances in chitins and chitosans useful for the Formulation of biopharmaceuticals in Sarmento B, Neves J. (ed.) Chitosan-based systems for biopharmaceuticals: Delivery, Targeting and Polymer Therapeutics. 2012 John Wiley & Sons, Ltd. 2012; pp. 3-21.

[58] Kittur F, Kumar A, Tharanathan R. Low molecular weight chitosans preparation by depolymerization with Aspergillus niger pectinase, and characterization, Carbohydr. Res. 2003; 338, 1283-1290.

[59] Kumar A, Tharanathan, R. A comparative study on depolymerization of chitosan by proteolytic enzymes, Carbohyd Polym. 2004; 58, 275–283.

[60] Hai L, Bang Diep T, Nagasawa N, Yoshii F, Kume T. Radiation depolymerization of chitosan to prepare oligomers, Nuclear Instruments and Methods in Physics Research B 2003; 208, 466–470.

[61] Cravotto G, Tagliapietra S, Robaldo B, Michele Trotta M. Chemical modification of chitosan under high-intensity ultrasound, Ultrasonics Sonochemistry 2005; 12, 95–98.

[62] Tian F, Liu Y, Hu K, Zhao B. Study of the depolymerization behavior of chitosan by hydrogen peroxide, Carbohydr. Polym. 2004; 57, 31–37.

[63] Mao S, Shuai X, Unger F, Simona M, Bi D, Kissel T. The depolymerization of chitosan: effects on physicochemical and biological properties, Int. J. Pharm. 2004; 281: 45–54.

[64] George M, Abraham T.E. Polyionic hydrocolloids for the intestinal delivery of protein drugs: alginate and chitosan--a review, J. Control Release 2006; 114: 1-14.

[65] Gan Q. Wang T. Chitosan nanoparticle as protein delivery carrier--systematic examination of fabrication conditions for efficient loading and release, Colloids Surf. B Biointerfaces 2007; 59: 24-34.

[66] Chaudhury A, Surajit Das. Recent advancement of chitosan-based nanoparticles for oral controlled delivery of insulin and other therapeutic agents. AAPS PharmSciTech, 2011; 12 (1) 10-20.

[67] Ma Z, Lim T, Lim, L. Pharmacological activity of peroral chitosan-insulin nanoparticles in diabetic rats, Int. J. Pharm. 2005; 293, 271-280.

[68] Makhlof A, Tozukaa Y, Takeuchi H. Design and evaluation of novel pH-sensitive chitosan nanoparticles for oral insulin delivery. European Journal of Pharmaceutical Sciences 2011; 42, 445–451.

[69] Sonaje K, Lin YH, Juang JH, Wey SP, Chen CT, Sung HW. In vivo evaluation of safety and efficacy of self-assembled nanoparticles for oral insulin delivery. Biomaterials 2009;30(12):2329–2339

[70] Sonaje K, Chen YJ, Chen HL, Shiaw-Pyng Wey, SP, Juang JH, Nguyen HN, Hsu CW, Lin KJ, Sung HW. Enteric-coated capsules filled with freeze-dried chitosan/poly(g-glutamic acid) nanoparticles for oral insulin delivery. Biomaterials 2010; 31, 3384-3394.

[71] Su FY, Lin KJ, Sonaje K, Wey SP, Yen TC, Ho YC, Panda N, Chuang EY, Barnali Maiti B, Sung HW. Protease inhibition and absorption enhancement by functional nanoparticles for effective oral insulin delivery. Biomaterials 2012; 33, 2801-2811.

[72] Mukhopadhyay P, Mishra R, Rana D, Kundu P. Strategies for effective oral insulin delivery with modified chitosan nanoparticles: A review. Progress in Polymer Science. 2012; doi:10.1016/j.progpolymsci.2012.04.004.

[73] Jin Y, Song Y, Zhu X, Zhou D, Chen C, Zhang Z, Huang Y. Goblet cell-targeting nanoparticles for oral insulin delivery and the influence of mucus on insulin transport. Biomaterials 2012; 33, 1573-1582.

[74] Yin L, Ding J, He C, Cui L, Tang C, Yin C. Drug permeability and mucoadhesion properties of thiolated trimethyl chitosan nanoparticles in oral insulin delivery. Biomaterials 2009; 30, 5691–5700.

[75] Sonia T, Sharma C. In vitro evaluation of N-(2-hydroxy) propyl-3-trimethyl ammonium chitosan for oral insulin delivery. Carbohydrate Polymers 2011; 84, 103–109.

[76] Zhu S, Qian F, Zhang Y, Tang C, Yin C. Synthesis and characterization of PEG modified N-trimethylaminoethylmethacrylate chitosan nanoparticles. European Polymer Journal 2007; 43, 2244–2253.

[77] Mao S, Bakowsky U, Jintapattanakit A, Kissel T. Self-assembled polyelectrolyte nanocomplexes between chitosan derivatives and insulin. Int. J. Pharm. 2008; 355, 299-306.

[78] Shelm R, Paul W, Sharma C. Development and characterization of self-aggregated nanoparticles from anacardoylated chitosan as a carrier for insulin. Carbohydrate Polymers 2010; 80, 285–290.

[79] Pouton C, Porter C. Formulation of lipid-based delivery systems for oral administration: Materials, methods and strategies. Adv. Drug Deliv. Rev. 2008; 60, 625–637.

[80] O'Driscoll C, Griffin B. (2008). Biopharmaceutical challenges associated with drugs with low aqueous solubility—The potential impact of lipid-based formulations. Adv. Drug Deliv. Rev. 2008; 60, 617–624.

[81] Morishita M, Matsuzawa A, Takayama K, Isowa K, Nagai T. Improving insulin enteral absorption using water-in-oil-in-water emulsion. Int. J. Pharm. 1998; 172, 189-198.

[82] Shima M, Tanaka M, Fujii T, Egawa K, Kimura Y, Adachi S. Matsuno, R. Oral administration of insulin included in fine W/O/W emulsions to rats. Food Hydrocolloids 2006; 20, 523–531.

[83] Lawrence M, Rees G. Microemulsion-based media as novel drug delivery systems. Adv. Drug Deliv. Rev. 2000; 45, 89–121.

[84] Moulik S, Paul, B. Structure, dynamics and transport properties of microemulsions, Advances in Colloid and Interface Science 1998; 78, 99-195.

[85] Sharma G, Wilson K, van der Walle C, Sattar N, Petrie J, Kumar M. Microemulsions for oral delivery of insulin: Design, development and evaluation in streptozotocin induced diabetic rats. European Journal of Pharmaceutics and Biopharmaceutics 2010; 76 159–169.

[86] Cilek A, Celebi N, Tirnaksiz F, Tay A. A lecithin-based microemulsion of rh-insulin with aprotinin for oral administration: Investigation of hypoglycemic effects in non-diabetic and STZ-induced diabetic rats. Int. J. Pharm. 2005; 298,176-185.

[87] Kraaling M, Ritschel W. Development of a colonic release capsule dosage form and the absorption of insulin, Methods Find. Exp. Clin. Pharmacol. 1992; 14, 199–209.

[88] Cho Y. Flynn M. Oral delivery of insulin. Lancet 1989; 2, 1518–1519.

[89] Ma E, Ma H, Zheng G, Duan M. In vitro and in vivo evaluation of a novel oral insulin formulation. Acta Pharmacol Sin. 2006; 27 (10) 1382-1388.

[90] Toorisaka E, Hashida M, Kamiya N, Ono H, Kokazu Y, and Goto M. Hypoglycemic effect of surfactant-coated insulin solubilized in a novel solid-in-oil-in-water (S/O/W) emulsion. Int.J.Pharm. 2003; 252 (1) 271-274.

[91] Toorisaka E, Hashida M, Kamiya N, Ono H, Kokazu Y, and Goto M. An enteric-coated dry emulsion formulation for oral insulin delivery. J. Control. Release 2005; 107, 91–96.

[92] O'Driscoll, C. Lipid-based formulations for intestinal lymphatic delivery. Eur. J. Pharm Sci.2002; 15, 405-415.

[93] Lin YH, Mi FL, Chen CT, Chang WC, Peng SF, Liang HF, Sung HW. Preparation and characterization of nanoparticles shelled with chitosan for oral insulin delivery. Biomacromolecules 2007; 8, 146-152.

[94] Ma Z, Yeoh HH, Lim LY, Formulation pH modulates the interaction of insulin with chitosan nanoparticles. J. Pharm. Sci. 2002; 91, 1396-1404.

[95] Sarciaux J, Acar L, and Sado P. Using microemulsion formulations for oral delivery of therapeutic peptides. Int. J. Pharm. 1995; 120, 127-136.

[96] Lyons K, Charman W, Miller R, Porter C. Factors limiting the oral bioavailability of N-acetylglucosaminyl-N-acetylmuramyl dipeptide (GMDP) and enhancement of absorption in rats by delivery in a water-in-oil microemulsion. Int. J. Pharm. 2000; 199, 17-28.

[97] Assaf S, Al-Jbour N, Eftaiha A, Elsayed A, Al Remawi M, Qinna N, Chowdhry B, Leharne S Badwan A. Factors involved in formulation of oily delivery system for proteins based on PEG-8 caprylic/capric glycerides and polyglyceryl-6 dioleate in a mixture of oleic acid with chitosan. Journal of Dispersion Science and Technology 2011; 32, 623–633.

[98] Chae S, Jang M, Nah J. Influence of molecular weight on oral absorption of water soluble chitosans, J. Control. Release 2005; 102: 383-394.

[99] Badwan A, Al-Remawi M, Eltaher N, Elsayed A. Nanocapsules for oral delivery of proteins. European Patent (EP2042166) date of publication, 1 April 2009.

[100] Badwan A, Al-Remawi M, Eltaher N, Elsayed A. Oral delivery of protein drug using microemulsion. International patent (WO2007/068311) date of publication, 21 June 2007.

[101] Elsayed A, Al-Remawi M, Qinna N, Farouk A, Badwan A. Formulation and characterization of an oily-based system for oral delivery of insulin. Euro. J. Pharm. Biopharm. 2009; 73: 269-279.

[102] Badwan A, Remawi M, Qinna N, Elsayed A, Arafat T, Melhim M, Abu Hijleh M, Idkaidek N. Enhancement of oral bioavailability of insulin in humans. Neuroendocrinology Letters 2009; 30: 101-105.

[103] Elsayed A, Al-Remawi M, Qinna N, Farouk A, Al-Sou'od K, Badwan A. Chitosan–sodium Lauryl sulphate nanoparticles as a carrier system for the in Vivo delivery of oral insulin. AAPS Pharm.Sci.Tech. 2011; 12, 958-964.

[104] Richardson S, Kolbe H, Duncan, R. Potential of low molecular mass chitosan as a DNA delivery system: biocompatibility, body distribution and ability to complex and protect DNA. Int. J. Pharm. 1999; 178, 231-243.

[105] Jeon YJ, Park P, Kim S. Antimicrobial effect of chitooligosaccharides produced by bioreactor. Carbohdr. Polym. 2001; 44, 71-76.

[106] Kondo Y, Nakatani A, Hayashi k, Ito M. (2000). Low molecular weight chitosan prevents the progression of low dose streptozotocin-induced slowly progressive diabetes mellitus in mice. Biol. Pharm. Bull. 2000; 23, 1458-1464.

[107] Qin C, Li H, Xiao Q, Liu Y, Zhu J, Du Y. Water-solubility of chitosan and its antimicrobial activity, Carbohydr. Polym. 2006; 63: 367–374.

[108] Elsayed AM. Oral Insulin Delivery System: Design, Development and Evaluation. PhD thesis. Faculty of Pharmacy, University of Gezira, Wad Medani; 2009.

[109] Morishita M, Matsuzawa A, Takayama K, Isowa K, and Nagai T. Improving insulin enteral absorption using water-in-oil-in-water emulsion. Int. J. Pharm. 1998; 172, 189-198.

[110] Araujo L, Sheppard M, Lobenberg R, Kreuter J. Uptake of PMMA nanoparticles from the gastrointestinal tract after oral administration to rats: modification of the body distribution after suspension in surfactant solutions and in oil vehicles. Int. J. Pharm. 1999; 176,209-224.

[111] Prasad Y, Minamimoto T, Yoshikawa Y, Shibata N, Mori S, Matsuura A, Takada K. In situ intestinal absorption studies on low molecular weight heparin in rats using Labrasol as absorption enhancer, Int. J. Pharm. 2004; 271, 225-232.

[112] Koga K, Kusawake Y, Ito Y, Sugioka N, Shibata N, Takada K. Enhancing mechanism of Labrasol on intestinal membrane permeability of the hydrophilic drug gentamicin sulphate. Eur. J. Pharm. Biopharm. 2006; 64, 82-91.

[113] Clement S, ; Dandona P, Still J, Kosutic G. Oral modified insulin (HIM2) in patients with type 1 diabetes mellitus: results from a phase I/II clinical trial, Metabolism. 2004; 53: 54.

[114] Calceti P, Salmaso S, Walker G, Bernkop-Schnurch A. Development and in vivo evaluation of an oral insulin-PEG delivery system. Eur. J. Pharm. Sci. 2004; 22, 315-323.

[115] Dave N, Hazra P, Khedkar A, Manjunath H, Iyer H, Suryanarayanan S. Process and purification for manufacture of a modified insulin intended for oral delivery. J. Chromatography A 2008; 1177, 282–286.

[116] Malkov D, Angelo R, Wang H, Flanders E, Tang H, and Gomez-Orellana I. (2005). Oral delivery of insulin with the eligen technology: mechanistic studies. Curr Drug Deliv. 2005; 2, 191-197.

[117] Sabetsky V, Ekblom J. Insulin: A new era for an old hormone. Pharmacological Research 2010; 61, 1–4.

[118] Luzio S, Dunseath G, Lockett A, Broke-Smith T, New R, Owens D. The glucose lowering effect of an oral insulin (Capsulin) during an isoglycaemic clamp study in persons with type 2 diabetes. Diabetes, Obesity and Metabolism 2010; 12, 82–87.

Chapter 3

Novel Mucoadhesive Polymers for Nasal Drug Delivery

Utkarshini Anand, Tiam Feridooni and Remigius U. Agu

Additional information is available at the end of the chapter

1. Introduction

The use of nasal cavity as a route of administration of drugs, specifically systemically acting drugs that pose a delivery challenge, have become an area of great interest to the pharmaceutical companies in the past decade. The physiology of the nasal cavity allows for variety of drug delivery possibilities and destinations which include local, systemic, vaccine, and access to the central nervous system (CNS)[1]

Anatomically, the nasal cavity can be divided into three functional regions (**Figure 1**):

1. Vestibular region having an area of 10 to 20 sq.cm and is situated just inside the nostrils. It is covered with stratified, keratinised and squamous epithelium.
2. Respiratory region having an area of about 130 sq.cm and occupies majority of the nasal cavity and consists of three turbinates namely inferior, middle and superior.
3. Olfactory region has an area of about 10 - 20 sq.cm. It is located in the roof of the nasal cavity and on the upper part of the nasal septum. It contains the receptors for the sense of smell. Local delivery of drugs in the nasal cavity can be used to treat allergies, congestion and infection. Systemic delivery of the drugs can be used for crisis treatments during a rapid onset of symptoms, daily administration of drugs for long-term treatment of disorders or delivery of peptides or proteins that may be difficult to administer. The nasal cavity can also be used to deliver vaccines including antigens (whole cells, split cells, and surface antigens) and DNA vaccines [1]. The nasal cavity also allows access to the CNS, thus allowing drugs to circumvent the blood-brain barrier (BBB) [1]. It has been suggested that there is free communication between the nasal submucosal interstitial space and the olfactory perinueronal space, which appears to be continuous with a subarachnoid extension that surrounds the olfactory nerve [2].

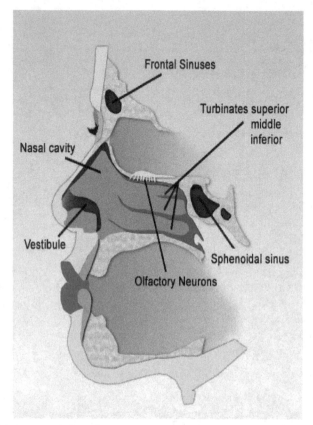

Figure 1. Nasal Anatomy and Physiology

The pharmaceutical companies are increasingly marketing drugs as nasal formulations, drugs such as sumatriptan, estradiol, buserelin, and calcitonin, all which have shown to have faster onset of action, improved bioavailability, and a better delivery method [3].

There are a number of advantages in using nasal cavity for administration of drugs. Some of the advantages are: avoidance of the gastrointestinal tract along with hepatic first pass metabolism, increased absorption and bioavailability of small and larger drug molecules[4]. Furthermore, drugs that have low oral bioavailability have been shown to be successfully delivered systemically using the nasal route; studies have suggested that the nasal route is a great alternative to parenteral route for delivery of protein and peptide drugs [4]. Also due to direct delivery of drugs to the systemic circulation, the onset of pharmacological action is rapid [5].

Administration of lower drug doses through the nasal route, may lead to lower side effects. The convenient delivery of drugs via the nasal route, especially in long-term therapies has proven to increase patience compliance compared to parenteral and injection methods [4].

Lipophilic drugs generally have no trouble being absorbed through the nasal cavity. In fact, the bioavailability of lipophilic drugs been shown to be very close to those of intravenous injection (100% bioavailability), for instance, fentanyl has been shown to have an 80% bioavailability for nasal administration [1].

Even though the nasal cavity has a large surface area along with extensive blood supply, it has been shown that the permeability of the nasal mucosa is low for polar molecules. The limiting-factor for nasal absorption of polar drugs such as peptides and proteins is epithelial membrane permeability. Drugs with molecular weights lower than 1000Da can generally pass the epithelial membrane via transcellular route, receptor mediated transport, vesicular transport, use of concentration gradient force [6], or travelling in the paracellular route through the tight junction between the cells. In fact tight junctions seem to have finite permeability to molecules with molecular radii less than or equal 3.6 A and are essentially impermeable to those with molecular radii greater than or equal to 15 A [7]. Despite the advantages of nasal drug delivery, some of the drugs may also cause inconvenience due to potential for nasal irritation. Pathological conditions such as cold and allergies may alter nasal bioavailability significantly, which can have an effect on the intended pharmacological action [8].

Another factor that plays an imperative role in low membrane transport of nasally administered drug therapeutics is rapid drug clearance by the mucociliary clearance mechanism. This problem is common with drugs that are not easily absorbed across the nasal membrane. It has been shown that drugs that do not readily cross the nasal membrane, whether liquid or power form are removed from the nasal cavity in 15-20 min [9]. Mucociliary clearance tends to decrease the residence time of the administered drug. This problem can be overcome using formulation strategies. Novel delivery platforms based on polymeric drug carriers along with variety of methods that can be used to improve the absorption of drugs through the nasal route will be discussed in the following paper. These delivery systems work by attaching themselves to the mucus layer and thus preventing clearance of the drug delivery system. Some of these delivery systems are still experimental, whereas others have advanced to clinical use. **Figure 2** summarizes the various mechanisms involved in mucoadhesion of the main drug carriers discussed in this chapter.

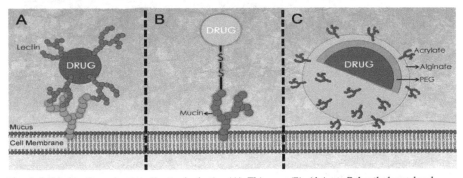

Figure 2. Mechanisms of mucoadhesion by lectins (A), Thiomers (B), Alginate Poly ethylene glycol acrylate (C).

2. Lectins

Lectins are classified as a group of structurally diverse proteins [10] that are found in plants as well as in the animal kingdom. They are also found in some microorganisms [11]. Lectins have the capability to identify and bind to specific sugar moieties. The sugar-binding moiety of most lectins is only a small part of the lectin, i.e., a major portion of lectin is not involved in the recognition and binding to the receptor[12]. Lectins also cause agglutination due to their ability to cross link sugar containing macromolecules. Primarily they identify only specific sugars like mannose, glucose, galactose, N-acetyl-glucosamine, N-acetyl galactosmaine, furose and N-acetyl neuramic acid [13]. The various lectins which have shown specific binding to the mucosa include lectins extracted from *Ulex europaeus* I, soybean, peanut and *Lens culinarius*. The use of wheat germ agglutinin has been on the rise due to its least immunogenic reactions, amongst available lectins [2]. Lectins have the ability to stay on the cell surface or become internalized via a process called endocytosis if the adhesion is receptor mediated. In this manner lectins offer twin functionality of not only allowing target specific attachment but also a means of delivering the drug through a controlled process to the cells by active cell mediated drug uptake [1]. Lectins have potential to be used in Nasal Drug Delivery, especially where internalization of the drug encapsulated nanoparticles is of particular importance such as DNA delivery[14]. Inspite of lectins offering significant advantages, it is worth noting that such polymers suffer at least in part from premature inactivation by shed off mucus. This phenomenon has been reported to be advantageous, given that the mucus layer provides an initial yet fully reversible binding site followed by distribution of lectin-mediated drug delivery systems to the cell layer[15].

There are three types of lectins - classified based on their molecular structure:

1. *Merolectins*: lectins which have one carbohydrate recognising domain [1].
2. *Hololectins*: lectins which have two or more carbohydrate recognising domains [1].
3. *Chimerolectins*: lectins with additional unrelated domains [1].

Lectins are involved in various biological processes: cell-to-cell recognition and communication, particularly in the mammalian immune system (transendothelial migration), adhesion and attack of infectious agents on host cells, and clearance of glycoproteins from the blood circulation [16]. Lectins are used in conjugation with other mucoadhesive polymers as drug delivery vehicles to the brain or systemic circulation through the nasal cavity. It was observed that negligible penetration of nanoparticles takes place between cells in the nasal epithelium when administered on their own. Secondly, mucociliary clearance reduced the residence time of the particles in the nasal cavity (particles cleared within the nose every 15 to 20min, thus, resulting in incomplete absorption of the formulation. Also it was found that, unmodified nanoparticles distributed in the nasal cavity without selectivity. This resulted in poor brain targeting efficiency of the formulation. To deal with these problems, novel lectin-modified nanoparticles were constructed. The lectin used was wheat germ agglutinin (WGA), which specifically binds to N-acetyl-D-glucosamine and sialic acid moieties, both of which were abundantly observed in the nasal cavity especially in the olfactory mucosa [17].

Factors like low ciliary irritation and high permeability among other considerations favour the potential use of lectins for nasal drug delivery [18]. Studies in animals concluded that lectins have minimal acute irritancy and can be thus be used for further in vivo studies[19]. However, many lectins are toxic or immunogenic especially those obtained from *Ricinus communis, Phaseolus vulgaris* and *Lycopersicon esculentum* and *Canavalia ensiformis*[5] .There is a probability that lectins promote the production of antibodies which could lead to the blockage of lectin-based delivery vehicles. These antibodies may also expose patients to the risk of systemic anaphylaxis on successive exposure. But, by using truncated varieties of lectin molecules as mucoadhesives this potential risk of toxicity may be triumphed over [20].

Mucoadhesive Polymer	Dosage Formulation	Active Ingredient	Reference
Odorranalectin	Liquid	coumarin-6	Wu H et al[21]
wheat germ agglutinin conjugated PEG-PLA nanoparticles	Liquid	coumarin-6	Liu Q et al[22]
Solanum tuberosum lectin-conjugated PLGA nanoparticles	Powder	coumarin-6	Chen J et al [18]

Table 1. Synopsis of the studies on the use of Lectins in formulations for nasal drug delivery

3. Thiomers

Thiomers are mucoadhesive polymers that have side chains carrying thiols which lead to formation of covalent bonds between the cystiene groups in the mucus and the polymer by thiol/disulphide exchange reactions or simple oxidation process. These bonds are also known as disulphide bridges. These bridges sometimes improve mucoadhesion by 100 folds. They also have permeability enhancing effect and ability to control the rate at which drugs are released. This property and increased mucoadhesion leads to higher residence time of the drugs administered in combination with thiomers hence improving their bioavailability [23]. Thiomers are also used in combination with other polymers like chitosan, poly acrylic acid, etc. Due to immobilization of thiol groups, mucoadhesive properties of these polymers are increased by 140 folds and 20 folds respectively [12]. Thus, thiomers are one of the most mucoadhesive polymers known at the present [24]. Thiomers enhance the permeability of drugs with the potential advantage of not being absorbed through the nasal mucosa compared to low molecular weight permeation enhancers. Thus their permeation enhancing effects can be maintained over a longer period of time while excluding systemic toxic effects.[25] Thiomers tend to cause reversible opening of the tight junctions with glutathione as permeation mediator [26]. Thiolated polymers display in situ gelling properties due to the oxidation of thiol groups at physiological pH-values, which results in the formation of inter- and intramolecular disulfide bonds[12]. This increases the viscosity of the formulation coupled with extensive crosslinking due to formation of disulphide bonds with the nasal mucosa, which increases the residence time of the formulation tremendously [27].

Other studies on thiomer combinations with other polymers by Bernkop-Schnurch led to formation of thiolated polycarbophil which increases the uptake of Leu-enkephalin from the nasal mucosa by 82 folds, thus a promising excipient for delivery of Leu-enkephalin through the nasal mucosa[28]. In another study, thiolated polyacrylate microparticles were generated for the nasal delivery of human growth hormone (hGH). The intranasal administration of this microparticulate formulation to rats resulted in a relative bioavailability of $8.11 \pm 2.15\%$ that represents a 3-fold improvement compared to microparticles comprising the corresponding unmodified polymer[29].

The nasal route is an attractive alternative to parenteral delivery for a number of therapeutic peptides such as calcitonin, insulin, desmopressin, buserelin and octreotide. However, membrane permeability is low for nasally administered peptides leading to low bioavailabilities, a short local residence time at the site of absorption and a high metabolic turnover in the epithelium. The three major approaches to increase the bioavailability of intranasally administered peptide drugs are (i) the use of permeation enhancers, (ii) incorporation of enzyme inhibitors and (iii) increasing local drug residence time using mucoadhesive polymers. Thiomers are capable of combining most of these strategies. Therefore, thiomers can be used as multifunctional vehicles for systemic nasal peptide delivery[30]. Due to their high molecular mass, thiomers are not absorbed from the nasal mucosa thus systemic toxic effects can be excluded. Ciliary Beat Frequency (CBF) studies with human nasal epithelium cells show that thiomers do not cause any alteration or impact on CBF. Thiomers have also been found in various studies to not cause any irritation to mucosal cells[31]. Table 2 summarizes nasal drug delivery studies with thiomers.

Mucoadhesive Polymer	Dosage Formulation	Active Ingredient	Reference
Thiomer (polycarbophil-cysteine)	Gel	Leu-enkephalin	Bernkop-Schnürch A et al.[28]
Thiomer (polycarbophil-cysteine /glutathione gel)	Gel	Human growth Hormone	Leitner VM et al.[32]
Thiomer (polycarbophil-cysteine)	Microparticles	phosphorothioate antisense oligonucleotide	Vetter A et al[33]
Thiolated chitosan	Microparticles	insulin	Krauland AH et al[34]

Table 2. Use of thiomers in mucoadhesive nasal formulations for systemic delivery

4. Alginate poly-ethylene glycol acrylate

Alginate Polyethylene glycol Acrylate is also known by the acronym Alginate-PEGAc. It has an alginate backbone with acrylated polyethylenglycol groups attached to it. This polymer meshes the properties of alginates (strength, simplicity and gelation) with characteristics specific to the acrylate functionality of PEG like mucoadhesion. PEG's have the ability to penetrate the mucus surface while the acrylate group of the polymer reacts with the sulphide group of glycoproteins present in the mucus. This results in a strong interaction between the mucus and the polymer [35]. It is expected to be cross-linkable by two different paths: chemically via the acrylate end groups and physically through the alginate backbone [36]. Alginate is a mucoadhesive polysaccharide of 1 →4 linked α-l-glucuronic acid and β-d-mannuronic acid which binds to the glycoproteins in the mucus through carboxyl–hydroxyl interactions [37]. It is anionic in nature. It is known to undergo ionic sol to gel transition (gelation) upon interaction with multivalent ions such as $Ca2^+$, $Fe2^+$ [38], thus reducing its adhesion to mucosal tissues [39]. On the other hand Poly-Ethylene Glycol (PEG) is an FDA approved polymer. It is non-toxic, non-immunogenic and non-antigenic. It has high solubility in water and rapid in vivo clearance. It also has the ability to form hydrogen bonds with sugar moieties on glycosylated proteins. This causes PEG to form strong bonds with mucus leading to increased mucoadhesion [25].

Poly Acrylic Acid forms hydrogen bonds between its carboxylic acid groups and sialic acid-carboxylic acid groups present in the mucus [40]. The most recent method for synthesis of Alginate PEG-Ac is a two stage procedure. First the synthesis of alginate thiol takes place. In the second stage, a Michael type addition reaction takes place where a nucleophilic addition between PEG-Diacrylate and alginate backbone occurs conjugating the two [25].

Modification of Alginates with addition of acrylic acid is done to optimize its shortcomings such as erosion in neutral pH. Addition of acrylic acid controls the release rate of drugs and also improves its adhesive properties [29]. Also it has been found that at physiological pH of 7.4 both poly acrylic acid and sialic acid undergo ionization, thus repelling each other. This leads to rapid removal of this polymer-based drug delivery system. Addition of PEG results in H-bonding with PAA enhancing the viscosity of the resulting drug delivery vehicle. Addition of PEG to the polymer increases the viscosity of the resulting polymer complex retarding disintegration and removal of the polymer from the mucosal surface thus increasing mucoadhesion [30]. The combination of the three functional moieties of Alginate Polyethylene glycol Acrylate leads to an improved novel polymer that can be used mucoadhesive nasal drug delivery.

5. Poloxamer (Pluronics)

There is a great interest in Poloxamer based formulations. A number of reviews have been published describing in detail poloxamer formulations like gels, poloxamer-coated nanoparticles, o/w and w/o emulsions, and solid polymer blends [41]. Poloxamers are made up of non-ionic difunctional triblock[42] copolymers containing a centrally located hydrophobic polypropylene oxide between hydrophilic polyethylene oxides [43,44]. Aqueous solutions of poloxamers are extremely stable in the presence of acids, alkalis and metal ions. These polymers are readily soluble in aqueous, polar and non-polar organic solvents. Hence, they are widely preferred choice as excipients in formulations [45]. Poloxamers are said to contain thermoreversible property and will convert from a liquid to a gel at body temperature, thus, causing in situ gelation at the site of interest [1] preventing the drug to be removed from the nasal cavity due to mucociliary clearance. This vastly improves the bioavailability of the drug administered. The formation of the gel can be explained as follows. When the poloxamer is cooled, the hydration layer surrounds the poloxamer molecule and hydrophobic portions are separated due to hydrogen bonding. As the temperature increases, desolvation of the hydrophilic chains occurs as the result of breakage of hydrogen bonds. This results into hydrophobic interactions amongst the polypropylene oxide domains and gel gets formed. Hydroxyl groups of the copolymer become more accessible due to hydration[46]. Thus, desolvation caused by increase in temperature and subsequently micellization results in formation of a more closely packed viscous gel [47] Various combinations of poloxamers and other mucoadhesive polymers like polycarbophil and polyethylene oxide have been found to be more advantageous since their combination tends to reduce the gelation temperature of poloxamer. This can help in making a polymer that can gel at the temperature observed in the nasal mucosa[5]. Poloxamers are also known as Pluronics. Pluronics have also been chemically combined with poly(acrylic acid)s like Dihydroxyphenylalanine (DOPA)[31] to produce systems with enhanced adhesion and retention in the nasal cavity.

One of the most promising poloxamer is Poloxamer 407 (Pluronic F127) because of its low toxicity, high solubility, bioadhesion characteristics, and   acceptability as drug delivery vehicle [48]. Some of the other investigated combination of poloxamers are polymer pluronic PF127 along with benzalkonium chloride which helped decreased the gelation onset temperature. This combination was prepared for the nasal delivery of Vitamin B12[49]. In another study, poloxamer 407 was combined with a mucoadhesive polymer or polyethylene glycol. The combination allowed the manipulation of the temperature at which the conversion of sol to gel would take place as well as decreasing and increasing the in vitro release of the drug respectively[50]. But work still needs to be done on reducing irritability which is one of the major limitations of these formulations[51]. Controlled release nasal formulations of propranolol have been made using a combination of poloxamers and other mucoadhesive polymers for such as Carbopol 934P. By controlling the release of the drug and by increasing its residence time in the nasal cavity, there was a significant increase in bioavailability of the drug[52]. Poloxamer properties are said to be affected by addition of various additives. Concentration can greatly affect the thermodynamic properties of poloxamer. Water soluble additives also affect the thermodynamic properties. The range at which gelation occurs increases with polymer concentration, whereas addition of sorbitol and PEG 15000 narrows the gel range. Significant enthalpy change occurs in gels containing sorbitol and PEG, indicative of interactions with the polymer during the phase transitions. As the concentration of the polymer increases, the aqueous gels display non-Newtonian characteristics. The hydrophobic interaction of Benzalkonium Chloride and pluronic produces a gel with higher viscosity. Addition of PEG 15000 helps achieve desired gelation characteristics for increased drug loading and use of desired formulation additives [41]. Poloxamers at low concentrations, when dispersed in liquid exist individually as monomolecular micelles. As the concentration of the pluronic in the system increases, it forms multi-molecular aggregates[53]. Different aggregate forms of poloxamers are seen depending on the molecular weight, solvent composition, and temperature[54]. Micellar behavior changes with changes in solvent composition and temperature. Various salts and additives like surfactants, polymers, cosolvents have marked effect on the micellar properties, clouding and solubilization characteristics of pluronic solutions[55]. Salts in the order of $Na_3PO_4 > Na_2SO_4 > NaCl$ have been found to lower the critical micellar temperature significantly[56]. Pluronic block copolymers are amongst the most potent drug targeting systems. Recent research on pluronics has generated new findings indicating immuno-modulation and cytotoxicity-promoting properties of Poloxamer 407 revealing significant pharmacological interest. Human trials are in progress based on these results [57]. Along with these new findings and favourable properties, poloxamers have generated immense interest as one of the most promising novel mucoadhesive drug delivery systems. Table 3 shows most of the published studies involving nasal drug delivery with this polymer.

Mucoadhesive Polymer	Dosage Formulation	Active Ingredient	Reference
Poloxamer 188 or 407	Nanovescicles	olanzapine	Salama HA et al[58]
Poloxamer-Chitosan	Gel	(32)P-siRNA dendriplexes	Perez AP et al[59]
poloxamer 407/ hydroxypropyl-β-cyclodextrin/chitosan	Gel	fexofenadine hydrochloride	Cho HJ et al[47]
chitosan-poloxamer 188	Spray	fentanyl	Fisher A et al[60]
PLGA: Pluronic F68	Nanoparticles	plasmid DNA	Csaba N et al[61]
Pluronic F127 (PF127)/ Carbopol 934P	Gel	sumatriptan	Majithiya RJ et al[62]
poloxamer 407/Polyethylene glycol	Liquid	metoclopramide hydrochloride	Zaki NM et al[63]
Poloxamer 407 /PEG 4000	Liquid	Radix Bupleuri	Chen E et al[64]
Poloxamer 407	Liquid	tetracosactide	Wüthrich P et al[65]
Pluronic F127	Microspheres	Bordetella bronchiseptica multiple antigens containing dermonecrotoxin	Kang ML et al[66]
Pluronic F127 (F127)/ chitosan	Liquid	tetanus toxoid	Westerink MA et al[67]
Pluronic PF 127	Gel	Vitamin B(12)	Pisal SS et al[68]
poloxamer 188	Liquid	isosorbide dinitrate	Na L et al[69]

Table 3. Application of Poloxamer (pluronics) in formulations for nasal drug delivery

6. Future prospects

Although several novel strategies are currently used for nasal drug delivery using bio-and muco-adhesion strategies, the potential exists to improve these methods using other strategies such as nanoparticles, bacterial adhesion, altered amino acid sequence, and antibody mechanism. A graphic representation of these methods is shown in Figure 3. Each of these methods is discussed below.

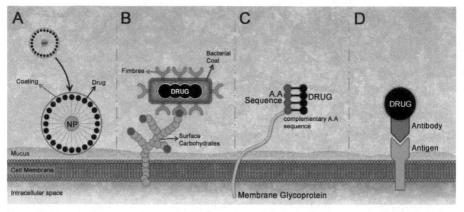

Figure 3. Potential future novel strategies for muco-/bio-adhesive drug delivery using Mucoadhesive Nanoparticles (A), Bacterial Adhesion (B), Altered Amino Acid Sequence (C) and Antibody mechanism (D).

7. Mucoadhesive nanoparticles

Nanoparticles generally vary in size from 10-1000nm. Biodegradable nanoparticles have been used frequently as drug delivery vehicles due to its better encapsulation efficiency, control release and less toxic properties[70]. They offer enhanced biocompatibility, superior drug/vaccine encapsulation, and convenient release profiles for a number of drugs, vaccines and biomolecules to be used in a variety of applications in the field of medicine[71]. The average pore size of viscoelastic mucus is around 150 ± 50 nm. Thus, formulations of mucoadhesive nanopolymers can lead to effective drug delivery to the target site. Commonly used materials for formulating nanoparticles are poly(lactide-co-glycolide) (PLGA) and Pluronics [55]. PEG coatings have been widely used in the development of polymeric drug carriers, including particles composed of biodegradable polyesters and polyanhydrides. PEG coatings reduce aggregation and enhance the blood circulation times of biodegradable nanoparticles designed for drug delivery[72]. Nanoparticles up to 200 nm in diameter that are coated with a dense layer of non-mucoadhesive PEG polymers, including drug carriers composed entirely of Generally Regarded As Safe(GRAS) components, readily penetrate nasal mucus. The development of polymeric particles with improved sinus mucus penetration capability should encourage the commercial development of new generations of nanoparticle-based intranasal drug delivery systems [46].

8. Bacterial adhesion

Non-denatured bacterial cell envelopes, also known as bacterial ghosts, are produced as a result of plasmid-encoded lysis gene *E* of bacteriophage in gram-negative bacteria[73]. Due to its hydrophobic nature, gene *E* product integrates into the inner membrane, resulting in fusion of inner and outer membrane. This leads to the formation of a trans-membrane tunnel[74]. The generated trans-membrane tunnel ranges between 40-80 nm in diameter, through which all cytoplasmic contents are expelled[75]. It is imperative to note that the process of Protein E-specific lysis does not result in physical or chemical denaturation of bacterial surface structures. The bacterial ghosts have been suggested to be a great alternative method for inactivated non-living whole-cell vaccination [76]. Depending on the site-directed sequences included in the fusion, a variety of foreign proteins can be expressed within or on the cell envelop of bacterial ghosts [77]. The advantage of using bacterial ghosts is, bacterial ghosts can be produced in large quantities, do not require the cold-chain-storage system, and are stable for a long time. Further, the size of the foreign protein insert can be very large (>600 amino acids) thus allowing the presence of multiple epitopes simultaneously[78].

The attachment of synthetic or natural macromolecules to mucus or epithelial surface is defined as bioadhesion. Bacteria are capable of adhering to the epithelium surface with aid of fimbriae, which are long, lectin-like proteins found on the surface of many bacterial strains[79]. There is a correlation between the pathogenicity of bacteria and the presence of fimbriae, thus, the adhesion of bacteria to epithelial surfaces can be used as an efficient method of efficient drug-delivery[80].

Bacterial ghosts have been shown to display bio-recognitive abilities which allow their attachment to different surfaces of numerous body tissues depending on the species chosen[81]. Many of these bacterial ghosts are able to bind to surfaces due to the presence of long fimbriae which facilitate the penetration of the mucus covering epithelial tissues[65]. Thus, as a result of the properties of fimbriae a bioadhesive drug delivery system has been developed by using the ghost bacteria with a therapeutic agent coupled to *E. coli* K99 fimbriae[62]. This strategy may be applied to nasal drug delivery with the intention of reducing mucociliary clearance.

9. Altered amino acid sequence and antibodies

Certain amino acid sequences can be used to promote binding of drug molecules to specific cell surface glycoproteins due to the amino acids having complementary sequences present to these glycoproteins[82]. In certain disease conditions the sequence of glycoproteins is altered. This altered state can be used as a target by complementary amino acid sequences by attaching them to a drug delivery device [66]. Antibodies can be produced against selected molecules present on mucosal surfaces. Due to their high specificity, antibodies can be a rational choice as a polymeric ligand for designing site-specific mucoadhesives. This approach can be useful for targeting drugs to tumour tissues[66] or even normal cells.

10. Conclusion

There is no question that the nasal route has a great potential for systemic drug delivery. The physiology of the nasal cavity creates a variety of opportunities for drug companies to develop local and systemic drugs. As nose- to- brain delivery makes it possible to by-pass the blood-brain-barrier for certain drugs; administration of drugs via this route for treatment of neurological diseases presents exciting opportunities. Despite the advantages of nasal drug delivery, the absorption and permeability of polar drugs through the nasal mucosa remains a challenge. The mucociliary clearance system compounds the problem by limiting how long the drug stays in the nasal cavity for absorption to take place. Hence several strategies have been developed to enable the drug molecules to attach onto the mucus or epithelial layer, thus preventing them from being cleared from the nasal cavity. The application of lectins, thiomers, alginate poly-ethylene glycol acrylate and poloxamers were discussed in this chapter. These polymers are not the only polymers used for nasal delivery. However, they are among the least reviewed polymers for systemic drug delivery via the nasal route. Other bioadhesive strategies including nanoparticles, bacterial adhesion, altered sequence and antibody strategies can further improve the bioavailability of polar drug molecules delivered via the nasal route. However, a lot of work remains to be done in this area.

Author details

Utkarshini Anand, Tiam Feridooni and Remigius U. Agu

Biopharmaceutics and Drug Delivery Laboratory, College of Pharmacy,
Faculty of Health Professions, Dalhousie University, Halifax, NS, Canada

11. References

[1] Illum L (2003) Nasal drug delivery--possibilities, problems and solutions J Control Release. 87(1-3):187-98.

[2] Graff CL, Pollack GM (2005) Nasal drug administration: potential for targeted central nervous system delivery. J Pharm Sci. 94(6):1187-95.

[3] Illum L (2002) Nasal drug delivery: new developments and strategies. Drug Discov Today. 7(23):1184-9.

[4] Upadhyay S, Parikh A, Joshi P, Upadhyay U.N, Chotai N. P (2011) Intranasal drug delivery system- A glimpse to become maestro. JAPS. 34-44

[5] Pires A, Fortuna A, Alves G, Falcão A (2009) Intranasal drug delivery: how, why and what for? J Pharm Pharm Sci. 12(3):288-311.

[6] McMartin C, Hutchinson LE, Hyde R, Peters GE (1987) Analysis of structural requirements for the absorption of drugs and macromolecules from the nasal cavity. J Pharm Sci. 76(7):535-40.

[7] Madara JL, Dharmsathaphorn K (1985) Occluding junction structure-function relationships in a cultured epithelial monolayer. J Cell Biol. 101(6):2124-33.

[8] Talegaonkar S, Mishra PR (2004) Intranasal delivery: An approach to bypass the blood brain barrier Indian J Pharmacol. 36(3): 140-147

[9] Illum L, Jørgensen H, Bisgaard H, Krogsgaard O, Rossing N (1987) Bioadhesive microspheres as a potential nasal drug delivery system. Int. J. Pharm. 39: 189–199.

[10] Mythri G, K Kavitha, M Rupesh, Singh J (2011) Novel Mucoadhesive Polymers –A Review. JAPS. 01 (08): 37-42

[11] Roy. S, Pal K, Anis A, Pramanik K, et al (2009) Polymers in Mucoadhesive Drug Delivery System: A Brief Note. Monomers and Polymers. 12 :483-495

[12] Lehr CM (2000) Lectin-mediated drug delivery: The second generation of bioadhesives. J Control Release. 65(1-2):19-29.
[13] Nathan Sharon, Halina Lis (2007) Introduction. Lectins. Springer
[14] Ugwoke M, Agu R, Verbeke N, Kinget R (2005) Nasal mucoadhesive drug delivery: Background, applications, trends and future perspectives Adv Drug Deliv Rev. 57(11):1640-65
[15] Andrews G, Laverty T, Jones D (2009) Mucoadhesive polymeric platforms for controlled drug delivery Eur J Pharm Biopharm. 71(3):505-18.
[16] Gavrovic-Jankulovic M, Prodanovic R (2011) Drug Delivery: Plant Lectins as Bioadhesive Drug Delivery Systems Journal of Biomaterials and Nanobiotechnology 2: 614-621
[17] Lectin-conjugated Nanoparticles for Drugs Delivery into Brain Following Intranasal Administration http://www.res-medical.com/pharmacy/15442 doa- 22nd January 2012
[18] Chen J, Zhang C, Liu Q, Shao X, et al, Solanum tuberosum lectin-conjugated PLGA nanoparticles for nose-to-brain delivery: in vivo and in vitro evaluations. J Drug Target. 2012 ;20(2):174-84
[19] Smart JD, Nicholls TJ, Green KL, Rogers DJ, Cook JD (1999) Lectins in drug delivery: a study of the acute local irritancy of the lectins from Solanum tuberosum and Helix pomatia.. Eur J Pharm Sci. 9(1):93-8.
[20] Clarka MA, Hirsta B, Jepson M (2000) Lectin-mediated mucosal delivery of drugs and microparticles Adv Drug Deliv Rev. 43(2-3):207-23.
[21] Wu H, Li J, Zhang Q, Yan X., et al (2012) A novel small Odorranalectin-bearing cubosomes: preparation, brain delivery and pharmacodynamic study on amyloid-β_{25-35}-treated rats following intranasal administration. Eur J Pharm Biopharm. 80(2):368-78
[22] Liu Q, Shen Y, Chen J, Gao X, et al (2012) Nose-to-brain transport pathways of wheat germ agglutinin conjugated PEG-PLA nanoparticles. Pharm Res. 29(2):546-58
[23] Bernkop-Schnürch A (2005) Thiomers: A new generation of mucoadhesive polymers. Adv Drug Deliv Rev. 57(11):1569-82.
[24] Grabovac V, Guggi D, Bernkop-Schnürch A (2005) Comparison of the mucoadhesive properties of various polymers. Adv Drug Deliv Rev. 57(11):1713-23.
[25] Bernkop-Schnürch A, Krauland AH, Leitner VM, Palmberger T (2004) Thiomers: potential excipients for non-invasive peptide delivery systems. Eur J Pharm Biopharm. 58(2):253-63.
[26] Clausen AE, Kast CE, Bernkop-Schnürch A (2002) The role of glutathione in the permeation enhancing effect of thiolated polymers. Pharm Res.19(5):602-8.
[27] Bernkop-Schnürch A, Hornof M, Zoidl T (2003) Thiolated polymers--thiomers: synthesis and in vitro evaluation of chitosan-2-iminothiolane conjugates. Int J Pharm. 260(2):229-37.
[28] Bernkop-Schnürch A, Obermair K, Greimel A, Palmberger TF (2006) In vitro evaluation of the potential of thiomers for the nasal administration of Leu-enkephalin. Amino Acids. 30(4):417-23.
[29] Leitner V, Guggi D, Bernkop-Schnürch A (2004) Thiomers in non-invasive peptide delivery: in vitro and in vivo characterisation of a polycarbophil–cysteine/glutathione gel formulation for hGH. J Pharm Sci. 93(7):1682-91.

[30] Bernkop-Schnürch A, Krauland AH, Leitner VM, Palmberger T (2004) Thiomers: potential excipients for non-invasive peptide delivery systems. Eur J Pharm Biopharm. 58(2):253-63.

[31] Hornof M, Weyenberg W, Ludwig A, Bernkop-Schnürch A (2003) Mucoadhesive ocular insert based on thiolated poly(acrylic acid): development and in vivo evaluation in humans. J Control Release. 89(3):419-28.

[32] Leitner VM, Guggi D, Bernkop-Schnürch A (2004) Thiomers in noninvasive polypeptide delivery: in vitro and in vivo characterization of a polycarbophil-cysteine/glutathione gel formulation for human growth hormone. J Pharm Sci. 93(7):1682-91.

[33] Vetter A, Bernkop-Schnürch A (2010) Nasal delivery of antisense oligonucleotides: in vitro evaluation of a thiomer/glutathione microparticulate delivery system. J Drug Target.18(4):303-12.

[34] Krauland AH, Leitner VM, Grabovac V, Bernkop-Schnürch A (2006) In vivo evaluation of a nasal insulin delivery system based on thiolated chitosan. J Pharm Sci. 95(11):2463-72.

[35] Davidovich-Pinhas M, Bianco-Peled H (2011) Alginate–PEGAc: A new mucoadhesive polymer. Acta Biomater. 7(2):625-33.

[36] Davidovich-Pinhas M, Bianco-Peled H (2011) Physical and structural characteristics of acrylated poly(ethylene glycol)–alginate conjugates. Acta Biomater. 7(7):2817-25.

[37] Bernkop-Schnürch A (2005) Mucoadhesive polymers: strategies, achievements and future challenges. Adv. Drug Del. Rev. 57: 1553-1555.

[38] Smidsrod O, Draget KI (1997) Alginate gelation technologies. Special Publication Royal Society of Chemistry. 192:279-294

[39] Laurienzo P, Malinconico M, Mattia G, Russo R, et al (2006) Novel alginate–acrylic polymers as a platform for drug delivery. J Biomed Mater Res A. 78(3):523-31.

[40] Lele BS, Hoffman AS (2000) Mucoadhesive drug carriers based on complexes of poly(acrylic acid) and PEGylated drugs having hydrolysable PEG–anhydride–drug linkages J Control Release. 69(2):237-48.

[41] Kabanov AV, Batrakova EV, Alakhov VY (2002) Pluronic block copolymers as novel polymer therapeutics for drug and gene delivery. J Control Release. 82(2-3):189-212.

[42] Schmolka IR (1972) Artificial skin, Preparation and properties of pluronic F127 gels for the treatment of burns. J. Biomed. Mater. Res. 6: 571-582.

[43] Chu, B, Zhou, Z (1996) Nonionic Surfactants: Polyoxyalkylene Block Copolymers, ed. Nace, V. M. (Marcel Dekker, New York): 67-143.

[44] Kabanov A, Batraoka E, Alakhov V (2002) Pluronic block copolymers as novel polymer therapeutics for oral and gene delivery. J. Control. Rel. 82:189-212

[45] Miller SC, Drabik BR (1984) Rheological properties of Poloxamer vehicles. Int. J. Pharm. 18:269-276.

[46] Cho HJ, Balakrishnan P, Park EK, Song KW (2011) Poloxamer/cyclodextrin/chitosan-based thermoreversible gel for intranasal delivery of fexofenadine hydrochloride. J Pharm Sci. 100(2):681-91.

[47] Katakam M., Ravis W., Banga A., Controlled release of human growth hormone in rats following parenteral administration of poloxamer gels. J. Control. Release 1997; 49(1) : 21–26

[48] Sambhaji S.P, Anant R.P, Kakasaheb R.M, Shivajirao S.K, Pluronic gels for nasal delivery of vitamin B12. *Int J Pharm*. 2004 ; 270(1-2):37-45.

[49] Noha M.Z, Gehanne A.A, Nahed D.M, Seham S, et al., Enhance bioavailability of metoclopramide HCl by intranasal administration of a mucoadhesive in situ gel with modulated rheological and mucociliary transport properties. *Eur J Pharm Sci*. 2007 ;32(4-5):296-307.

[50] Sharma N, Sharma A, Sharma PK, Garg G, et al (2010) Mucoadhesive Thermoreversible nasal delivery system. J Pharm Research. 3(5): 991-997

[51] Gonjari ID, Kasture PV (2007) Liposomes of propranolol hydrochloride dispersed in thermoreversible mucoadhesive gel for nasal drug delivery. Current Pharma Research Journal. 95(1-9)

[52] Guzman M, Aberturas MR, Garcia F, Molperceres J (1994) Gelatin gels and polyoxyethylene-polyoxypropylene gels: comparative study of their properties. Drug Dev. Ind. Pharm. 20:2041-2048.

[53] Wanka G, Hoffmann H, Ulbricht W (1990) The aggregation of poly (ethylene oxide)-poly (propylene oxide)-poly (ethylene oxide)-block-copolymers in aqueous solution. Colloid Polym. Sci. 268: 101-117.

[54] Desai PR, Jain NJ, Sharma RK, Bahadur P (2001) Effects of additives on micellization of PEO/PPO/PEO block copolymer F127 in aqueous solution. Colloids and surfaces A: Physicochem. Eng. Aspects. 178: 57-69.

[55] Pandit N, Trygstad T, Croy S, Bohorquez M, et al (2000) Effect of salts on micellization, clouding, and solubilization behavior of pluronic F127 solutions. J. Colloid and Interface Sci. 222: 213-220.

[56] Dumortier G, Grossiord JL, Agnely F, Chaumeil JC, (2006) A review of poloxamer 407 pharmaceutical and pharmacological characteristics. Pharm Res. 23(12): 2709-28.

[57] Salama HA, Mahmoud AA, Kamel AO, Abdel Hady M (2012) Phospholipid based colloidal poloxamer-nanocubic vesicles for brain targeting via the nasal route. Colloids Surf B Biointerfaces. 100:146-54.

[58] Perez AP, Mundiña-Weilenmann C, Romero EL, Morilla MJ (2012) Increased brain radioactivity by intranasal P-labeled siRNA dendriplexes within in situ-forming mucoadhesive gels. Int J Nanomedicine.7:1373-85

[59] Fisher A, Watling M, Smith A, Knight A (2010) Pharmacokinetic comparisons of three nasal fentanyl formulations; pectin, chitosan and chitosan-poloxamer 188. Int J Clin Pharmacol Ther. 48(2):138-45.

[60] Csaba N, Sánchez A, Alonso MJ (2006) PLGA:poloxamer and PLGA:poloxamine blend nanostructures as carriers for nasal gene delivery. J Control Release. 113(2):164-72.

[61] Majithiya RJ, Ghosh PK, Umrethia ML, Murthy RS (2006) Thermoreversible-mucoadhesive gel for nasal delivery of sumatriptan. AAPS PharmSciTech. 7(3):67.

[62] Zaki NM, Awad GA, Mortada ND, Abd Elhady SS (2007) Enhanced bioavailability of metoclopramide HCl by intranasal administration of a mucoadhesive in situ gel with modulated rheological and mucociliary transport properties. Eur J Pharm Sci. 32(4-5):296-307

[63] Chen E, Chen J, Cao SL, Zhang QZ, et al (2010) Preparation of nasal temperature-sensitive in situ gel of Radix Bupleuri and evaluation of the febrile response mechanism. Drug Dev Ind Pharm. 36(4):490-6.

[64] Wüthrich P, Martenet M, Buri P (1994) Effect of formulation additives upon the intranasal bioavailability of a peptide drug: tetracosactide (ACTH1-24). Pharm Res. 11(2):278-82

[65] Kang ML, Jiang HL, Kang SG, Guo DD, et al (2007) Pluronic F127 enhances the effect as an adjuvant of chitosan microspheres in the intranasal delivery of Bordetella bronchiseptica antigens containing dermonecrotoxin. Vaccine. 25(23):4602-10

[66] Westerink MA, Smithson SL, Srivastava N, Blonder J, et al (2001) ProJuvant (Pluronic F127/chitosan) enhances the immune response to intranasally administered tetanus toxoid. Vaccine. 20(5-6):711-23.

[67] Pisal SS, Paradkar AR, Mahadik KR, Kadam SS (2004) Pluronic gels for nasal delivery of Vitamin B12. Part I: preformulation study. Int J Pharm. 270(1-2):37-45.

[68] Na L, Mao S, Wang J, Sun W (2010) Comparison of different absorption enhancers on the intranasal absorption of isosorbide dinitrate in rats. Int J Pharm. 397(1-2):59-66

[69] Lai SK, Suk JS, Pace A, Wang YY (2011) Drug carrier nanoparticles that penetrate human chronic rhinosinusitis mucus. Biomaterials. 32(26): 6285-90

[70] Mahapatro A, Singh DK (2011) Biodegradable nanoparticles are excellent vehicle for site directed in-vivo delivery of drugs and vaccines. J. Nanobiotechnology. ; 9:55

[71] Tang BC, Dawson M, Lai SK, Wang YY, et al (2009) Biodegradable polymer nanoparticles that rapidly penetrate the human mucus barrier. Proc Natl Acad Sci U S A. 106(46): 19268–19273.

[72] Witte A, Wanner G, Lubitz W, Höltje JV (1998) Effect of phi X174 protein E-mediated lysis on murein composition of Escherichia coli. FEMS Microbiol Lett. 164(1):149-57.

[73] Witte A, Wanner G, Sulzner M, Lubitz W (1992) Dynamics of PhiX174 protein E-mediated lysis of Escherichia coli. Arch Microbiol. 157(4):381-8.

[74] Witte A, Wanner G, Bläsi U, Halfmann G, et al (1990) Endogenous transmembrane tunnel formation mediated by phi X174 lysis protein E. J Bacteriol. 172(7): 4109-14.

[75] Szostak MP, Mader H, Truppe M, Kamal M, et al (1997) Bacterial ghosts as multifunctional vaccine particles. Behring Inst Mitt. (98): 191-6.

[76] Walcher P, Cui X, Arrow JA, Scobie S, et al (2008) Bacterial ghosts as a delivery system for zona pellucida-2 fertility control vaccines for brushtail possums (Trichosurus vulpecula). Vaccine. 26(52): 6832-8.

[77] Walcher P, Mayr UB, Azimpour-Tabrizi C, Eko FO, et al (2004) Antigen discovery and delivery of subunit vaccines by nonliving bacterial ghost vectors. Expert Rev Vaccines. 3(6): 681-91.

[78] Bernkop-Schnürch A, Gabor F, Spiegl P (1997) Bacterial adhesins as a drug carrier: covalent attachment of K99 fimbriae to 6-methylprednisolone. Pharmazie. 52(1): 41-4.

[79] Lee JW, Park JH, Robinson JR (2000) Bioadhesive-based dosage forms: the next generation. J Pharm Sci. 89(7): 850-66.

[80] Huter V, Szostak MP, Gampfer J, Prethaler S, et al (1999) Bacterial ghosts as drug carrier and targeting vehicles. J Control Release. 61(1-2): 51-63.

[81] Vasir JK, Tambwekar K, Garg S (2003) Bioadhesive microspheres as a controlled drug delivery system. Int J Pharm. 255(1-2): 13-32.

Chapter 4

Novel Drug Delivery Systems for Modulation of Gastrointestinal Transit Time

Yousef Javadzadeh and Sanaz Hamedeyazdan

Additional information is available at the end of the chapter

1. Introduction

In view of from recent advancements, in a time of augmented remarks to the efficacy and safety of the medicines embedded in dosage forms, it seems as important as ever to study the pharmaceutical concept of the latter in different aspects, prerequisite for a successful pharmacotherapy.

Despite tremendous advancements in drug delivery, oral administration of therapeutic agents still remains the favored rout for majority of clinical applications, due to the excellent accessibility, and patient compliance as well as the preferred alternative route of drug administration for non-invasive drug delivery among the other various routes [Mollekar & Youan, 2006]. Although there have been several limitations in oral administration of drugs like non-uniform drug absorption profiles, incomplete drug release, shorter residence time of dosage forms in absorption window and etc. to systemic circulation it has come a long way. Now, it has turned towards modifying and manipulating oral dosage forms to exploit from different conditions of the gastrointestinal (GI) tract for drug delivery in various ways [Hirtz, 1985].

In view of the fact that the correlation between drug intake and a clinical response is complex enough, the choice and design of the ideal pharmaceutical dosage form of a drug delivery system would be critically important to reach a progress in superior drug development. Variations between drug response within individuals could be attributed either to product bioavailability (like the rate and extent of drug absorption), drug pharmacokinetics (which includes the metabolism, distribution, and elimination of a drug), or the particular concentration-effect relationship, which in turn could potentially be influenced through a mixture of intrinsic and extrinsic variables [Hirtz, 1985; Martinez & Amidon, 2002; Javadzadeh et al., 2010].

With reference to the Biopharmaceutical Classification System, introduced by the Food and Drug Administration (FDA) in 1995, drugs have been categorized in terms of their solubility and intestinal permeability in four primary groups (Figure 1).

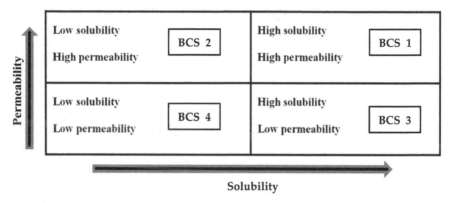

Figure 1. The Biopharmaceutical Classification System (BCS) as defined by the FDA

Drugs that are categorized in class one (BCS 1) are supposed to be well absorbed when taken orally, due to their high solubility and high permeability characteristics. Whereas, all other drugs in BSCs 2 to 4 suffer from low solubility, low permeability or both, and would present challenges to the drug developments. Drugs that are classified in low solubility groups keep drug absorption via the GI tract as the limiting factor for reaching in suitable blood-levels of drugs [Martinez & Amidon, 2002; Javadzadeh et al., 2007].

As far as we know, absorption of drugs from intake (e.g., oral delivery systems) to its site of action is a complex process, or more accurately, a combination or succession of complicated processes which is schematically presented in Figure 2.

After oral administration, drug leaves the formulation and dissolves in the aqueous digestive fluids. It reacthes and crosses the GI mucosal membrane before passing into blood, moving along the GI tract with the luminal content at a variable speed. Once the drug is reached into the blood circulation, processes of drug metabolism and elimination starts, whilst, it is also possible for some drug degradation or metabolism to occur sooner than the absorption is completed leading for a decrease in drug efficiency [Riley et al., 1992].

In general, absorption of drugs through GI tract varies on account of many factors like the nature and surface area of the GI mucosal membrane varying from the stomach to the rectum, as well as the physicochemical properties of the pharmaceutical dosage form along with the luminal content. Hence, a balance among these factors would have a notable effect on how much of the administered drug reaches to the bloodstream that is summed up by the term bioavailability. Considering the pharmacokinetics and disciplines of drug discovery and drug delivery, it has become obvious that a deep understanding of the biology and anatomy of the GI tract is of substantial value for optimizing the bioavailability of orally administered drugs.

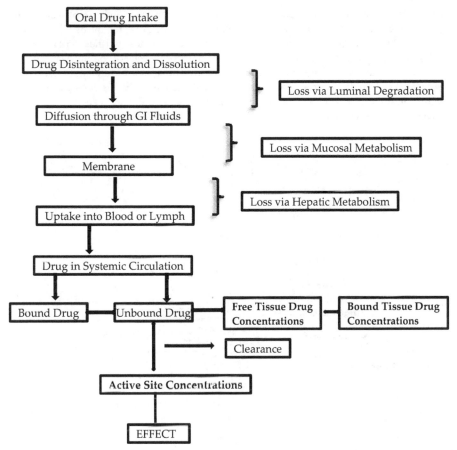

Figure 2. Schematic representation of the relationship between an oral dosage form of a drug and its ultimate effect.

2. GI anatomy and dynamics

GI tract is a group of organs joined in a long tube which is divided into several sections, each of that fulfills a specific function. The tract begins with oral cavity, follows pharynx, esophagus, stomach, small intestine and large intestine ending with rectum to anus part (Figure 3).

Each segment has certain morphological and physiological features, but there is almost a common structure for all parts of GI with muscular walls comprising four different layers: inner mucosa, submucosa, muscularis externa, and the serosa.

Stomach serves the most primarily mixing area and a reservoir that secretes pepsinogen, gastric lipase, hydrochloric acid, and the intrinsic factor. This section of the GI tract is normally impermeable for absorption of most materials into the blood except water, ions, alcohol, and certain drugs such as aspirin. It follows small intestine, the major digestive and absorptive site of the GI tract, providing an extended surface area by the circular folds of about 10 mm height through the microvilli on the absorptive cells of the mucosa. The last part of the GI tract is the large intestine extending from the ileum to the anus with 1.5 m long and 6.35 cm in diameter serving mainly the fecal storage and water absorptive roles. It is significant that no enzymes are secreted in the mucosa, and the last stage of digestion is primarily conducted by the resident bacteria [McConnell et al., 2008].

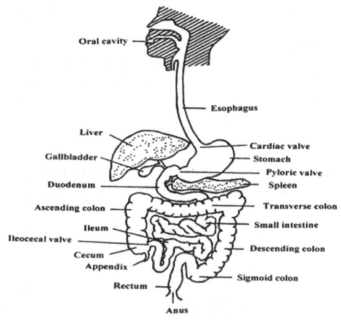

Figure 3. Anatomy of the human gastrointestinal tract [Friend & Tozer, 1992).

Not surprisingly, these anatomical and physiological parameters of the GI tract remarkably affect the rate and level of drug absorptions and should be assessed. There are several difficulties and rules in designing controlled release systems to be considered for better absorption and enhanced bioavailability of drugs embedded in the orally administered dosage forms. One principal requisite for the successful performance of orally administered drugs is that the drug should have good absorption throughout the GI tract, to certify continuous absorption of the released drug [Davis, 2005]. Regarding the BCS classification of drugs, this could be a major constraint in oral controlled drug delivery systems that not all drugs are evenly absorbed throughout the GI tract. Seeing as, most of the orally administered drugs display region-specific absorption that could be related to differential drug solubility and stability in different regions of the GI tract as a result of changes in environmental pH, degradation by enzymes present in the lumen of the intestine or interaction with endogenous compounds (Table 1). Furthermore, drugs that are substrates of certain enzymes in particular regions of the GI tract might have regional variability in their absorption along the GI tract. One should consider this region specific drug absorption concept for designing the ideal drug formulation. It has been widely accepted that about 90% of all absorption of nutrients takes place in the small intestine, and the rest occurs in the stomach and large intestine, depending on the defining characteristics of GI fluids and membrane surface area at different locations [Davis, 2005]. Consequently, transit time of a pharmaceutical dosage form through the GI tract would determine how long a drug will be in contact with its preferred absorptive region.

Section	Length (cm)	Diameter (cm)	pH	Major constituents	Transit time (h)
Oral cavity	15- 20	10	5.2- 6.8	Amylase, Maltase, Ptyalin, Mucins	Short
Esophagus	25	2.5	5- 6	-	Very short
Stomach	20	15	1.2– 3.5	Hydrochloric acid, Pepsin, Rennin, Lipase, Intrinsic factor	0.25- 3
Duodenum	25	5	4.6– 6.0	Bile, Trypsin, Chymotrypsin, Amylase, Maltase, Lipase, Nuclease, CYP3A4	1- 2
Jejunum	300	5	6.3– 7.3	Amylase, Maltase, Lactase, Sucrase, CYP3A5	-
Ileum	300	2.5- 5	7.6	Lipase, Nuclease, Nucleotidase, Enterokinase	1- 10
Cecum	10- 30	7	7.5 - 8	-	Short
Colon	150	5	7.9 - 8	-	4- 20
Rectum	15- 19	2.5	7.5 - 8	-	Variable

Table 1. Anatomical and physiological features of the human GI tract

The usual transit time for a drug formulation or for a nutrient to pass from the stomach to the ileocecal valve (through the small intestine) is around three hours and transit time for colon is much longer up to twenty hours or more. Subsequently, the time a drug will have in its absorption site would be fairly short, more so if the drug is preferentially absorbed in the proximal small intestine rather than throughout the small intestine. Accordingly, a drug that is largely or solely absorbed from the upper GI tract would have variable bioavailability distressed by factors that change GI transit. Moreover, GI transit time of a drug formulation as the most limiting physiological factor in the development of oral drug delivery systems might be altered by the physiological properties of the GI tract too. The patterns of GI transit and gastric emptying depend on whether the person is in a fasted or fed state, and the physical state of the drug delivery system, either a solid or a liquid form [Bode et al., 2004].

Gastric emptying of liquids in the fasted state is a function of the volume administered, whereas, indigestible solids are emptied from the stomach as a function of their physical size [Bardonnet et al., 2006; Khobragade et al., 2009].

There also exist several issues affecting motility of the GI tract such as systemic disease, drug therapy and intrinsic GI disorders. Diabetes, idiopathic intestinal muscle disease, Chaga's disease, muscular dystrophy, gastroparesis and etc. are characterized by delayed gastric emptying and a reduction in GI motions. On the contrary, in the case of diarrhea, infectious diseases, thyrotoxicosis and irritable bowel syndrome an increased GI motion is usually detected [McConnell, Fadda et al., 2008]. Even though, increasing the rate of gastric emptying and GI motility increases the rate of drug absorption, for digoxin and riboflavin, increased GI motility is associated with a decrease in the rate of drug absorption. It is of note to be reminiscent of the fact that, a failure in therapeutic efficiency of drugs is inevitable due to the delayed drug absorption issued from altered gastric emptying if the drug has a short biological half-life.

Anticholinergic medications, tricyclic antidepressants, levodopa, and β-adrenergic agonists are famous groups of medicine that suppress GI motility. Alternatively, drugs that enhance GI motility by increasing contractile force and accelerating intraluminal transit are called prokinetics like metoclopramide, cisapride, tegaserod, and erythromycin (macrolide antibiotic). Other groups of medical preparations (proton pump inhibitors, antacids, histamine receptors type 2 antagonists, etc.) that are used to treat a wide variety of stomach and duodenal diseases associated with hyper-acidity by raising the intragastric pH would alter the pH-dependent solubility and stability level of a certain kind of drugs administered orally. Most drugs are absorbed via passive diffusion of the nonionized form, so the amount of ionization at the different physiological pH values encountered in the GI tract would bring about non-uniform drug absorption and bioavailability [McConnell, Fadda et al., 2008].

Although it is not possible to predict accurately the magnitude and clinical relevance of all drug absorption interactions through the GI tract, designing a suitable dosage form that would function independent of the digestive state, clinical condition, or GI motility of the individuals is an imperative fundamental of the drug delivery system dominating these constraints. So the important requisite for the successful performance of oral drug delivery systems is that the drug should have good absorption throughout the GI tract. Since, all the orally controlled-release drug delivery systems would show limited utilization in the GI controlled administration of drugs if the systems cannot remain in the absorption site for the lifetime of the dosage form, establishing a prolonged GI transit time of orally administered drugs appears to be logical.

3. Prolongation of GI retention

It is clear from the recent scientific literatures that an increased interest among the academic and industrial research groups still exists in formulating novel dosage forms that are retained in the stomach for a prolonged and predictable period of time.

The most feasible method for achieving a prolonged and predictable drug delivery in the GI tract is to control the gastric residence time by gastro retentive and sustained release dosage forms that have some beneficial in safety and efficacy over normal release systems. This method of application is especially helpful in delivery of sparingly soluble and insoluble drugs. It is acknowledged that, as the solubility of a drug decreases, the time available for drug dissolution becomes less adequate and so the transit time becomes an important factor affecting drug absorption in drugs with lower solubility. Other drug candidates suitable for gastroretentive drug delivery systems include those drugs that are locally active in the stomach, drugs with narrow absorption window in GI tract, drugs that are unstable in the intestinal or colonic environment, drugs that act locally in the proximal part of GI tract or disturb normal colonic microbes like antibiotics and also drugs that exhibit low solubility at high pH values. Concerning the pharmacotherapy of the stomach through local drug release of gastroretentive dosage forms, bringing about high levels of drug concentrations at the gastric mucosa (eradication of *Helicobacter pylori* from the submucosal tissue of the stomach), and treating stomach and duodenal ulcers, gastritis and oesophagitis, the risk of gastric carcinoma would be drastically reduced. In contrast, there are drugs that do not fit in gastroretentive drug delivery systems; Drugs that have very limited acid solubility, drugs that suffer instability in the gastric environment, and drugs intended for selective release in the colon should follow other techniques of drug delivery to reach for their intended site of action. Hence, gastroretentive dosage forms despite providing rather constant drug concentrations in the bloodstream for longer periods of time do not fulfill this benefit with several groups of drugs.

One of the advantages of the sustained release dosage forms is that medication are administered less often than other dosage forms reducing fluctuations of drug concentration in the bloodstream. As a result, patients are not repeatedly subjected to different levels of drug which are less or more than adequate. Nor does the blood chemistry undergo frequent chemical imbalances, which might be risky to the patient's health. Additionally, through gastroretentive dosage forms not only the bioavailability and therapeutic efficacy of drugs are improved but also it may allow for a possible reduction in the dose because of the steady therapeutic levels of drugs. Drugs that have poor solubility in higher pH, absorption windows in stomach, and the ones requiring locall delivery in stomach could be delivered ideally to the site of action by these gastroretentive formulations. On the other hand, drugs that cause irritation to gastric mucosa and the ones meet first-pass metabolism or have stability problems in gastric fluids are not appropriate for these kinds of drug delivery systems.

In brief, gastric retention is a means to enable a delivery strategy that will function irrespective of the digestive state, clinical condition, or GI motility of the individuals with longer drug residence time in the stomach being advantageous in superior drug bioavailabilities and also in certifying local action of some drugs in the upper part of the GI tract. Various approaches that have currently become leading methodologies for increasing the resistance time of a dosage form in the stomach would be highlighted in this section forward. Nevertheless, the early reports on gastroretentive systems have been well-reviewed in pervious literatures, only the more recent development and strategies will be discussed here.

3.1. Intragastric floating drug delivery systems

3.1.1. Introduction

Design of floating pharmaceutical dosage forms with a bulk density less than gastric fluid is one of the thriving trends for enhancing drug residence in the stomach. These systems would act independent of the highly variable nature of the gastric emptying process resulting in reduced fluctuations of drug bioavailabilities.

Apart from the commented benefits established by these floating systems, they could also have their limitations given that they require a satisfactory level of fluid in the stomach to float. Likewise, in the fed state a change in body position to supine could have a direct effect on the floating system. In order to design a more systematic and intellectual floating system it is as important as ever to study different aspects of these systems to have a deeper insight to the buoyancy, drug release mechanisms, effectiveness and reliability of these floating systems as an strategy for establishing an efficient gastroretentive drug delivery system [Blanquet et al., 2004].

In this regard, different approaches have been followed to support the buoyancy of dosage forms in the stomach. Based on the mechanism of floatation, two obviously different technologies are employed in development of floating dosage forms, effervescent and non-effervescent systems

3.1.2. Effervescent systems

These buoyant systems are usually matrices of swellable polymers along with effervescent components that generate carbon dioxide (CO_2) entrapped in swollen hydrocolloids of the dosage forms. In these systems floatation is achieved through the incorporating of a gas within the formulation lessoning density of the system and making it float on the gastric fluids [Krogel & Bodmeier, 1999; Sungthongjeen et al., 2008].

Acid - base reactions have been utilized for decades to produce various pharmaceutical preparations which effervesce as contacting with water. Sources affording the acidity in effervescent reactions are essentially provided by acids, acid anhydrides, and acid salts where organic acids, citric and acetic acids are the most commonly used materials. In contrast, carbonates and bicarbonates in contact with acids are used typically as CO_2 generation sources. Carbonates not only play critical role in making the dosage form buoyant but also provide the initial alkaline micro environment for the polymers to gel [Sungthongjeen, Sriamornsak et al., 2008; Patel et al., 2009; Rajab et al., 2010]. These carbon dioxide generating components could be intimately mixed within the matrix to produce a single-layered dosage form or a multi-layered formulation which might contain the gas generating mechanism in one hydrocolloid containing layer and the drug in the other layer formulated for the sustained release effect (Figure 4). The matrices are fabricated so that upon contact with gastric fluid, carbon dioxide is liberated with an upward motion of the dosage form maintaining its buoyancy in the gellified hydrocolloid. Totally, the reaction is due to the CO_2 generated by neutralization in the effervescent layer with the diffusion of water through the swellable membrane layer. However, there may be a lag time relying on the duration of gas generation reaction that could end in gastric emptying of the dosage form before floatation. More reliable gastric emptying patterns are attained for multi particulate formulations consisting loads of small discrete units as compared with single unit formulations containing one unit suffering from "all or none concept" [Sungthongjeen et al., 2006]. These multi particulate formulations are also better distributed in the GI tract and are less likely to cause local irritation. Recently, much more emphasis is being laid on the development of multi particulate dosage forms rather than single unit systems to their potential benefits like increased bioavailability, reduced risk of systemic toxicity, reduced risk of local irritation and predictable gastric emptying manners.

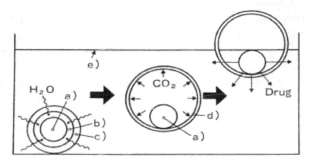

Figure 4. Mechanism of action in effervescent floating drug delivery system.

This view is supported by a variety of papers developing effervescent systems using different polymers and drugs, all agreed in the practicality and feasibility of the approach. In this regard, Pahwa et al. formulated effervescent floating tablets of famotidine with an effective and safe therapy for stomach ulcers in a reduced dose manner [Pahwa et al., 2012]. Hydroxypropyl methylcellulose K15M and hydroxypropyl methylcellulose K100M as gel forming agents along with sodium bicarbonate and citric acid as gas generating agents were used in the research. Concerning the results of the study, it was concluded that the addition of gel-forming polymers, methocel and gas generating agent, sodium bicarbonate along with citric acid were essential to achieve in vitro buoyancy profile. Faster and higher CO_2 generation caused by increasing the concentration of effervescent agents resulted in higher swelling of polymeric membrane according to a higher gas pressure [Pahwa, Chhabra et al., 2012]. Additionally, expansion of the hydrated matrices increased the surface area available for dissolution and presence of gas bubbles hindered the diffusion path, decreasing the release constant values. Concisely, in these systems generation of the CO_2, entrapped in the matrix is the constant principle rule that has been widely established in studies of this category.

3.1.3. Non-effervescent systems

Non-effervescent systems incorporate a high level of one or more gel forming, highly swellable, cellulosic hydrocolloids, poly saccharides or matrics forming polymers into the formulations employing no gas forming agents during the procedures. These gel formers, polysaccharides and polymers hydrate in contact with gastric fluids and form a colloidal gel barrier resulting in the floatation of the dosage form. Practical approaches in formulating non-effervescent floating dosage forms are listed below.

3.1.3.1. Hydrodynamically Balanced Systems (HBS)

The HBS systems are developed with gel-forming hydrocolloids forming a hydrated gel layer in the outer exposed surface of the dosage form on contact with gastric fluids imparting buoyancy for a long period of time. Gel-forming or highly swellable cellulose type hydrocolloids such as hydroxypropyl cellulose, hydoxyethyl cellulose, hydroxypropyl methyl cellulose, polysaccharides, matrix forming polymers and the drug that is with gel-forming hydrocolloids are homogeneously thoroughly mixed within the HBS formulations [Khattar et al., 1990; Dorozynski et al., 2004]. Hydration of the inner layers brings about surface hydration and a soft gelatinous barrier around the dosage form. This soft gelatinous mass on the surface of the formulation provides a water-impermeable colloid gel barrier on the surface of the tablets. Consequently, the hydrated gel controls the rate of water penetration into the dosage form and the rate of drug release from the HBS. Different varieties of polymers could be utilized in the floating drug delivery systems as well in the HBS. Kumar et al. studied effect of different excipients and polymers on floating behavior and drug release from floating HBS matrices. It was found that the selection of suitable excipients depending on polarity of drug modulates the floatability and drug release profiles where water uptake in the floating matrix increased with the increase in the loading of polar drugs and decreased with non-polar drugs [Kumar et al., 2004]. Elsewhere, a hydrodynamically balanced delivery system of clarithromycin was developed by Nama et al. to prolong gastric residence time with a desired in vitro release profile for the localized action in the stomach, with the intention of *Helicobacter pylori* mediated peptic ulcer treatment. Different kinds of polymers with various possible concentrations were assessed to establish the optimum formulation with 66.2% clarithromycin, 12% HPMC K4M polymer, 8% sodium bicarbonate offered improved floating lag time less than 3 min and 12 h duration of floating [Nama et al., 2008].

In general, use of HBS is desirable which swell to create a gel-like structure after administration and attain a density less than that of gastric fluids where a prolonged drug delivery is required. Not many practical reports were found on the non-effervescent HBS drug formulations as compared to the effervescent systems. As a matter of fact, considering the all or none gastric emptying of HBS dosage forms, development of floating drug delivery system using multiple-unit devices to distribute uniformly within the gastric content and gradually pass through the GI tract still is one of the challenges in this field.

3.1.3.2. Porous systems

Porous materials are emerging day by day as a new category of drug delivery systems due to the several alternative features such as stable uniform porous structure, high surface area, and tunable pore sizes with narrow distribution and well defined surface properties. Theses porous carriers have been playing one of the key roles in the pharmaceutical industries including development of novel drug delivery systems such as floating and sustained drug delivery systems in improving the solubility of poorly water soluble drugs [Ahuja & Pathak, 2009; Sher et al., 2009]. Porous structures such as silica, porous ceramic, ethylene vinyl acetate, polypropylene foam powder and titanium dioxide allow the inclusion of drugs inside a porous compartment possessing a relatively lower density than the gastric juice thus remaining buoyant in the stomach [Streubel et al., 2002]. This approach of flotation is based on the principle of the encapsulation of a drug reservoir inside a microporous compartment with pores along its top and bottom walls. Any other polymer that may be added to the dosage form would moderately cover the pores and entrap air within the system. However, the peripheral walls might get completely sealed to prevent any direct contact of the gastric surface with the drug bringing about delayed release of drugs. Besides, the entrapped air would gradually removed from the formularion in exposure to gastric medium, leading to an extended floating times with a more reproducible and predictable drug release manner. After all, interests and notable surveys have been directed in recent years towards the porous carriers as controlled drug delivery matrices.

A multi particulate floating delivery system, consisting of highly porous carrier material calcium silicate, glipizide as the drug, and eudragit S as the polymer, was developed by Pandya et al. Glipizide as a second-generation sulfonylurea with short biological half-life (3-4 h) and the site of the absorption in the stomach was an excellent candidate for development of controlled-release dosage forms that are retained in the stomach increasing the absorption, drug efficiency, along with decrease in dose requirements. In this regard, they evaluated effects of various formulation variables on the internal and external particle morphology, micromeritic properties, in vitro floating behavior, and in vitro drug release. The designed system, showed excellent buoyancy and suitable drug release pattern, possibly being advantageous in terms of increased bioavailability of glipizide over an extended period of time [Pandya et al., 2011].

More recently, Yao et al. developed a simple and rapid method of floatation to prepare a novel kind of inner-porous floating beads using foam solution using poloxamer 188 as foaming agents and alginate as foaming stabilizer. Riboflavin, a water-soluble vitamin was used as a model drug which has a narrow absorption window in the upper part of the intestine and a saturable absorption mechanism. In this method poloxamer 188 was used as an effective amphiphilic surfactant which could lower the water surface tension significantly. In addition, foam solution was formed by stirring in the presence of poloxamer 188, winding microbubbles in the alginate and stabilizing the foam solution. Findings of the study revealed that addition of the non-ionic surfactants poloxamer 188 lead to the formation of a surfactant–polymer complex through interactions between polymer and surfactant contributing in the foamability and foam stability of the formulations. Moreover, higher concentration of the poloxamer 188 increased the foamability and foam stability of the mixed solution. These results were verified through scanning electron microscopy cross-section pictures of the beads showing inner-porous with fully bubbled nature of the beads with very thin wall bubbles stacked together. Additionally, gamma scintigraphic images and pharmacokinetic studies in vivo showed that the beads could retain in the stomach for over 6 h and improved bioavailability of the drug [Yao et al., 2012].

3.1.3.3. Alginate beads

Lately, both natural and synthetic hydrophilic polyionic systems like alginates have been a center of attention for preparation of floating systems. The interest in alginates is chiefly due to their high biocompatibility and nontoxic nature in oral administration that also demonstrate protective effect on the mucous membranes of the upper GI tract. Alginate beads with the structure of spherical gels are taken shaped through dropwise addition of aqueous alginate solution to the aqueous solution containing calcium ions and/or other di and polyvalent cations [Javadzadeh et al., 2010]. The pH dependent reswelling property of dried alginate beads let them to be administrated as a unique vehicle as the multi unit floating dosage forms in GI tract as early as 1980s [Murata et al., 2000].

In recent years, the amount of literature published on development of these alginate beads providing satisfactory data for a variety of applications has been grown remarkably. In a study, cinnarizine, a piperazine derivative as a Ca channel blocking and anti- histaminic drug suffering from incomplete and variable oral absorption which occurs mainly in the proximal small intestine was formulated as a floating multiple unit dosage form of alginate beads. Ghareeb et al. formulated floating cinnarizine olive oil-entrapped emulsion gel beads by the emulsion–gelation method. They came into conclusion that formulation variables greatly influenced the mean particle size and in vitro drug release characteristics of the prepared beads. Ultimately, the experimental observations suggested cinnarizine loaded alginate beads could potentially be useful in drug delivery systems for making controlled release gastroretentive floating beads of drugs via the ionotropic gelation technique [Ghareeb et al., 2012]. Furthermore, in our previously published paper, we prepared floating beads of metronidazole via the ionotropic gelation method employing gas forming (sodium bicarbonate) and porous (calcium silicate) agents followed by a physicochemical evaluations. It was found that the kind and amount of agents used to make the beads floated, i.e., sodium bicarbonate and calcium silicate, had a profound effect on the beads size, morphology, and floating ability as well as drug release profile [Javadzadeh, Hamedeyazdan et al., 2010]. In general, high compatibility of the alginate beads in achieving a suitable floating dosage form controlling the drug release from the beads with a definite kinetic of release was clear enough to be supported.

Novel prospects for application of floating alginate beads were accomplished by emphasizes on advantages and future potential of probiotic loaded beads in the treatment of GI disorders. As we know, probiotics are live microbial feed supplements that beneficially affect the host by improving its intestinal microbial balance that may undergo antagonistic interactions with pathogenic bacteria. However, significance of probiotics survival in the GI tract, their translocation, colonization and the fate of probiotic derived active components indicate a need and scope of packaging them into a suitable delivery system to increase the viability of the probiotics, both outside and inside the body. Singh et al. developed a floating drug delivery system of *Lactobacillus acidophilus* via orifice ionic gelation method in alginate beads. They evaluated the efficacy of the approach in experimental model of cold restraint stress induced gastric ulcer in terms of ulcer index; hemorrhagic streak length; mucus content and histopathological examinations. According to the authors, the developed formulations not only efficiently protected the entrapped probiotic cells, but also effectively delivered and retained viable bacteria in the stomach [Singh et al., 2012]. The prolonged and continuous release of the probiotic in the gastric mucosa allowed them for an ensured therapeutic efficacy of the developed floating system against ulcers post-induction, thus suggesting an efficient line of treatment.

3.1.3.4. Hollow microspheres / microballoons

One of the renowned approaches in devising multiple unit floating systems are the hollow microspheres (microballoons), spherical empty particles without core that are designed to float on gastric juice [Gholap et al., 2010]. Hollow microspheres incorporating a drug dispersed or dissolved throughout particle matrix have the potential for controlled release of drugs. These microspheres are characteristically prepared by solvent diffusion and evaporation methods where the relative polymer is dissolved in an organic solvent and the drug dissolved or dispersed in the polymer solution is emulsified into an aqueous phase containing suitable additive (surfactants / polymer) to form oil in water emulsion (Figure 5). After removal of the organic solvent, polymer precipitates at the oil/water interface of droplets, forming cavity and thus making them hollow to impart the floating properties. Frequently used polymers in developing hollow microspheres are polycarbonate, chitosan, methocil, polyvinyl acetate, carbopol cellulose acetate, calcium alginate, eudragit, agar and also pectin [Soppimath et al., 2006].

In general, hollow microspheres are believed to be prominent buoyant systems as they provide a multi-unit system with an improved floating property. This view is supported by scores of reports on development of the emulsion solvent diffusion method to form hollow microspheres employing different polymers and drugs to follow a promising drug delivery system floating on the gastric juice. Rosiglitazone hollow microspheres were prepared through modified quasi-emulsion solvent diffusion method by Gangadharappa et al. to improve the oral hypoglycemic agent's bioavailability. The formulated dosage form controlled the drug release, avoiding dose dumping, in an extended floating duration [Gangadharappa et al., 2011]. Elsewhere, Rane et al. prepared hollow microspheres of rosiglitazone were by O/W emulsion-solvent diffusion technique using biodegradable anionic acrylic resin as a polymer. They provided evidence that a modification of external aqueous phase with salt ($CaCl_2$ and $NaCl$) improved the drug entrapment efficiency for moderately soluble drug by 45–50% as a result of salting out effect. Predominantly, the release mechanism for formulations was diffusion controlled and followed the first order kinetics [Rane et al., 2012].

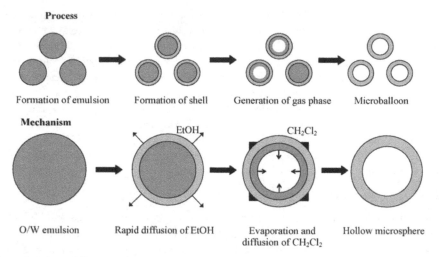

Figure 5. Solvent diffusion and evaporation technique in formation of the hollow inner core microspheres.

3.1.4. Physicochemical evaluations

In development phase for floating dosage forms, designing a selection of suitable control principles is of crucial importance. This would be beneficial in preventing the development efforts to costly late stage product failures throughout the manufacture and administration periods too. Besides, health authorities worldwide necessitate accurate adjustment of the physicochemical parameters of the formulation for all individually administered dosage forms in advance to clinical phase [Parikh & Amin, 2008].

3.1.4.1. In vitro buoyancy and drug release properties

Not surprisingly, insufficient and inconsistent formulation buoyancy, drug dissolution and the subsequent inadequate drug efficacy are some of the routine challenges to be coped with during the development of floating drug delivery systems when they are administrated orally. It is of essential for these kinds of dosage forms to have a satisfactory floating activity, for giving the drug a chance for sufficient dissolution rate, absorption, and a suitable clinical efficacy, as well. Since, different physiological situations may affect the results for buoyancy and dissolution and drug release from pharmaceutical dosage form, in vitro tests for buoyancy and drug release studies are usually carried out in close proximity to the physiological conditions of the human body to lessen the variation derive from altered dissolution medium. The apparatus and procedures of USP are preferred the best to make a better correlation between in vitro and in vivo results of the floating and drug release tests. Generally, the tests are determined in 900 mL of simulated gastric fluid (HCl/NaCl with 0.02% Tween 80, pH 1.2) maintained at 37°C using basket or paddle stirring elements of the USP dissolution apparatus [Mudie et al., 2010]. Besides, the time needed for the dosage form to float and duration of the buoyancy are noted as the floating lag-time and flotation time are evaluated as the floating behavior of the formulations.

There have been numerous published reports on diverse challenges of the floating drug delivery systems applying a variety of floating agents to encourage buoyancy of the pharmaceutical dosage forms with a controlled drug release. Gupta at al. prepared floating microspheres of clopidogrel bisulfate using different viscosities of ethyl cellulose and triethyl citrate as a plasticizer using emulsion solvent diffusion technique. It was detected that the drug release from the floating microspheres matrix was completely controlled by the polymer as the polymer proportion in the formulation was increased, a decrease in drug loading, drug release was observed. The floating ability of different formulations was found to be altered according to polymer ratio. Overall, the prepared formulations showed appropriate balance between buoyancy and drug release rate dependent on the amount of formulation variables [Gupta & Rajpoot, 2012]. Most of the relative papers dealing with the development and optimization of the buoyancy lag time and duration of drug release employed both swellable polymers and gas generating systems to increase the buoyancy and lag times. Several studies in this filed have shown that different factors influence the buoyancy and drug release from a pharmaceutical dosage form and contributing in different patterns of drug release in similar floatation preparation methods.

Accordingly, different factors influence the buoyancy and drug release from a pharmaceutical dosage form. Solubility of the drug in dissolution medium as well as the formulation variables in the dosage form are the dynamic items, contributing distinctively in drug release differences of the floating dosage forms with similar basic floatation preparation methods. It has always been a great challenge to modify the drug release in an expected manner and assess the efficiency of the dosage form in an in vivo environment. Even if the more or less standardized in vitro methods described in the pharmacopeial monographs are used in different studies, the correlation between in vivo and in vitro results must be confirmed from case to case in individuals prior to the clinical application.

3.1.4.2. In vivo assessments

Very early on, in the development phase of drugs a reliable relationship has to be established between in vitro and in vivo test, in order to expose therapeutically relevant discrepancies first between different formulations and later also between drug production batches. This correlation is most likely if the test conditions are in close proximity to the physiological circumstances. Hardly ever, do the in vitro assessments fully counterpart the in vivo results, since the standard USP methods have not been a reliable predictors of in vivo performance of the floating pharmaceutical dosage forms [Kaus et al., 1999]. Apart from the drug release pattern of the dosage form, it is the absorption, distribution, metabolization and excretion influence the in vivo drug concentration at the site of action. In view of the fact that interplay of the pharmacokinetic and pharmacodynamic parameters for a particular drug also has a noteworthy effect on the efficiency of the floating dosage form, in vivo evaluations appear to be requisite. Tracking the in vivo floating behavior and location of dosage form through GI tract providing a broad insight for formulating the optimal floating drug delivery system could be established via radiography, gamma scintigraphy, gastroscopy, ultrasonography and magnetic resonance imaging. Considering the majority of the surveys in this case, not only the relevant correlation between in vivo and invitro assessments was confirmed but also effectiveness and reliability of these floating systems as an excellent strategy for controlled delivery of drugs was ascertained [Jain et al., 2006; Ali et al., 2007; Wei & Zhao, 2008; Guguloth et al., 2011].

3.1.4.3. Drug release kinetic for the floating drug delivery systems

Over the past few decades, the large variety of formulations devoted to floating drug delivery systems with varied physicochemical properties have become manifested which influence the drug release patterns of these formulations. In the same way as the ideal purpose of any drug delivery system is to maintain drug concentration in the blood or in target tissues at a desired value as long as possible, focusing on the drug release profiles to design a more systematic and intellectual floating system is has become even more rational. Accordingly, study of the drug release kinetics is often useful in obtaining one or two physically meaningful parameters which are employed for comparative purposes and relating the release parameter with important parameters such as bioavailability [Wagner, 1969; Barzegar-Jalali et al., 2008; Dash et al., 2010].

There are number of kinetic models, which described the overall release of drug from the dosage forms. Seeing as both qualitative and quantitative changes in a formulation could alter drug release and in vivo performance of the dosage form, developing tools that facilitate drug development by reducing the necessity of bio-studies is always desirable [Arifin et al., 2006; Javadzadeh, Hamedeyazdan et al., 2010]. Referring our former studies on drug release mechanisms from floating drug delivery systems, no a single kinetic model is customary for the floating dosage forms, even if the flotation strategies were the same [Adibkia et al., 2011]. Formulation variables, approaches in establishing formulation buoyancy and the kinetic models in analyzing the drug release data should have chosen parallel to present a suitable model fitting for these systems. In general, evaluating the mechanism behind drug release profile from floating dosage forms is complicated, and requires careful observance of the physicochemical properties of the dosage form.

3.2. Mucoadhesive gastrointestinal drug delivery systems

3.2.1. Introduction

For years pharmaceutical scientists have been fascinated by the concept of bioadhesion. The term bioadhesion implies attachment of a drug carrier system to a specific biological location like epithelial tissue. This bioadhesion phenomenon is referred to as mucoadhesion if the adhesive attachment is to a mucus coat [Davidovich-Pinhas & Bianco-Peled, 2010]. Mucoadhesive drug delivery systems are used to localize a delivery device within the lumen to enhance the drug absorption in a site-specific manner since the luminal surface of the GI tract is a richly glycosylated tissue that presents considerable advantages in the use of formulations with mucoadhesive properties.

3.2.2. Factors affecting mucoadhesion

Mucoadhesive characteristics are affected by a factor of both the bioadhesive polymer and the medium in which the polymer will exist in. The mucoadhesive properties of polymers themselves are concerned by diversity of factors such as molecular weight, flexibility, hydrogen bonding capacity, cross-linking density, charge, concentration, and hydration (swelling) of a polymer, which is briefly discussed below [Lahoti et al., 2011].

3.2.2.1. Polymer-related factors

Molecular weight: In general, it has been revealed that the bioadhesive strength of a polymer increases with molecular weights above 100,000.

Flexibility: Bioadhesion could be result of the diffusion of the polymer chains in the interfacial region. Then, containing of a substantial degree of flexibility is essential in order to get the desired entanglement with the mucus. In general, mobility and flexibility of polymers can be related to their viscosities and diffusion coefficients, where in the case of higher flexibility, greater diffusion into the mucus network was seen.

Hydrogen bonding ability: It was found that for occurring of mucoadhesion, polymers must contain functional groups that are able to form hydrogen bonds. It was also showed that flexibility of the polymer is imperative to advance this hydrogen bonding potential.

Cross-linking density: It gives the impressions that with increasing density of cross-linking, diffusion of water into the polymer network take place at a lower rate resulting an inadequate swelling of the polymer and a decreased rate of interpenetration between polymer and mucin.

Charge: Nonionic polymers show a smaller degree of adhesion compared to anionic polymers. It was also shown that some cationic polymers display superior mucoadhesive properties, especially in a neutral or slightly alkaline medium. Furthermore, some cationic polymers such as chitosan that has high molecular weight have shown good adhesive properties.

Concentration: In the lower concentration of the polymer, the number of penetrating polymer chains per unit volume of the mucus is small, and then the interaction between polymer and mucus is unstable. In general, the more concentrated polymer would result in a longer penetrating chain length and better adhesion. However, there is a critical concentration, above which the polymer generates an "unperturbed" situation due to a significantly coiled structure. As a result, the accessibility of the solvent to the polymer decreases, and chain penetration of the polymer is considerably reduced. Therefore, higher concentrations of polymers do not necessarily improve mucoadhesive properties and, in some cases, diminished effect was seen.

Hydration (swelling): For any polymer in order to develop the interpenetration process between polymer and mucin, hydration is required to expand and create a proper "macromolecular mesh" of sufficient size, and also to induce mobility in the polymer chains.

3.2.2.2. *Environmental factors*

The mucoadhesion of a polymer not only depends on its molecular properties, but also on the environmental factors adjacent to the polymer (pH, feed condition, and movement of the GI tissues while eating, drinking, or talking). Therefore, an optimum time period for the administration of the dosage form is necessary in order to avoid many of these interfering factors [Lahoti, Shep et al., 2011].

3.2.3. *Polymers used for mucoadhesive drug delivery*

Polymers have played an important role in designing mucoadhesive drug delivery systems. Customarily, in these systems mucoadhesive polymers adhere to the mucin layer on the mucosal epithelium followed by a decrease in drug clearance rate from the GI absorption site, thereby increasing the time available for drug absorption [Rajput et al., 2010]. Polymers used in such system may have natural or synthetic origin. These polymers are classified as:

3.2.3.1. *Hydrophilic polymers*

These polymers are soluble in water. When put into an aqueous media, start to swell and subsequent dissolution of the matrix is occurred. The polyelectrolytes show superior mucoadhesive property in comparison with neutral polymers. Anionic polyelectrolytes, e.g. poly (acrylic acid) and carboxymethyl cellulose, have been broadly used for preparation of mucoadhesive formulations for their ability to exhibit strong hydrogen bonding with the mucin. Chitosan has been widely used as a cationic polyelectrolyte mucoadhesive polymer developing mucoadhesive property of these systems via electrostatic interactions with the negatively charged mucin chains. Moreover, these ionic polymers might have a drug delivery matrix exhibiting mucoadhesive property by developing ionic complex with the counter-ionic drug molecules. Alternatively, non-ionic polymers, such as poloxamer, hydroxypropyl methyl cellulose, methyl cellulose, poly (vinyl alcohol) and poly (vinyl pyrrolidone), have been used for mucoadhesive properties, as well. The hydrophilic polymers would be used as viscosity modifying/enhancing agents in the development of liquid ocular delivery systems for increasing the bioavailability of active agents by reducing the drainage of the administered formulations since they form viscous solutions when dissolved in water. Accordingly, a mucoadhesive drug delivery system would be established by these polymers when they are directly compressed in the presence of drugs. Polymers that are used frequently in ocular mucoadhesive delivery systems are usual polysaccharides and its derivatives like chitosan, methyl cellulose, hyaluronic acid, hydroxypropyl methylcellulose, hydroxypropyl cellulose, xanthan gum, gellan gum, guar gum, and carrageenan [Roy et al., 2009]. Besides, sustained release of drugs through these hydrophilic mucoadhesive polymers is accomplished in combination of the cationic cellulose derivatives (e.g. cationic hydroxyethyl celluloses) with various anionic polymers.

3.2.3.2. *Hydrogels*

Three-dimensionally crosslinked polymer chains have the ability to hold water within its porous structure forming hydrogels that are usually characterized with the presence of hydrophilic functional groups like hydroxyl, amino and carboxyl groups bringing about the water holding capacity of these hydrogels. However, it is of value to note that with increase in the crosslinking density of hydrogels a decrease in the mucoadhesion would be inevitable. Preparation of the hydrogels by the condensation reaction of poly (acrylic acid) and sucrose pointed out an increase in the mucoadhesive property with the increase in the crosslinking density that was attributed to the rise in the poly (acrylic acid) chain density per unit area. In this regard, Wood and Peppas developed a system in which ethylene glycol chains were grafted on methacrylic acid hydrogels and were functionalized with wheat germ agglutinin. In this system the intestinal residence time of the delivery system was improved by binding of the wheat germ agglutinin with the specific carbohydrate moieties present in the intestinal mucosa. Mucoadhesive hydrogel based formulations not only have beneficial in drug targeting but also they are of use in improving the bioavailability of the poorly water soluble drug. Typically, Muller and Jacobs prepared a nanosuspension of buparvaquone, a poorly water soluble drug, by incorporating it within carbopol and chitosan based hydrogels [Muller & Jacobs, 2002]. Improved bioavailability of the drug in mucoadhesive delivery systems was determined when compared over the nanosuspension indicating the increased retention time of the delivery system within the GI tract.

3.2.3.3. Thiolated polymers

The mucoadhesive properties of the polymers (e.g. poly (acrylic acid) and chitosan) along with the paracellular uptake of the bioactive agents would be significantly improved through the presence of free thiol groups in polymeric skeleton which could help in the formation of disulphide bonds with that of the cysteine-rich sub-domains present in mucin. Some of the polymers including thiol groups are chitosan–iminothiolane, poly (acrylic acid)–cysteine, poly(acrylic acid)–homocysteine, chitosan–thioglycolic acid, chitosan–thioethylamidine, alginate cysteine, poly(methacrylic acid)–cysteine and sodium carboxymethylcellulose–cysteine [Roy, Pal et al., 2009].

3.2.3.4. Lectin-based polymers

Lectins that are found in both animal and plant kingdom in addition to various microorganisms, are the proteins which have ability to reversibly bind with specific sugar or carbohydrate residues, providing with specific cyto-adhesive property for targeted delivery systems. Lectins extracted from *Ulex europueus I*, soybean, peanut and *Lens culinarius* have demonstrated specific binding to the mucosa. Additionally, wheat germ agglutinin amongst other available lectins has shown limited immunogenic reactions exhibiting potential capacity to bind to the intestinal and alveolar epithelium as the favorable muccoadhesive polymer [Roy, Pal et al., 2009].

3.2.4. Methods of evaluation

Mucoadhesive polymers and drug delivery systems can be evaluated by testing their adhesion strength by both in vitro and in vivo tests (Table 2).

In vitro / ex vivo methods	In vivo methods
• Methods determining tensile strength	• Use of radioisotopes
• Methods determining shear stress	• Use of gamma scintigraphy
• Adhesion weight method	• Use of pharmacoscintigraphy
• Fluorescent probe method	• Use of electron paramagnetic resonance (EPR) oximetry
• Flow channel method	• X ray studies
• Mechanical spectroscopic method	• Isolated loop technique
• Falling liquid film method	
• Colloidal gold staining method	
• Viscometer method	
• Thumb method	
• Adhesion number	
• Electrical conductance	
• Swelling properties	
• In vitro drug release studies	
• Mucoretentability studies	

Table 2. Variety of in vitro / in vivo tests for evaluation of the adhesion strength in mucoadhesive sustems

The GI transit time of these dosage forms could be measured by using one of the many radio opaque markers like barium sulphate which is coated to the bioadhesive dosage form so as to assess the GI transit by means of X-ray inspection. Both the distribution and retention can be studied by using of gamma scintigraphy. Using a non invasive technique to determine the transit time of mucoadhesive polymers is also popular and this could be imaged via labeling of the polymer with a gamma emitting nucleotide determining with the help of gamma scintigraphy. Another recent technique is to use magnetic resonance imaging to localize the point of release of thiolated polymers from dosage forms via the use of gadolinium determining by ascertaining the residence time of the fluorescently tagged thiomer on intestinal mucosa of rats after 3 hours [Tangri et al., 2011]). Although, considering the high cost, time consuming and ethical factors, these techniques are less usual common, evaluating the true mucoadhesive potential of the pharmaceutical dosage form is of essential [Shaikh et al., 2011].

Accordingly, there have been several successful attempts in identifying these putative bioadhesive or mucoadhesive materials using in vitro and in vivo tests but success usually has failed in translating to human studies in the stomach and small intestine [Sohrabi et al., 2009; Movassaghian et al., 2011]. It may be due to the lack of correlation between mucosal conditions in the GI tract, and test models that are not in close proximity to the physiological circumstances. This phenomenon reinforces the note that appropriate testing methods are required to be developed, with suitable compositions and mechanical forces. Moreover, the continuous production of mucous by the gastric mucosa to replace the mucous that is lost through peristaltic contractions seems to limit the potential of mucoadhesion as a gastroretentive force. On the contrary, colonic mucoadhesion due to the lower mucus turnover and sensitivity to mucus secretory stimulus is much more successful than small intestinal or gastric approaches, due to a thicker mucus layer and lower disruptive colonic motility.

On the whole, it is suggested that this system normalizes the overall variations in drug GI transit time and allows for a more consistent performance of the formulations within and between individuals, improving the overall efficacy of drugs. However, the high turnover rate of gastric mucus and the probable local irritation by these drug formulations has remained challenging in this approach.

3.3. Conclusion

Ever since, the pharmaceutical concept of a dosage form seriously manipulate the stability, solubility, bioavailability, and other features of a medicine identifying these potential liabilities allows us to predict, control and avoid any complexities that may arise during pharmacotherapy. Hence, acquiring a clear notion of the assorted characteristics of drug delivery systems will not only allow proficient design of drug formulation, but also an improved in vitro and pre-clinical in vivo behavior of the drug, better in vitro - in vivo correlations, as well as opening new features in administrating drugs via novel drug delivery systems.

Author details

Yousef Javadzadeh and Sanaz Hamedeyazdan
Biotechnology Research Center and Faculty of Pharmacy, Tabriz University of Medical Sciences, Iran

4. References

Adibkia, K.; Hamedeyazdan, S. & Javadzadeh, Y. (2011). Drug release kinetics and physicochemical characteristics of floating drug delivery systems. *Expert Opin Drug Deliv*, Vol. 8, No. 7, pp. 891-903, ISSN: 1744-7593.

Ahuja, G. & Pathak, K. (2009). Porous carriers for controlled/modulated drug delivery. *Indian J Pharm Sci*, Vol. 71, No. 6, pp. 599-607, ISSN: 1998-3743.

Ali, J.; Arora, S.; Ahuja, A.; Babbar, A. K.; Sharma, R. K.; Khar, R. K. & Baboota, S. (2007). Formulation and development of hydrodynamically balanced system for metformin: in vitro and in vivo evaluation. *Eur J Pharm Biopharm*, Vol. 67, No. 1, pp. 196-201, ISSN: 0939-6411.

Arifin, D. Y.; Lee, L. Y. & Wang, C. H. (2006). Mathematical modeling and simulation of drug release from microspheres: Implications to drug delivery systems. *Adv Drug Deliv Rev*, Vol. 58, No. 12-13, pp. 1274-1325, ISSN: 0169-409X.

Asnaashari, S.; Khoei, N. S.; Zarrintan, M. H.; Adibkia, K. & Javadzadeh, Y. (2011). Preparation and evaluation of novel metronidazole sustained release and floating matrix tablets. *Pharm Dev Technol*, Vol. 16, No. 4, pp. 400-407, ISSN: 1097-9867.

Badhan, A. C.; Mashru, R. C.; Shah, P. P.; Thakkar, A. R. & Dobaria, N. B. (2009). Development and Evaluation of Sustained Release Gastroretentive Minimatrices for Effective Treatment of H. pylori Infection. *AAPS PharmSciTech*, Vol. 10, No. 2, pp. 459-467, ISSN: 1530-9932.

Bardonnet, P. L.; Faivre, V.; Pugh, W. J.; Piffaretti, J. C. & Falson, F. (2006). Gastroretentive dosage forms: overview and special case of Helicobacter pylori. *J Control Release*, Vol. 111, No. 1-2, pp. 1-18, ISSN: 0168-3659.

Barzegar-Jalali, M.; Adibkia, K.; Valizadeh, H.; Shadbad, M. R.; Nokhodchi, A.; Omidi, Y.; Mohammadi, G.; Nezhadi, S. H. & Hasan, M. (2008). Kinetic analysis of drug release from nanoparticles. *J Pharm Pharm Sci*, Vol. 11, No. 1, pp. 167-177, ISSN: 1482-1826.

Blanquet, S.; Zeijdner, E.; Beyssac, E.; Meunier, J. P.; Denis, S.; Havenaar, R. & Alric, M. (2004). A dynamic artificial gastrointestinal system for studying the behavior of orally administered drug dosage forms under various physiological conditions. *Pharm Res*, Vol. 21, No. 4, pp. 585-591, ISSN: 0724-8741.

Bode, S.; Dreyer, M. & Greisen, G. (2004). Gastric emptying and small intestinal transit time in preterm infants: a scintigraphic method. *J Pediatr Gastroenterol Nutr*, Vol. 39, No. 4, pp. 378-382, ISSN: 1536-4801.

Dash, S.; Murthy, P. N.; Nath, L. & Chowdhury, P. (2010). Kinetic modeling on drug release from controlled drug delivery systems. *Acta Pol Pharm*, Vol. 67, No. 3, pp. 217-223, ISSN: 0001-6837.

Davidovich-Pinhas, M. & Bianco-Peled, H. (2010). Mucoadhesion: a review of characterization techniques. *Expert Opin Drug Deliv*, Vol. 7, No. 2, pp. 259-271, ISSN: 1744-7593.

Davis, S. S. (2005). Formulation strategies for absorption windows. *Drug Discov Today*, Vol. 10, No. 4, pp. 249-257, ISSN: 1359-6446.

Dorozynski, P.; Jachowicz, R.; Kulinowski, P.; Kwiecinski, S.; Szybinski, K.; Skorka, T. & Jasinski, A. (2004). The macromolecular polymers for the preparation of hydrodynamically balanced systems--methods of evaluation. *Drug Dev Ind Pharm*, Vol. 30, No. 9, pp. 947-957, ISSN: 0363-9045.

Gangadharappa, H. V.; Biswas, S.; Getyala, A.; Vishal Gupta, N. & Pramod Kumar, T. M. (2011). Development, In vitro and In vivo Evaluation of Novel Floating Hollow Microspheres of Rosiglitazone Maleate. *Der Pharmacia Lettre*, Vol. 3, No. 4, pp. 299-316, ISSN: 0975-5071.

Ghareeb, M.; Issa, A. & Hussein, A. (2012). Prepared and characterized cinnarizine floating oil entrapped calcium alginate beads. *IJPSR*, Vol. 3, No. 2, pp. 501-508, ISSN: 0975-8232.

Gholap, S. B.; Banarjee, S. K.; Gaikwad, D. D.; Jadhav, S. L. & Thorat, R. M. (2010). Hollow microsphere: A Review. *International Journal of Pharmaceutical Sciences Review and Research*, Vol. 1, pp. 74-79, ISSN: 2231-2781.

Guguloth, M.; Bomma, R. & Veerabrahma, K. (2011). Development of sustained release floating drug delivery system for norfloxacin: in vitro and in vivo evaluation. *PDA J Pharm Sci Technol*, Vol. 65, No. 3, pp. 198-206, ISSN: 1948-2124.

Gupta, J. & Rajpoot, A. (2012). Formulation development and in-vitro evaluation of floating microspheres of clopidogrel bisulfate. *IJBTR*, Vol. 2, No. 1, pp. 212-218, ISSN: 2249 - 4871.

Hirtz, J. (1985). The gastrointestinal absorption of drugs in man: a review of current concepts and methods of investigation. *Br J Clin Pharmacol*, Vol. 19 Suppl 2, pp. 77S-83S, ISSN: 0306-5251.

Jain, S. K.; Agrawal, G. P. & Jain, N. K. (2006). A novel calcium silicate based microspheres of repaglinide: in vivo investigations. *J Control Release*, Vol. 113, No. 2, pp. 111-116, ISSN: 0168-3659.

Javadzadeh, Y.; Hamedeyazdan, S.; Adibkia, K.; Kiafar, F.; Zarrintan, M. H. & Barzegar-Jalali, M. (2010). Evaluation of drug release kinetics and physico-chemical characteristics of metronidazole floating beads based on calcium silicate and gas-forming agents. *Pharm Dev Technol*, Vol. 15, No. 4, pp. 329-338, ISSN: 1097-9867.

Javadzadeh, Y.; Shokri, J.; Hallaj-Nezhadi, S.; Hamishehkar, H. & Nokhodchi, A. (2010). Enhancement of percutaneous absorption of finasteride by cosolvents, cosurfactant and surfactants. *Pharm Dev Technol*, Vol. 15, No. 6, pp. 619-625, ISSN: 1097-9867.

Javadzadeh, Y.; Siahi, M. R.; Asnaashari, S. & Nokhodchi, A. (2007). Liquisolid technique as a tool for enhancement of poorly water-soluble drugs and evaluation of their physicochemical properties. *Acta Pharm*, Vol. 57, No. 1, pp. 99-109, ISSN: 1330-0075.

Kaus, L. C.; Gillespie, W. R.; Hussain, A. S. & Amidon, G. L. (1999). The effect of in vivo dissolution, gastric emptying rate, and intestinal transit time on the peak concentration and area-under-the-curve of drugs with different gastrointestinal permeabilities. *Pharm Res*, Vol. 16, No. 2, pp. 272-280, ISSN: 0724-8741.

Khattar, D.; Ahuja, A. & Khar, R. K. (1990). Hydrodynamically balanced systems as sustained release dosage forms for propranolol hydrochloride. *Pharmazie*, Vol. 45, No. 5, pp. 356-358, ISSN: 0031-7144.

Khobragade, D. S.; Parshuramkar, P. R.; Ujjainkar, A. P.; Mahendra, A. M.; Phapal, S. M. & Patil, A. T. (2009). Conception and evaluation of sustained release polymeric matrix beads for enhanced gastric retention. *Curr Drug Deliv*, Vol. 6, No. 3, pp. 249-254, ISSN: 1567-2018.

Klausner, E. A.; Lavy, E.; Friedman, M. & Hoffman, A. (2003). Expandable gastroretentive dosage forms. *J Control Release*, Vol. 90, No. 2, pp. 143-162, ISSN: 0168-3659.

Krogel, I. & Bodmeier, R. (1999). Floating or pulsatile drug delivery systems based on coated effervescent cores. *Int J Pharm*, Vol. 187, No. 2, pp. 175-184, ISSN: 0378-5173.

Kumar, K. M.; Shah, M. H.; Ketkar, A.; Mahadik, K. R. & Paradkar, A. (2004). Effect of drug solubility and different excipients on floating behaviour and release from glyceryl monooleate matrices. *International Journal of Pharmaceutics*, Vol. 272, pp. 151–160, ISSN: 2249–3522.

Lahoti, S. S.; Shep, S. G.; Mayee, R. V. & Toshniwal, S. S. (2011). Mucoadhesive Drug Delivery System: A Review. *Indo-Global Journal of Pharmaceutical Sciences*, Vol. 1, No. 3, pp. 243-251, ISSN: 2249- 1023.

Martinez, M. N. & Amidon, G. L. (2002). A mechanistic approach to understanding the factors affecting drug absorption: a review of fundamentals. *J Clin Pharmacol*, Vol. 42, No. 6, pp. 620-643, ISSN: 0091-2700.

McConnell, E. L.; Fadda, H. M. & Basit, A. W. (2008). Gut instincts: explorations in intestinal physiology and drug delivery. *Int J Pharm*, Vol. 364, No. 2, pp. 213-226, ISSN: 0378-5173.

Motlekar, N. A. & Youan, B. B. (2006). The quest for non-invasive delivery of bioactive macromolecules: a focus on heparins. *J Control Release*, Vol. 113, No. 2, pp. 91-101, ISSN: 0168-3659.

Movassaghian, S.; Barzegar-Jalali, M.; Alaeddini, M.; Hamedyazdan, S.; Afzalifar, R.; Zakeri-Milani, P.; Mohammadi, G. & Adibkia, K. (2011). Development of amitriptyline buccoadhesive tablets for management of pain in dental procedures. *Drug Dev Ind Pharm*, Vol. 37, No. 7, pp. 849-854, ISSN: 1520-5762.

Mudie, D. M.; Amidon, G. L. & Amidon, G. E. (2010). Physiological Parameters for Oral Delivery and in Vitro Testing. *Mol Pharm*, ISSN: 1543-8392.

Muller, R. H. & Jacobs, C. (2002). Buparvaquone mucoadhesive nanosuspension: preparation, optimisation and long-term stability. *Int J Pharm*, Vol. 237, No. 1-2, pp. 151-161, ISSN: 0378-5173.

Murata, Y.; Sasaki, N.; Miyamoto, E. & Kawashima, S. (2000). Use of floating alginate gel beads for stomach-specific drug delivery. *Eur J Pharm Biopharm*, Vol. 50, No. 2, pp. 221-226, ISSN: 0939-6411.

Nama, M.; Gonugunta, C. S. R. & Reddy Veerareddy, P. (2008). Formulation and Evaluation of Gastroretentive Dosage Forms of Clarithromycin. *AAPS PharmSciTech*, Vol. 9, No. 1, pp. 231-237, ISSN: 1530-9932.

Pahwa, R.; Chhabra, L.; Lamba, A.; Jindal, S. & Rathour, A. (2012). Formulation and in-vitro evaluation of effervescent floating tablets of an antiulcer agent. *J. Chem. Pharm. Res.*, Vol. 4, No. 2, pp. 1066-1073, ISSN: 0975-7384.

Pandya, N.; Pandya, M. & Bhaskar, V. H. (2011). Preparation and in vitro Characterization of Porous Carrier-Based Glipizide Floating Microspheres for Gastric Delivery. *J Young Pharm*, Vol. 3, No. 2, pp. 97-104, ISSN: 0975-1505.

Parikh, D. C. & Amin, A. F. (2008). In vitro and in vivo techniques to assess the performance of gastro-retentive drug delivery systems: a review. *Expert Opin Drug Deliv*, Vol. 5, No. 9, pp. 951-965, ISSN: 1742-5247.

Patel, A.; Modasiya, M.; Shah, D. & Patel, V. (2009). Development and in vivo floating behavior of verapamil HCl intragastric floating tablets. *AAPS PharmSciTech*, Vol. 10, No. 1, pp. 310-315, ISSN: 1530-9932.

Rajab, M.; Jouma, M.; Neubert, R. H. & Dittgen, M. (2010). Optimization of a metformin effervescent floating tablet containing hydroxypropylmethylcellulose and stearic acid. *Pharmazie*, Vol. 65, No. 2, pp. 97-101, ISSN: 0031-7144.

Rajput, G. C.; Majmudar, F. D.; Patel, J. K.; Patel, K. N.; Thakor, R. S.; Patel, B. P. & Rajgor, N. (2010). Stomach Specific Mucoadhesive Tablets As Controlled Drug Delivery System – A Review Work. *International Journal on Pharmaceutical and Biological Research*, Vol. 1, No. 1, pp. 30-41, ISSN: 0976- 285X.

Rane, B. R.; Gujarathi, N. A. & Patel, J. K. (2012). Biodegradable anionic acrylic resin based hollow microspheres of moderately water soluble drug Rosiglitazone Maleate: preparation and in vitro characterization. *Drug Dev Ind Pharm*, ISSN: 1520-5762.

Riley, S. A.; Sutcliffe, F.; Kim, M.; Kapas, M.; Rowland, M. & Turnberg, L. A. (1992). The influence of gastrointestinal transit on drug absorption in healthy volunteers. *Br J Clin Pharmacol*, Vol. 34, No. 1, pp. 32-39, ISSN: 0306-5251.

Roy, S.; Pal, K.; Anis, A.; Pramanik, K. & Prabhakar, B. (2009). Polymers in Mucoadhesive Drug Delivery System: A Brief Note. *Designed monomers and polymers*, Vol. 12, pp. 483-495, ISSN: 2158-7043.

Shaikh, R.; Raj Singh, T. R.; Garland, M. J.; Woolfson, A. D. & Donnelly, R. F. (2011). Mucoadhesive drug delivery systems. *J Pharm Bioallied Sci*, Vol. 3, No. 1, pp. 89-100, ISSN: 0975-7406.

Sher, P.; Ingavle, G.; Ponrathnam, S.; Poddar, P. & Pawar, A. P. (2009). Modulation and optimization of drug release from uncoated low density porous carrier based delivery system. *AAPS PharmSciTech*, Vol. 10, No. 2, pp. 547-558, ISSN: 1530-9932.

Singh, P. K.; Deol, P. K. & Kaur, I. P. (2012). Entrapment of Lactobacillus acidophilus into alginate beads for the effective treatment of cold restraint stress induced gastric ulcer. *Food & Function*, Vol. 3, No. 1, pp. 83, ISSN: 2042-6496.

Sohrabi, M.; Soleimani, J.; Roshangar, L.; Vatansever, S.; Arbabi, F.; Khaki, A. A.; Abbasi, M. M.; Dustar, Y. & Javadzadeh, Y. (2009). The effect of dietary and topical celecoxib on 4-nitroquinoline-1-oxide-induced lingual epithelium alternations in rat. *J Pak Med Assoc*, Vol. 59, No. 11, pp. 769-774, ISSN: 0030-9982.

Soppimath, K. S.; Aminabhavi, T. M.; Agnihotri, S. A.; Mallikarjuna, N. N. & Kulkarni, P. V. (2006). Effect of coexcipients on drug release and floating property of nifedipine hollow microspheres: A novel gastro retentive drug delivery system. *Journal of Applied Polymer Science*, Vol. 100, No. 1, pp. 486-494, ISSN: 0021-8995.

Streubel, A.; Siepmann, J. & Bodmeier, R. (2002). Floating microparticles based on low density foam powder. *Int J Pharm*, Vol. 241, No. 2, pp. 279-292, ISSN: 0378-5173.

Sungthongjeen, S.; Paeratakul, O.; Limmatvapirat, S. & Puttipipatkhachorn, S. (2006). Preparation and in vitro evaluation of a multiple-unit floating drug delivery system based on gas formation technique. *Int J Pharm*, Vol. 324, No. 2, pp. 136-143, ISSN: 0378-5173.

Sungthongjeen, S.; Sriamornsak, P. & Puttipipatkhachorn, S. (2008). Design and evaluation of floating multi-layer coated tablets based on gas formation. *Eur J Pharm Biopharm*, Vol. 69, No. 1, pp. 255-263, ISSN: 0939-6411.

Tangri, P.; Khurana, S. & Madhav, N. V. S. (2011). Mucoadhesive drug delivery: mechanism and methods of evaluation. *International Journal of Pharma and Bio Sciences*, Vol. 2, No. 1, pp. 458-467, ISSN: 0975-6299.

Wagner, J. G. (1969). Interpretation of percent dissolved-time plots derived from in vitro testing of conventional tablets and capsules. *J Pharm Sci*, Vol. 58, No. 10, pp. 1253-1257, ISSN: 0022-3549.

Wei, Y. M. & Zhao, L. (2008). In vitro and in vivo evaluation of ranitidine hydrochloride loaded hollow microspheres in rabbits. *Arch Pharm Res*, Vol. 31, No. 10, pp. 1369-1377, ISSN: 0253-6269.

Yao, H.; Zhu, J.; Yu, J. & Zhang, L. (2012). Preparation and evaluation of a novel gastric floating alginate/poloxamer inner-porous beads using foam solution. *Int J Pharm*, Vol. 422, No. 1-2, pp. 211-219, ISSN: 1873-3476.

Chapter 5

Processing and Templating of Bioactive-Loaded Polymeric Neural Architectures: Challenges and Innovative Strategies

Viness Pillay, Pradeep Kumar, Yahya E. Choonara, Girish Modi, Dinesh Naidoo and Lisa C. du Toit

Additional information is available at the end of the chapter

1. Introduction

The chapter highlights the current drug delivery strategies and phenomenon involved in the design of neural architectures employed for neuropharmaceutical applications attempting to replicate the nervous tissues. We seek to give an overview of the current drug delivery approaches such as degradable/diffusion-based delivery systems, affinity-based delivery systems, and immobilized drug delivery systems used to generate bioactive-release from scaffolds for neural tissue engineering applications. We talk about the combinatorial approach being employed in recent years in the form of "new generation of multifunctional biomaterials" which are - able to mimic the molecular regulatory characteristics by providing a three-dimensional architecture representing the native extracellular matrix and also able to sequester and deliver biomolecular moieties in highly specific manner. A special focus will be given to the micro- and nano-structured scaffolds which have been proved to be effective in axonal repairing, in guiding functional neurogenesis and in controlling stem cell differentiation. Emphasis will be given to the processing requirements for synthetic and natural polymers and biomaterials for producing potential scaffold materials as well as to the templating of the target drugs with their benefits and drawbacks. A detailed discussion will be provided for certain specialised and recently developed architectures in the form of injectable matrices, electrospun nanofibers, and hydrogels. Injectable scaffolds provide a very unique advantage of being a non-invasive approach for neural tissue engineering as further damage to the soft neural tissue due to surgery can be prevented. Current injectables in tissue engineering consists of gelation methods based on in situ chemical polymerization and crosslinking, photo-initiated polymerization and crosslinking, thermogelling injectable systems, ionic crosslinking, and self-assembling. Injectable scaffolds also provide opportunities for drug delivery in the form of composite materials with embedded micro- and nanoparticles. Additionally, the easy customization of the injectable architectures by modification of solidification, porosity, biofunctionalization, mechanical properties, and biodegradation is an added attribute. The electrospinning process, on the other hand can be used to engineer neural architectures having micro to nanoscale topographical cues as well as micromeritic properties similar to the extracellular matrix. Enhanced cell attachment, drug loading, and mass transfer properties can be easily obtained by changing the surface-to-volume ratio and by controlling the bulk mechanical properties of electrospun scaffolds where the fibers can also be oriented or arranged randomly, to regulate the biological response to the scaffold. Drugs ranging from anti-inflammatory and antibiotic agents to growth factors, proteins, DNA, and RNA, and even living cells can be incorporated into electrospun scaffolds. Interventionally, the current tissue engineering and therapeutic approaches pertaining to neural injuries will be analysed and critiqued in detail with respect to various strategies, perspectives, challenges and expanding opportunities. Considerable efforts have been carried out to enhance the properties of tissue engineering architectures via surface engineering and surface functionalization for providing an extracellular matrix mimicking environment for better cell adhesion and tissue in-growth. These modifications can be carried out through plasma treatment, wet chemical method, surface graft polymerization, and co-fabrication of surface active agents and polymers. These modifications can further be designed and customised to release bioactive molecules, such as growth factors, DNA, or drugs, in a sustained manner to facilitate tissue regeneration (**Figure 1**) [1]. Target molecules are usually loaded on the surface of scaffolds by physical adsorption, nanoparticles assembly on the surface, layer-by-layer multilayer assembly, and chemical immobilization. Tissue engineering scaffolds can deliver bioactives via certain signals such as interspersed signals, immobilized signals and signal delivery from cells and hence act as specialised and desired controlled release matrices.

Material choices for the fabrication of neural architectures will be elucidated among, but not limited to, synthetic polymers such as poly(lactic acid), poly(glycolic acid) and co-polymers; poly(lactic acid-co-ethylene glycol); synthetic polyesters (PLA, PLGA) and collagen blends; aliphatic/aromatic degradable polyesters; polyfumarates; poly(ethylene terephtalate)–poly(butylene terephtalate); polyhydroxyalkanoates; poly(glycerol sebacate); hydroxyl group containing polymers; amine group containing polymers; poly(amido-amines)s; N-succinimidyl tartarate monoamine–poly(ethylene glycol)-block poly(D,L-lactic acid); poly(depsipeptide-co-lactide); poly(urethane)s; pluronic F-127 (PEO–PPO–PEO); tyrosine-derived polycarbonates; polyorthoesters; polyphosphazenes; polyanhydrides; polypyrrole; and poly ether ester amides and natural polymers such as alginates, chitosan, hyaluronans, and carageenans as well as self-assembling peptides.

Specific and representing examples cited, but not limited to, are as follows: Incorporation of protein-eluting microspheres (poly(lactide-co-glycolide) (PLGA 50/50)) into biodegradable nerve guidance channels (chitin tubes) for controlled release of growth factor; sodium tripolyphosphate cross-linked chitosan microspheres for controlled release of bioactive nerve growth factor; multifunctional, multichannel bridges that deliver neurotrophin encoding lentivirus (encoding the neurotrophic factors NT-3 or BDNF) for regeneration following spinal cord injury (combining gene delivery with biomaterials); poly(2-hydroxyethyl methacrylate-co-methyl methacrylate) nerve guidance channels as nerve growth factor delivery vehicles; regrowth of axons in lesioned adult rat spinal cord: promotion by implants of cultured Schwann cells; and sustained release of dexamethasone from hydrophilic alginate hydrogel matrices using PLGA nanoparticles for neural drug delivery.

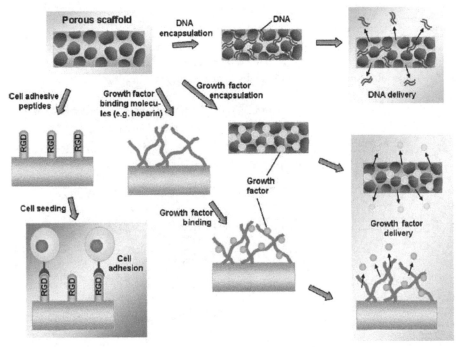

Figure 1. Surface engineered and growth factor releasing scaffolds for tissue engineering: Scaffolds can be either immobilized with cell specific ligands for cell adhesion, or encapsulated with growth factors or DNA to promote cell proliferation and morphogenesis [Adapted from Ref. 1 with permission © Elsevier Science BV].

2. Meta analysis of leading research reports

2.1. Local drug delivery for neuroprotection and tissue repair

In a series of studies, Shoichet et al., (2006, 2009a, 2009b) demonstrated the potential of hyaluronic acid-methyl cellulose (HAMC) blend as an injectable scaffold for the delivery of bioactives to an injured spinal cord, via an intrathecal injection, in conjugation with providing necessary support and microenvironment for the proliferation of neural cells. The studies were conducted in the backdrop of three most common strategies for localized intrathecal delivery viz. a bolus injection, a minipump delivery, and an injectable gel that localizes release to the site of injection. The first method pose a challenge in terms of the effects being short-lived due to washing-out of the therapeutic molecule by cerebrospinal fluid and the second one being invasive and may lead to complication ranging from device blockage to infection. The novel HAMC blends' strategy provided a potential solution (**Table 1**) through the design of a shear-thinning based gel with an inherent property of increase in gel strength with an increase in temperature fast gelling [**Figure 2**].

S. No.	Design criteria	Advantage
1.	Fast gelling	localized delivery to the site of injection; no spread-out with the cerebrospinal fluid (CSF) flow
2.	Injectable through 30G needle	minimally invasive surgery
3.	Non-cell adhesive	minimization of scar formation in the intrathecal space
4.	Degradable	no need for scaffold removal afterwards
5.	Biocompatible	minimized foreign body reaction

Table 1. Design criteria for an injectable scaffold architecture

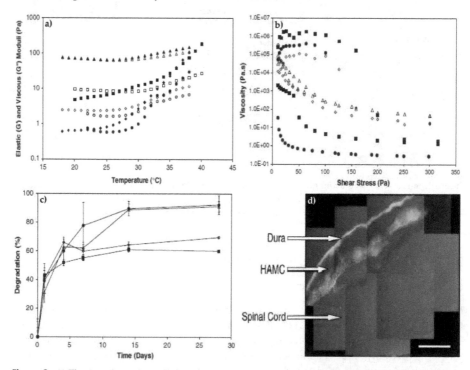

Figure 2. A) Elastic and viscous moduli of injectable gels at 1Hz using a rheometer with a cone and plate geometry (●) 7%MC G', (○) 7%MC G'', (■) 9%MC G', (□) 9%MC G'', (▲) HAMC G', (Δ) HAMC G'', (▼) acet-HAMC G', and (◊) acet-HAMC G''. B) Thixotropic loop of injectable gels at 37°C (●) 7%MC, (■)

9%MC, (Δ) HAMC, and (◊) acet-HAMC. C) *In vitro* degradation in aCSF of (●) 7%MC, (■) 9%MC, (Δ) HAMC, and (◊) acet-HAMC determined by change of dry mass over time. D) Parasagittal section of rat spinal cord rostral to site of injection shows that the fluorescent HAMC is localized in situ in the intrathecal space where it was injected [Adapted from Ref. 4 with permission © Elsevier Science BV].

In a typical experiment, 2% HA was blended with 7% MC and the gelation mechanism, degradation profile, and cell adhesion were studied in vitro. Additionally, in vivo studies were carried out for testing the injectability, biocompatibility and therapeutic efficacy (2006). Furthering the study, the potential of HAMC blend for the delivery of neuroprotectant such as nimodipine and erythropoietin were investigated experimentally. Specifically, nimodipine-loaded gels yielded particle size-dependent biphasic release profiles suggesting the accelerated delivery of poorly soluble drugs with tuneable release rates. In an another report, in vitro erythropoietin release studies revealed a 16 h release profile with the implant showing reduced cavitation after spinal cord injury along with enhanced neuronal number proving the potential of HAMC in neuroprotection after neural injury [2-4].

2.2. Multifunctional, multichannel bridges that deliver neurotrophin encoding lentivirus

Tuinstra at al., 2012, addressed the neural injury regeneration challenge by proposing a "gene delivery-biomaterial combination" strategy to surpass the "multiple barriers limiting regeneration". Spinal cord injury induced neuron and oligodendrocyte cell death, demyelination, inflammation, and deposition of a glial scar are attributed to insufficient trophic factor support, and up-regulation of axonal growth inhibitors. To overcome the deficiency of trophic factors, peripheral nerve implants are preferred due to their biograft-architecture and secretion of trophic factors by cells such as Schwann cells. However, the source limitation and the ill-defined contribution of the architecture and cell-secreted factors led to the requirement of systems and strategies capable of recapitulating their effects. To overcome the challenges, the delivery of lentiviral vectors (encoding neurotrophin-3 (NT-3) and brain derived neurotrophic factor (BDNF)) from multiple channel bridges was proposed as a combinatorial approach to promote regeneration in the injured SC. Interventionally, the lentivirus was immobilized to hydroxyapatite nanoparticles and then loaded into poly(lactic acid-co-glycolic acid) (PLGA) bridges for implantation into a rat spinal cord lateral hemisection and the axonal growth and myelination were characterized as a function of time, treatment, and location within the bridge. The strategy was aimed at (a) providing mechanical stability to the injured tissue, (b) channels directing the axonal elongation, (c) supporting cell infiltration, (d) preventing cavity formation secondary to the initial injury, (d) limiting scar formation. Interestingly, the cells were aligned with the major axis of the bridge providing a directional signal for regenerating axons [5].

2.3. In situ gelling hydrogels for local delivery of BDNF after spinal cord injury

Over the last decade, a research group led by Ravi V. Bellamkonda at Wallace H. Coulter Department of Biomedical Engineering, Georgia Institute of Technology and Emory

University, Atlanta, USA, has emerged as a leading authority working towards the development of neurological biomaterials and therapeutics especially focusing on neural injuries. Jain et al., 2006, developed an agarose in situ gelling three-dimensional (3D) scaffold capable of initiating axonal growth in 3D. To this 3D scaffold was added neurotrophic factor BDNF-loaded lipid microtubule (40μm in length and 0.5μm in diameter) for local release of the bioactive. The individual benefits incurred by the components are structured in **Table 2**. Spinal cords treated with agarose/BDNF displayed no axonal bulbed-up morphology and the axons crossed the interface into the hydrogel scaffold based on the NF-160kDa staining data analysis where NF-160 kDa intensity was significantly greater than the agarose-treated spinal cords at the interface [6].

Agarose scaffold	Brain derived neurotrophic factor
Biocompatible: does not cause an adverse reaction when implanted in vivo,	encouraged neurite growth into the scaffolds
can be optimized for maximum axonal outgrowth through manipulation of the porosity and mechanical properties,	reduced the reactivity of the astrocytes and the production of chondroitin sulfate proteoglycans (CSPGs)
Support cell migration	enhanced the ability of regenerating fibers to enter the permissive hydrogel scaffold
can be utilized as part of a trophic factor delivery system with embedded sustained release vehicles,	acted as a chemo-attractant for the axons to cross the interface
can be used to bind protein to its backbone for spatial control	reduces the minimal inflammatory response agarose gels generate in vivo

Table 2. Salient features of the in situ gelling hydrogel components

2.4. Neurite extension in anisotropic LN-1 scaffolds

An in vitro study by Dodla and Bellamkonda, the importance of directional cues for neural regeneration was proposed. The hypothesis was based on the performance outcomes of autografts where the researchers theorized that "anisotropic hydrogel scaffolds with gradients of a growth-promoting glycoprotein/extracellular matrix protein, laminin-1 (LN-1), may promote directional neurite extension and enhance regeneration". The scaffolds were fabricated via photochemical coupling approach wherein LN-1 was immobilized onto three-dimensional (3D) agarose scaffolds in gradients of differing slopes. A significant increase in the Dorsal root ganglia (DRG) neurite extension rates were observed in case of anisotropic scaffolds as compared to their isotropic analogues proving the importance and potential of built-in directional cues for guided tissue or nerve regeneration [7]. In line with the functionalized scaffold properties developed above, Crompton et al., 2007, described the potential of Polylysine-functionalized chitosan as an in vitro substrate, scaffold for cortical cells, and for neural tissue engineering as an injectable scaffold. The functionalized polysaccharide polymer was rendered thermoresponsive by ionic gelation mechanism of glycerophosphate. In first of its kind study of chitosan-GP network gels on neural tissue, the 3D culture model showed that the survival of cells on chitosan/GP was less than the PDL-modified chitosan/GP justifying the inclusion of PDL as functionality for neural applications [8].

2.5. Topical delivery of Tx-MP-NPs into the contusion injured spinal cord

The delivery of bioactives on the site of neural injury can be achieved by various means including intravenous delivery eventually passing through blood brain barrier and reaching the site of action or through intrathecal/intracranial injection for localized delivery. Targeted delivery is an additional option but not much tried and tested for CNS injuries. The i.v. strategy encompasses the probability of inefficiency as compared to the localised delivery but invasiveness is a drawback for the later intervention. Chvatal et al., 2008, and later Kim et al., 2009, reported the therapeutic effectiveness of nanoparticle-mediated localized methylprednisolone (MP) delivery for spinal cord injury intervention. These studies tested the therapeutic effect of MP-loaded PLGA nanoparticles, incorporated into an agarose gel, in in vivo models of spinal cord injury. The first study by Chvatal et al, 2008, concentrated on the spatial distribution of MP along with the acute anti-inflammatory effect. In a typical fabrication, the drug was first conjugated with Texas-red cadaverine (Tx, Biotium) allow its visualization in and around an injured spinal cord. Thereafter, the PLGA nanoparticles were prepared using a double emulsion method followed by their incorporation into the agarose gel. Two different types agarose gel were used: denser gel without nanoparticles (SeaKem) and gel containing nanoparticles (SeaPlaque) as shown in **Figure 3**.

According to **Figure 4**; the drug-indicator conjugate revealed a slow release over six days and the data was used to determine the amount of Tx-MP released from the gel-embedded NPs showing a continual release pattern. The release was probably due to the gradual degradation of PLGA polymeric structures. In this way, a continual delivery of MP can be provided to the injured spinal cord thereby exerting its anti-inflammatory action with a single administration and hence can provide much needed lipid-peroxidation inhibition during the initial and acute phase of secondary injury. To further simulate the in vivo environment, the in vitro release studies of Tx-MP from NPs embedded in agarose hydrogels was examined by co-incubation with LPS-stimulated primary rat microglia. The quantification of nitric oxide (NO) release from the microglia at different time points, 24, 72, and 96 h, showed that the cells treated with Tx-MP-NPs had significantly reduced NO production as compared to the cells treated with Saline NPs (as a negative control) further proving that the hydrogel-based delivery system (i.e., NPs embedded in agarose gel) can be used as an MP depot.

The quantification of spatial distribution of Tx-MP in the contusion injured spinal cord revealed that MP diffused up to 1.5mm deep and up to 3 mm laterally into the injured spinal cord within 2 days. Other significant observations of this study included decreased early inflammation, reduction in the number of ED-1þ macrophages/activated microglia, diminished expression of pro-inflammatory proteins such as Calpain and iNOS, and finally reduced lesion volume within 7 days after contusion injury [9].

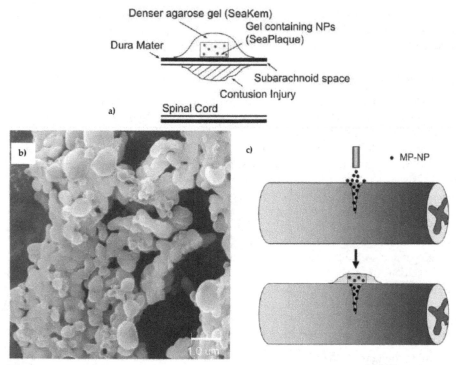

Figure 3. a) Schematic showing the Tx-MP-NP embedded gel is placed directly onto the injury site, on top of the dura. The denser gel is injected on top and quickly cooled to hold the NP embedded gel in place and minimize outward diffusion of Tx-MP. b) Methylprednisolone-encapsulating PLGA nanoparticles (MP-NP): SEM image of the lyophilized MP-NPs. c) Schematic of topical and local delivery of the MP-NPs onto dorsal over-hemisection lesioned spinal cord [Adapted from Ref. 9 with permission © Elsevier Science BV].

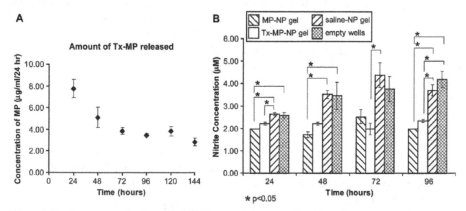

Figure 4. In vitro characterization of Tx-MP-NPs. (A) Release profile of Tx-MP over 6 days in vitro. Plotted is the amount of MP released every 24 h. (B) Bioassay showing the amount of nitrite in the

media surrounding LPS-activated microglia that had been treated with gels containing either MP-NP, Tx-MP-NP, Saline-NP, or nothing. This represents the amount of NO produced by microglia in each of these conditions for 4 days [Adapted from Ref. 9 with permission © Elsevier Science BV].

2.6. Nanoparticle-mediated local delivery of methylprednisolone

Further extending the above results, Kim et al., 2009, conducted a detailed histological and behavioural study of the developed local and sustained MP delivery through the use of biodegradable polymer-based nanoparticles. The following histological parameters were recorded:

1. reduced the reactivity of pro-apoptotic proteins (Calpain and Bax)
2. increased reactivity of anti-apoptotic protein (Bcl-2) at the lesion site
3. reduced iNOS (a key mediator of inflammation and neurotoxic effects expression
4. ratio of Bcl-2 to Bax, a key determinant of neuronal commitment to apoptosis, was increased indicating that MP treatment reduced the mitochondria-mediated cell death pathway.

These results suggest that sustained MP delivery by slow release MP-NP can reduce the reactivity of the injury-related proteins. Furthermore, MP-NP treatment produced significantly improved functional outcomes within one week after injury wherein MP-NP-treated groups performed significantly better in the beam walking test.

In conclusion, following advantages of MP-NP local delivery over conventional systemic delivery were proposed:

1. Better therapeutic effect as compared to systemic MP delivery;
2. More efficient, targeted delivery to the injury site as the MP delivery via systemic administration is influenced by the short pharmacokinetic half-life of intravenous MP (2.5–3 h) and P-glycoprotein-mediated exclusion of MP from the spinal cord necessitating a high-dose MP regimen. However, a significantly lower dose was required using nanoparticle-encapsulated MP (approximately 400 mg/ animal) and delivering this dose locally onto the target tissue. Additionally, this significantly enhanced the therapeutic effectiveness of MP by increasing the local dose levels at the target site;
3. Potential to adjust delivery rate or duration since the MP release profile from nanoparticles can be controlled through the composition of the biodegradable polymer, the rate, amount, or duration of delivery can be adjusted;
4. Stable formulation in form of injectable and lyophilized fine (submicron) powder formulation (unlike cell-based therapies). The formulation can be stored as a lyophilized fine powder and then easily suspended in saline or embedded in hydrogel and locally delivered onto the lesion site [10].

2.7. Sustained delivery of thermostabilized chABC

Furthering their study on the involvement of various axonal growth promoters and inhibitors, Bellamkonda and co-workers targeted Chondroitin sulfate proteoglycans, a major class of axon growth inhibitors that are up-regulated after spinal cord injury and contribute to regenerative failure, via the use of Chondroitinase ABC (chABC) capable of digesting glycosaminoglycan chains on CSPGs thereby overcoming the CSPG-mediated inhibition. The formulation problem concerned with chABC is the loss of its enzymatic activity 37 °C, necessitating the use of repeated injections or local infusions for a prolonged period making it clinically inefficient. Lee et al., 2010, designed a thermostabilized chABC and developed a system for its sustained local delivery in vivo thereby resolving the problem to a great extent as the novel thermostabilized chABC retained its biological activity at 37 °C in vitro for up to 4 weeks [Figure 5].

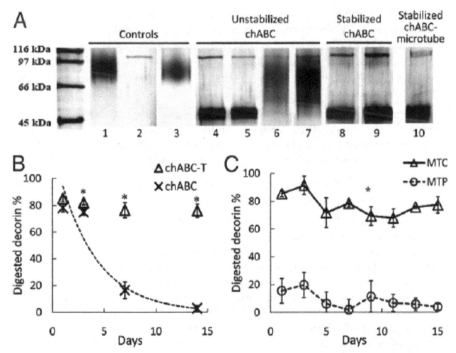

Figure 5. Enhanced thermal stability of chABC with trehalose, and sustained chABC release with lipidmicrotubes. (A) SDS-PAGE assay of enzymatic activity of chABC. (B) Kinetic analysis of chABC deactivation by DMMB assay. The dotted line represents the calculated deactivation curve of chABC in 1× PBS. (C) Enzymatic activity of post released chABC (Δ) and penicillinase (o) with trehalose/microtubes [Adapted from Ref. 11 © Proceedings of National Academy of Science (PNAS)].

Briefly, chABC was thermostabilize using the sugar trehalose and a hydrogel-microtube based delivery system was used for the sustained local delivery of chABC in vivo [11]. Key finding of the study included:

a. Trehalose Significantly Enhances chABC Thermal Stability and Prolongs Enzyme Activity

b.   Temperature stabilization of chabc by trehalose was due to conformational stability

c.   Thermostabilized chABC (TS-chABC) retains its ability to digest CSPGs in vivo 2 weeks post-injury,

d.   CS-GAG levels remain significantly depleted at the lesion site for at least 6 weeks post-SCI.

e.   Enhanced axonal sprouting and functional recovery is observed after topical delivery of agarose-microtube-chabc scaffolds after SCI

f.   Animals treated with thermostabilized chABC in combination with sustained neurotrophin-3 delivery showed significant improvement in locomotor function and enhanced growth of cholera toxin B subunit– positive sensory axons and sprouting of serotonergic fibers.

g.   chABC thermostability facilitates minimally invasive, sustained, local delivery of chABC that is potentially effective in overcoming CSPG-mediated regenerative failure.

2.8. Sustained delivery of activated Rho GTPases and BDNF

In the next stage of their Chondroitin sulfate proteoglycans targeting, Bellamkonda and co-workers fabricated constitutively active (CA) Rho GTPases, CA-Rac1 and CA-Cdc42, and BDNF loaded 1,2-bis-(tricosa-10,12-diynoyl)-sn-glycero-3-phosphocholine lipid microtubes for the sustained release of bioactives to the lesion site for the alleviation of CSPG-mediated inhibition of regenerating axons. The lipid tubules were further loaded into an *in situ* gelling agarose-protein architecture similar to previous studies where nanoparticles were incorporated into an agarose injectable gel. The sustained release characteristics of the developed system were characterised both in vitro and in vivo BDNF was conjugated to rhodamine for its in vivo quantification. As depicted in **Figure 6**, 3 mg of BDNF was released within the first 24 h followed by a cumulative release of 4mg within the first 3 days. After this initial burst release, approximately 3ng/day of BDNF was released for the subsequent 11 days. For in vivo release study, microtubes loaded with BDNF/Rhodamine embedded in the agarose were injected into the spinal cord cavity. Spatial quantification of BDNF/Rhodamine displayed its presence in the spinal cord tissue between 1 to 2 mm proximal to the lesion site (Fig. 1B). An overlap of ED-1+ cells (green) with the BDNF-Rhodamine demonstrated co-localization and subsequent engulfment of the BDNF-Rhodamine by the ED-1+ cells. Additionally, BDNF-Rhodamine was double labelled with DAPI to visualize cell nuclei confirmed the presence of neurotrophins [12]. In conclusion, the study utilized the hydrogel/microtubule scaffold delivery system to deliver BDNF, CA-Cdc42, or CA-Rac1 to decrease the sensitivity of growth cones to CSPGs, and promote axonal growth through CSPG-rich regions at the lesion site based on following three phenomena:

1.   The use of the in situ gelling hydrogel allows the lesion cavity to be conformally filled.

2.   The lipid microtubes allow slow release of therapeutics from the hydrogel over time.

3.   This strategy allows neuroprotective or axonal migration stimulators to be delivered locally over time.

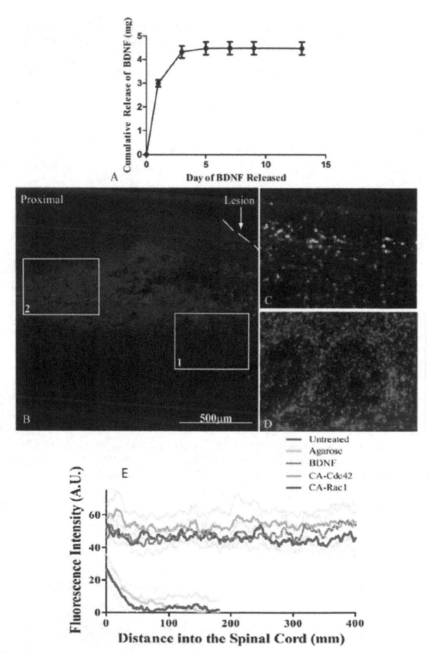

Figure 6. In Vitro and In Vivo Diffusion of BDNF. A. In vitro release assay of BDNF over the first 2 weeks. The graph shows that an initial burst released 4 mg of BDNF within the first 3 days. An average

of 3 ng/day of BDNF was released for the following 11 days. The data represent mean 6 SEM B. An image of the proximal region of a spinal cord section after delivery of BDNF/Rhodamine at 46. The 206images labelled 1 and 2 are outlined with white boxes in A and demonstrate that BDNF/Rhodamine diffused approximately 2 mm proximal to the lesion site. The dashed line represents the interface between the spinal cord and scaffold. White arrows indicate BDNF/Rhodamine. C. A 206image of ED-1+ cells (green) and BDNF-Rhodamine (red). The image shows some overlap demonstrating engulfment of the BDNF-Rhodamine by the ED-1+ cells. D. A 206image of DAPI (blue) and BDNF-Rhodamine (red) demonstrates that not all of the BDNF-Rhodamine is taken up by resident and migrating cells. Quantitative analysis of NF-160 intensity for the stained spinal cords. The spinal cords treated with CA-Cdc42, CA-Rac1, and BDNF had significantly higher fluorescent intensity and also had extended further into the scaffold filled spinal cord cavity than the untreated and agarose controls [Adapted from Ref. 12 © PLoS ONE].

2.9. Multiple-channel scaffolds to promote spinal cord axon regeneration

Moore et al., 2006, introduced a proposition regarding the use of a conjugation of molecular, cellular, and tissue-level treatments for spinal cord injury to elicit functional recovery in animal models or patients. In a tri-component study, multiple-channel biodegradable scaffolds were tested as a platform to investigate the effects scaffold architecture, transplanted cells, and locally delivered molecular agents on axon regeneration. Biodegradable polymers such as PLGA can provide a tissue scaffold, a cell delivery vehicle, and a reservoir for sustained drug delivery. Therefore, PLGA scaffolds were fabricated using injection moulding with rapid solvent evaporation.

The scaffolds so formed have characteristic plurality of distinct channels running parallel along the length of the scaffolds with various customized channel sizes and geometries. Inherent to the channels were void fractions (as high as 89%) with accessible void fractions as high as 90% through connections 220mm or larger. Scaffolds degradation and bioactive release in vitro accounted for over a period of 30 weeks and 12 weeks, respectively. The degradation profile of PLGA scaffold demonstrated typical polyhydroxy acid characteristics as the scaffold molecular weight decreased steadily from 100% of the initial molecular weight down to 5% by 26 weeks of degradation. Interestingly, minimal mass loss was observed for the first 20 weeks. The next ten weeks culminated into a more precipitous mass loss generating a sigmoidal mass loss behavior typical for PLGA degradation. The negligible change in mass during initial phase corroborated well with the slight changes in morphology. However, the morphology of the degrading scaffolds changed drastically during the precipitous phase. The model drug, Fluorescein isothiocyanate (FITC-D), was incorporated using, mechanical mixing within the polymer scaffolds. However the method was quite effective for scaffold loading, an inhomogeneous dispersal appeared in the final fabricated scaffolds. A drug release-scaffold degradation comparison in **Figure 7** compared the mass and molecular weight degradation profiles with model drug release. An initial burst over the first 48 h was followed by a period of more steady release for 4 weeks. The sustained release continued for next 8 weeks after which little or no release was detected for the remainder of the degradation period.

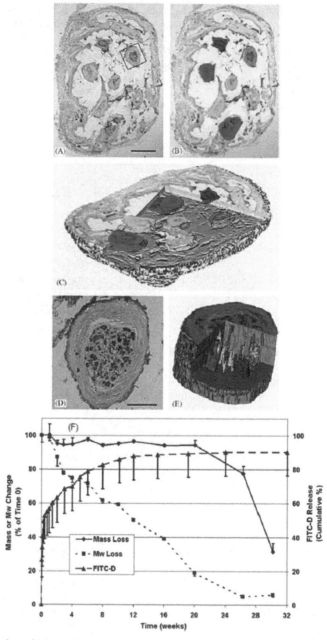

Figure 7. Histological images of tissue cables within scaffold channels. (A) Histological cross section near rostral end of scaffold showing tissue cables within all seven channels. Boxed region is shown in

greater detail in D. (B) Histological cross section shown in A with channels segmented and displayed in
color. (C) Orthographic, wedged view of 16 serial slices registered, segmented, and reconstructed to
reveal 3-D structure of channels. (D) Histological cross section of boxed region in A; (E) Orthographic,
wedged view of reconstructed channel shown in D, with segmented axon bundles displayed in color.
(F) Degradation and FITC-D release profile. Mass or molecular weight change is indicated as a
percentage of initial value at time zero. FITC-D release is indicated as a cumulative percentage of
loaded drug [Adapted from Ref. 13 with permission © Elsevier Science BV].

The release of the drug progressed in corroboration with scaffold degradation. However,
the inhomogeneity played its role as a very high variability was observed. The polymeric
architecture was designed to act as a template for the arrangement of cells that may attract
and guide regenerating axons rather than for guiding the regenerating fibers by providing
an oriented surface. The delivery system was proposed to be flexible enough to provide
incorporation of various drugs/biomolecule/bioactives that may add tropic attraction,
neuroprotection, or reduce the inhibitory effects of secondary injury. Another important
aspect of the study was to attest the effect of incorporation of Schwann cell in the scaffold
as their harvesting, suspension, and distribution into scaffold channels is of critical
importance in this field. Results indicated that Schwann cells were successfully harvested,
suspended in Matrigel, and loaded into distinct channels, and that cells survived in
culture under physiologic conditions within the scaffold. Axon regeneration was
visualized by 3-D reconstruction of serial histological sections, an approach that appears
useful for evaluation of regenerating tissue architecture as shown in **Figure 7**. The 3-D
reconstructions demonstrated the arrangement of the seven channels containing
regenerating axons, as well as live axon bundles within the channels. This novel depiction
corroborated well with the channels which were found distributed as arranged by the
scaffold, with scaffold and tissue in the spaces separating the channels, approximately. An
important finding revealed that channels generally contained a centralized core of tissue
containing axons and capillaries, surrounded by circumferential fibrous tissue.
Furthermore, macrophages could be identified, due to their engulfment of neurofilament-
stained material [13].

2.10. Laminin and nerve growth factor-laden three-dimensional scaffold

Yu et al., 1999, engineered Leminin-functionalized agarose hydrogel scaffolds for the
stimulation of neuronal process extension based on the hypothesis that "substrate-bound
neurite promoting extracellular matrix (ECM) proteins and chemo-attractive diffusible
trophic factors influence and stimulate axon guidance and neurite extension". The study
indicated that the effect of LN-modified agarose gels on DRG/PC12 cell neurite outgrowth
involves receptors for YIGSR/integrin/31 subunits, respectively. Additionally, 1,2-bis(10,12-
tricosadiynoyl)-sn-glycero-3-phosphocholine based lipid micro-cylinders were loaded with
nerve growth factor (NGF), and embedded into agarose hydrogels which resulted in a
directional neurite extension from DRGs in agarose hydrogels due to the presence of trophic
factor gradients. The NGF-loaded lipid micro-cylinders released physiologically relevant
amounts of NGF for at least 7 days *in vitro* based on a PC12 cell-based bioassay confirming

that the agarose hydrogel scaffolds can be used as biosynthetic 3D bridges capable of promoting regeneration across severed nerve gaps [14].

2.11. Agarose and methylcellulose hydrogel blends for nerve regeneration applications

Taking leads from the research done by Shoichet and co workers and from Bellamkonda and co workers, Martin et al., 2009, designed injectable scaffold consisting of agarose and methylcellulose (MC) as the responsive polymers. The following rationale was cited in support of using a blend of MC and agarose instead of using agarose alone: the low melting point of agarose makes it difficult to use *in vivo* and hence need to be cooled after injection wherein blowing of gases onto nervous system tissue could potentially be harmful to neurons that survived the initial injury. The release of bioactive from such gelling mixtures was related to the dissolution of the scaffold itself under physiological conditions. In an interesting experiment the percentage of hydrogel dissolved was measured on day 1, 4, 7, 14 and 28. Plain agarose dissolved completely when left in PBS in a 37 °C incubator for only 7 days, making it difficult to record the percentage dissolved due to hydrogel instability. However, the blends were approximately 70% dissolved by the end of 28 days in the cycled PBS solution. Pristine 7% methylcellulose proved to be a weaker hydrogel that dissolves more rapidly than the hydrogel blends, dissolving over 75% in 28 days. This confirmed the applicability of the blend in comparison to individual polymers. Furthermore, the authors pointed that "the ease of creation, simplicity of delivery and use of natural biocompatible components that solidify naturally without the use of ultraviolet light or cross linkers add to the advantages of utilizing this blend" [15].

2.12. An injectable, biodegradable hydrogel for trophic factor delivery

Piantino et al., 2006, devised a new method for an injectable based drug delivery system for the delivery of trophic factors to the injured neural tissues. The method utilized an injectable liquid polymer solution that crosslinks into a biodegradable, water-swollen hydrogel when photo-activated under visible light. The investigators described the uniqueness of their system over other systems as follows:(1) the system can provide constant and tailorable delivery of one or more growth factors to the precise site where needed; (2) reduce the possibility of host–graft rejection, as may occur with the use of live tissue or cell preparations; (3) does not involve viral vectors, which may induce an inflammatory response and which may require prolonged delays in achieving high levels of gene expression; and (4) does not involve the use of devices that can malfunction or cause infections (e.g., pumps or catheters). Briefly, degradable poly(ethylene glycol) hydrogels are formed from the radical polymerization of acrylated poly(lactic acid)-b-poly(ethylene glycol)-b-(poly lactic acid) (PLA-b-PEG-b-PLA) macromers. The network degradation and subsequent molecular release properties can be controlled by altering the network chemistry of these injectable hydrogels such as the number of degradable units and network crosslinking density by changing the macromer concentration). The degradation of the hydrogels was postulated to be due to hydrolysis in the network crosslinks. The release profile of NT-3 *in vivo* was determined using ELISA and a peak was reported at the site of injury as early as 3 h after hydrogel administration. High concentrations over a distance of 1 cm and more were cited site on day 6 followed by a decline to approx. one-third of maximum after 14 at 14 days. The NT-3 levels within the first few millimetres of the lesion site were in the range of 50 ng/ml/g of tissue when averaged over the entire tissue sample. In vitro release studies corroborated well with the inv vivo data with a burst release of ~40% over first 24 hours and a sustained release thereafter. Interventionally, NT-3, delivered via hydrogel in the vicinity of injured nerve terminals, was presumed to be transported retrogradely to cortical pyramidal cells thereby promoting axonal branching along with promoting plasticity of the raphespinal tract and finally promoting the outgrowth of descending pathways involved in locomotor control leading to the lesion size being slightly smaller in NT-3-treated vs. control animals as early as 1 day and 1 week post-lesion [16].

2.13. Hydrogel scaffold and microspheres for supporting survival of neural stem cells

To develop a biomaterial composite for promoting proliferation and migration of neural stem cells (NSCs) and to rescue central nervous system (CNS) injuries, Wang et al., 2011 constructed a NSCs-cultured delivery system based on crosslinked hyaluronic acid (HA) hydrogels, containing embedded BDNF and vascular endothelial growth factor (VEGF)-loaded poly(lactic-co-glycolic acid) (PLGA) microspheres for controlled delivery as well as angiogenesis on the materials. The study was designed on the drawbacks of previous studies that have shown an intrinsic ability of neural stem cells (NSCs) to regenerate in various neurological diseases' intervention. The most important among these were the low viability and undesired differentiation of the grafted NSCs and also the glial scar formation. In addition to these, the deficiency of neurotrophic factors and growth factors following the CNS may also contribute to failure of neural regeneration. The in vitro release kinetics study by ELISA measured the loading of BDNF and VEGF in microspheres as 0.10 and 0.34 μg/mg microspheres, respectively, corresponding to 52% and 84% loading efficiency making the loading efficiencies of HA gel composites in the range of 17.4 and 56.6 ng/mg, respectively, when embedded with microspheres. Interestingly, no burst release characteristic to the PLGA microspheres was within the period of 6 days wherein bioactives were released from the microspheres constantly and cumulatively. The thorough washing of the microspheres was believed to overcome the burst release of the proteins from the surface and provided a slow and linear release profile during the test period. During the first week of the study, about 20–30% of the loaded proteins were release possible by diffusion from areas near the surface as the degradation of PLGA was insignificant during initial phases. In contrast, the release of growth factors from the hydrogel embedded with microspheres revealed an initial "burst" followed by a stable release phase. This was attributed to the fact that released factors might have remained in the hydrogel during the cross-link processing leading to the diffusion through the hydrogel matrix. However, the cumulative amount of bioactive release was reduced to 12% and 13% of total loading as compared to 20-30% in case of microspheres alone which was postulated to be due to the presence of the surrounding HA hydrogel as a delayed or deposited effect on the release profile of the biofactors [17].

2.14. Controlled release of Neurotrophin-3 from fibrin-based tissue engineering scaffolds

Pathologically, the ability of chronically injured supraspinal axon tracts to regenerate decreases if intervention is delayed for too long. The barriers to axonal regeneration in case of a chronically injured spinal cord are reported to be overcome interventionally by using a combination of diffusible growth stimulating molecules and a favourable growth stimulating extracellular matrix such as the use of a continuous transgenic delivery of neurotrophic factors from engineered cells that also secrete extracellular matrix (ECM) is conducive to regeneration [18]. However, there is a limitation of this strategy as that the growth is limited to the regeneration of axons into the transplant site, the source of the growth stimulating neurotrophins, and the axons fail to regenerate back into host tissue. Sakiyama-Elbert and co workers, 2009, coined the need for temporary controlled release of growth-stimulating neurotrophins that not only promote axon growth into the lesion but also foster growth into healthy spinal cord tissue thereby connecting the newly grown tissue to the neural tissue that survived the injury. The intervention consisted of delayed treatment of SCI with controlled release of neurotrophin-3 (NT-3) from fibrin scaffolds providing a supportive regenerative environment, reducing the accumulation of reactive astrocytes surrounding the lesion and enhancing the presence of neural fibers within the lesion. The heparin-based delivery system (HBDS) developed earlier by the investigators [19], was utilized as it forms non-covalent interactions between neurotrophins, heparin, and a covalently linked bi-domain peptide (ATIII peptide), which can be incorporated into the fibrin scaffold and allow for the controlled release of growth factors from the scaffolds. The controlled released of the biofactor from the fibrin scaffold was assessed in terms of quantification of neural fiber density, astrocyte density, and chondroitin sulfate proteoglycan density along with macrophage/microglia immune profile analysis. The final results demonstrated that controlled release of NT-3 promotes increased neural fiber density within the lesion and decreased reactive astrocyte staining around the lesion of subacute SCI (2 weeks after the injury) at a dose of 500 ng/mL of NT-3 with HBDS [20]. These results were in corroboration with the earlier reports where the NT-3/HBDS was employed in an acute SCI (immediately after the injury) model wherein the it promoted a significant increase in the density of neural fibers sprouting [21-23].

2.15. Nerve guidance channels as drug delivery vehicles

However, safe and effective use of pro-regenerative molecules requires a localized, controlled and sustained delivery to the site of neural injury. However, there are many challenges pertaining to the various approaches available in the neural arena as described in Table 3.

To overcome the challenges shown in the table above, Piotrowicza and Shoichet, 2006, developed a liquid–liquid centrifugal casting process which enables the formation of nerve guidance channels (NGCs) from acrylate-based hydrogels such as poly(hydroxylethylmethacrylate-co-methylmethacrylate) or P(HEMA-co-MMA). The NGCs themselves were fabricated by a liquid–liquid centrifugal casting process and the protein incorporation strategies were compared in terms of protein distribution and nerve growth factor (NGF) release profile. The centrifugal casting process is based on the following phenomenon: Phase separation of the polymer phase from the monomer formulation during polymerization in a rotating cylindrical mould and hence the denser polymer phase is pushed to the periphery by centrifugal forces, where it gels forming a tube. The NGCs thus formed were semipermeable, soft and flexible, and matched the modulus of the nerve or spinal cord.

S. No.	Approaches	Challenge
1.	Systemic administration	short half-lives and high potency of many biomolecules, and delivery to the CNS is further limited by the blood–brain barrier
2.	osmotic mini-pumps	infections or tissue damage, pump failure due to catheter dislodgement or occlusion, as well as drug instability in the pump reservoir
3.	local administration as growth factor solutions	factors lose bioactivity in solution
4.	local administration as matrices saturated with growth factors	easily leak from the channel during the implantation procedure
5.	NGCs prepared by dip-coating or solution casting	the creation of a non-symmetric growth factor concentration profile within the lumen of the NGC

Table 3. Challenge inherent to various bioactive administration approaches

The investigators formulated three different approached for the delivery of nerve growth factor (NGF) using Nerve guidance channels (NGCs constituted with of poly(2-hydroxyethyl methacrylate-co-methyl methacrylate), P(HEMA-co-MMA) as the polymeric platform to facilitate regeneration after transection injury to the spinal cord: (1) NGF was encapsulated (with bovine serum albumin (BSA)) in biodegradable poly(D,L-lactide-co-glycolide) 85/15 microspheres, which were combined with a PHEMA polymerization formulation and coated on the inside of pre-formed NGCs by a second liquid–liquid centrifugal casting technique; (2) pre-formed NGCs were imbibed with a solution of NGF/BSA and (3) NGF/BSA alone was combined with a PHEMA formulation and coated on the inside of pre-formed NGCs by a second liquid–liquid centrifugal casting technique. The channels imbibed with NGF showed no sustained release of NGF as was achieved from NGCs with either NGF-loaded microspheres or NGF alone incorporated into the inner layer with values of 1040 pg/cm, 220 pg NGF/cm, and 8624 pg/cm, respectively, after 28 days [**Figure 8**]. As a key finding, the release of the bioactive from the conduits was dependent on the slow-degrading characteristic of the microspheric system as well as on the "maximum amount of microspheres" that could be incorporated into the cylindrical structure. Another important finding of the report was that the liquid–liquid centrifugal casting process demonstrated potential towards localized and controlled release of multiple factors key to tissue regeneration after neural injuries [24].

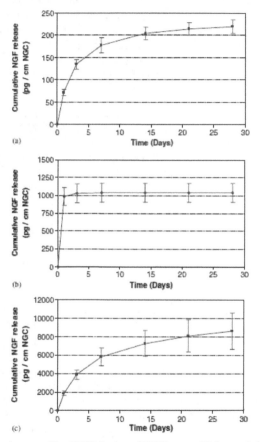

Figure 8. Cumulative release profile of NGF (pg/cm of NGC) over a 28-day period from NGCs (a) coated with an inner layer of PHEMA containing NGF-loaded PLGA 85/15 microspheres; (b) imbibed with NGF; and (c) coated with an inner layer of PHEMA containing directly entrapped NGF [Adapted from Ref. 24 with permission © Elsevier Science BV].

2.16. Self-assembling peptide nanofiber scaffold enhanced with RhoA inhibitor

In a recent study, Zhang et al., 2012, focused on two major targets for axonal regeneration after a spinal cord injury:

a. The reconstruction of the gap in the injured spinal cord
b. Inactivation of RhoA to ameliorate the hostile microenvironment perilesion

To achieve these targets, Zhang et al., 2012, transplanted self-assembling peptide nanofiber scaffold (SAPNS) based local delivery of RhoA inhibitor to the lesion sites after acute spinal cord injury centred on their previous reports wherein the SAPNS had shown multiple regeneration-facilitating properties to improve the recovery of the injured spinal cord and brain and that SAPNS has potential for controlled bioactive release. The study was based on the hypothesis that this novel combination might act by providing regrowth-promoting scaffold reducing the physical obstacles after injury (characteristic SAPNS capability of filling the cavities and alleviating glial scarring) and the RhoA inhibitor released from the combination implants may exert a therapeutic effect conducive for axonal regrowth.

As depicted in **Figure 9**, the SAPNS implants, with or without CT04 incorporation, reconstructed the injured spinal cord whereas a significant gap was developed in the lesion site in the saline group. Additionally, the implants integrated closely with the surrounding host tissue with no cavities or gaps occurring between the implants and host tissue. Another striking finding was the presence of the cells such as fibroblasts, which mainly clustered in the centre of the lesion area and formed collagen fibers, along with lymphocytes, macrophages, astrocytes, and microglias scattered among the fibroblasts. The growth of such cellular mass may further hindered the cavity or cysts formation- a major cause of anatomical disconnection after SCI. On the drug delivery note, SAPNS delivery of CT04 significantly improved the axonal regrowth. Based on fluorescent characteristics of dextran, it was incorporated into SAPNS to track the spread-out and diffusion of the bioactive in the lesion site. Seven days after the transplantation of the SAPNS incorporated with Dextran, significant fluorescence was observed into the surrounding host cord from the SAPNS, while the implant still retained high fluorescent signal confirming the release of chemicals from SAPNS and indication that SAPNS can effectively serve as a platform for further controlled release of exogenous therapeutic molecules of interest. In conclusion, the SAPNS delivery system proved to be capable of minimal risk of carrying biological pathogens or contaminants, providing 3-dimensional environment constructed for cell growth and migration, minimal cytotoxicity to the host, no apparent immune response, easy conformity to the various shape of lesion cavities, and immediate haemostatic and controlled drug release properties [25].

2.17. Sustained delivery of chondroitinase ABC from hydrogel system

As explained earlier in this report, chondroitin sulfate proteoglycans (CSPGs) are among the principal factors responsible of axon growth inhibition and they contribute to regenerative failure, promoting glial scar formation in an injured spinal cord. Chondroitinase ABC (chABC), although capable of digesting these proteoglycans leading to the degradation of glial scar and favoring axonal regrowth, suffers from delivery drawbacks such as administration being invasive, infection-prone and clinically problematic. Rossi et al., 2012, developed an agarose-carbomer (AC1) hydrogel, which they previously used in SCI repair strategies [26-28], as a delivery system capable of an effective chABC administration based on following considerations: ability to include chABC within its pores and the possibility to be injected into the target tissue; and release kinetics and the maintenance of enzymatic activity can be

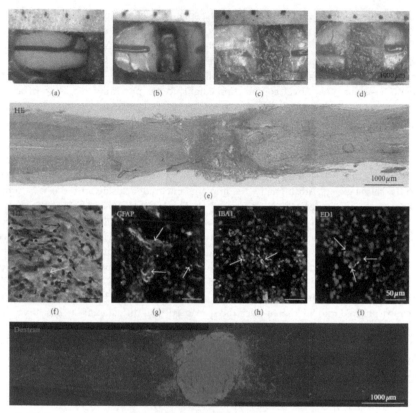

Figure 9. The implants of various SAPNS reconstructed the injured spinal cord. (a–d)Macroscopic observations of lesion sites immediately after surgery. (a) Sham surgery; (b) saline group; (c) SAPNS with vehicle group; (d) SAPNS+CT04 combination group. (e) HE staining shows the lesion area was reconstructed 12 weeks after SAPNS transplanted. (f) HE staining shows various cells in the grafted scaffold, which include fibroblast (black arrow), macrophage (yellow arrow), and lymphocyte (arrow head). (g–i) Immuno-staining shows the GFAP-positive astrocytes (g), IBA1 positive microglias (h) and ED1 positive macrophages (i) in the grafted scaffold. (j) shows the Dextran, a red fluorescent dye, was partially diffused from the mixture of SAPNS and Dextran at 7 days after transplantation [Adapted from Ref. 25 © Hindawi Publishing Corporation].

positively assessed. Additionally, being a hydrogel, AC1 had its own advantages in terms of (I) the ability to retain water; (II) mimicking living tissues; (III) high biocompatibility; and (IV) the possibility to allow precisely controlled release rates. As demonstrated in Figure 10, AC1 appeared to be a chemical gel synthesized through a statistical block polycondensation between Carbomer 974P and agarose. chABC was loaded before the sol/gel transition resulting in its physical entrapment within the three-dimensional polymeric network of the gel. Macroscopically, a highly entangled nanostructure was confirmed by ESEM analysis proving its ECM mimicking nature. In brief, Carbomer 974 P provided the main cross-linking properties via its carboxylic groups which in turn reacted with hydroxyl groups from agarose leading to the formation of a three dimensional matrix. The in vitro release kinetics displayed typical hydrogel characteristics wherein a rapid initial release of Tx was observed during the initial phases due to a high concentration gradient possible caused by: molecules placed near solvent-hydrogel interface that may rapidly escape into the supernatant solution; molecules diffusing through the large pores of the hydrogel in comparison to the molecules diffusing through smaller pores. The burst release was followed by slower release and eventually forming a plateau. After this initial burst, the release became slower and reached a plateau - steady state condition - after 7 days. Importantly, the whole amount of Tx loaded was release eventually confirming the absence of any stable bonds between hydrogel polymeric network and loaded Tx. Furthermore, it confirms the hydrogel's capacity to deliver even those molecules that are deeply entrapped in its core [29].

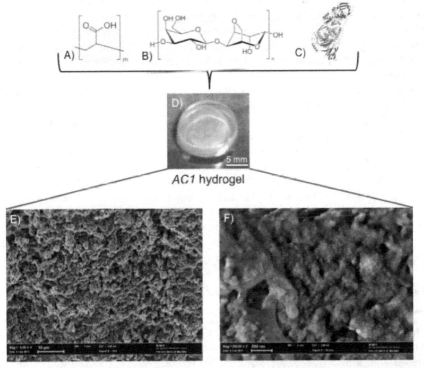

Figure 10. Carbomer 974P (A); agarose (B) were chemically cross-linked to form hydrogel in phosphate buffer saline solution. Esterification, hydrogen bonding and carboxylation bring polymer chains statistically closer, thus creating a stable heterogeneous structure. The gelling solution was homogenized together with chondroitinase ABC (chABC); (C) above sol-gel transition temperature. From a macroscopic point of view the resulting material appears as in (D). From a microscopic point of view the hydrogel is densely structured, as observable by ESEM analysis. [Adapted from Ref. 29 © MDPI Publishing]

2.18. Injectable functionalized self-assembling scaffold

Self-assembling peptides (SAPs) perfectly mimic the extra-cellular matrix's structural and conformational characteristics; can be injected into the lesion site; are reabsorbable; and have sites for biofunctionalizations making them a perfect nanomaterial for application in regenerative. Cigognini et al., 2011, explored the biofunctionalizability of self-assembling peptides to enhance the *in vitro* neural stem cells survival and differentiation. This injectable nanofibrous gel was composed of RADA16-I functionalized with a bone marrow homing motif (BMHP1) which was further optimized via the insertion of a 4-glycine-spacer for amelioration of scaffold stability and exposure of the biomotifs. The scaffold was injected immediately after contusion in the rat spinal cord was evaluated for its putative neuroregenerative properties in terms of early effects by semi-quantitative RT-PCR and the late effects by histological analysis. The axon regeneration/sprouting across the cyst was quantified by the presence of GAP-43 positive fibers and the relative value of GAP-43 immunopositive area was represented as percentage of the total cyst area (Figure 11Bi). Interestingly, a significantly greater synthesis of GAP-43 in 4G-BMHP1 group (12.946±2.03% of the whole cyst area) in comparison with saline (6.336±1.7% of the whole cyst area) and SCI control (5.846±1.29% of the whole cyst area) groups was originated (Figure Bii). The chronic inflammatory response, evaluated by counting macrophages into the lesion site (Figure 11Ci), revealed that several infiltrating CD68 immunopositive cells in all groups, indicating that at the late phase of the injury the scaffold didn't significantly affect the host immune response (Figure Cii). Similarly, cyst and cavities extent, measured on hematoxylin-eosin stained sections (Figure 11Ai), was similar in all groups (Figure Aii) wherein no significant differences were observed among treatment and both control groups when the cavities size within the cyst excluding strands of connective tissue (trabeculae) were measured (Figure Aiii). Conclusively, the injectable SAP based scaffold demonstrated potential for enhanced matrix remodelling, release of trophic factors, cell migration and basement membrane deposition leading to an increased number of regenerating/sprouting axons after incomplete SCI. Apart from the neuro-compatibility, the scaffolds were able to fill the cavities at SCI site with implications leading to a good matrix for the in vivo delivery of growth factors and/or stem cells into the injured CNS [30].

2.19. Effects of dibutyryl cyclic-AMP on survival and neuronal differentiation of neural stem/progenitor cells

Enthused by the poor control over transplant cell differentiation and survival, Kim et al., 2011, introduced a combinatorial approach wherein the cell transplantation therapy was adjoined with a bioactive release platform. Firstly, dibutyryl cyclic-AMP (dbcAMP) was encapsulated within poly(lactic-co-glycolic acid) (PLGA) microspheres and embedded within chitosan guidance channels. Secondly, neural stem/progenitor cells (NSPCs) were seeded in fibrin scaffolds within the channels (Figure 12). The idea behind the study was to determine whether dbcAMP, which can influence the in vitro differentiation of NSPCs into neurons, will be able to enhance survival of transplanted NSPCs through prolonged exposure either in vitro or in vivo through its controlled release from microspheres in

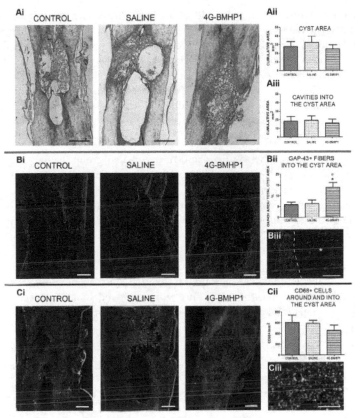

Figure 11. Quantitative histological analysis in the chronic phase of SCI. (A): lesion size was quantified on spinal cord longitudinal sections stained with hematoxylin/eosin (Ai) and it was reported as cumulative area (mm2). No significant differences among groups were found when measuring both the whole cyst area (Aii) and the cavities into the cyst area (Aiii). (B): GAP-43 positive fibers (Bi and Biii, red) were measured on six longitudinal sections after immunofluorescence staining and the values were expressed as percentage of the total area of the cyst. The GAP-43 immunopositive area was significantly higher in biomaterial-treated group (4G-BMHP1) than both control groups (saline and SCI control) (Bii). In Biii the positive GAP-43 signal is showed at higher magnification (asterisk and dotted line indicate the cyst and its border, respectively). (C): CD68 positive cells (Ci and Ciii, green) were counted on three longitudinal sections after immunofluorescence staining and reported as cumulative number per mm2. Nuclei were counterstained with DAPI. Macrophage infiltration was observed in the tissue surrounding the cyst and into the cavities of all groups (Cii). In Ciii, at higher magnification, an image representative of the CD68 positive cells (arrows) was observed in all groups [Adapted from Ref. 30 © PLoS ONE].

vicinity of NSPCs. The in vitro differentiation if NSPCs to betaIII-tubulin positive neurons was evaluated by immunostaining and mRNA expression. The in vivo studies were conducted by transplantation in spinal cord injured rats wherein the survival and differentiation of NSPCs was evaluated. For the greatest neuronal differentiation in the presence of constant dbcAMP, the dbcAMP release from PLGA microspheres was optimized to release the bioactive for a period of 1 week based on the preliminary in vitro data. As depicted in Figure 12, drug release from native microspheres was linear over 11 days while the release of dbcAMP occurred over approximately 5 days after incorporation into channels. The mass balance results cleared this anomaly in release profiles which showed that the there was less drug content in dbcAMP microsphere loaded channels than expected microsphere quantity which was further due to drug losses during the process of embedding microspheres into the channel. Two major results were reported for the NSPC survival and differentiation as follows:

a. NSPC survival was highest in the dbcAMP pre-treated group, having approximately 80% survival at both time points as compared to that of stem cell transplantation results of less than 1% survival at similar times.
b. The dbcAMP pre-treatment resulted in the greatest number of in vivo NSPCs differentiated into neurons (3764%), followed by dbcAMP-microsphere treated NSPCs (27614%) and untreated NSPCs (1567%).
c. The reverse trend was observed for NSPC-derived oligodendrocytes and astrocytes, with these populations being highest in untreated NSPCs.
d. Chitosan channels implanted in a fully transected spinal cord resulted in extensive axonal regeneration into the injury site, with improved functional recovery after 6 weeks in animals implanted with pre-differentiated stem cells in chitosan channels [31].

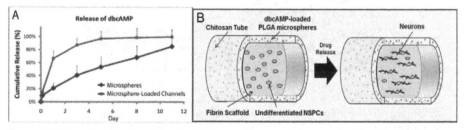

Figure 12. Microsphere-loaded channels effectively release dbcAMP in vitro. A) Cumulative release profiles of dbcAMP from free-floating microspheres and microsphere-loaded channels. The process of embedding microspheres into channel walls is likely responsible for early degradation of PLGA and faster drug release from channels. B) Schematic of the entubulation strategy. NSPCs are seeded on fibrin scaffold within a chitosan channel. Drug-loaded PLGA microspheres release the differentiation factor dibutyryl cyclic-AMP in a local and sustained manner, influencing NSPCs to preferentially differentiate into neurons [Adapted from Ref. 31 © PLoS ONE].

2.20. Local gene delivery from ECM-coated poly(lactide-co-glycolide) multiple channel bridges

In order to promote transgene expression in the injured spinal cord, Laporte et al., 2009, investigated the potential of surface immobilization to deliver complexed DNA (lipoplexes) from a multiple channel bridge in order to address the barriers related to cell survival, scar tissue formation, and axonal elongation and guidance by targeting a range of cellular processes. The report was based on the inherent low expression levels of lipoplexes due to the lipoplex instability upon injection in vivo. The authors postulated that the "local delivery of lipoplexes from a biomaterial may have the ability to maintain lipoplex stability, and therefore increase the number of transfected cells and transgene expression". Based on their previous study, multiple linear guidance channels were able to support cell infiltration and integrate effectively into the spinal cord wherein the channels induced cell orientation along its major axis and supported and directed axon elongation across the channels [32]. Strategically, lipoplexes were immobilized to the surface of the bridges as follows:

i.   incubation of DNA with extra cellular matrix (ECM)-coated PLGA surfaces (incubation),

ii.   drying of ECM onto PLGA and then drying of DNA onto ECM (2-step drying), and

iii.   drying a mixture of DNA and ECM proteins onto PLGA surfaces (1-step drying).

A series of in vitro studies were carried out to investigate the surface properties of the polymer, three ECM proteins (collagen, laminin, and fibronectin), and the immobilization strategies for their ability to bind and stabilize the vector, and to transfect cells. In vivo studies were performed with a rat spinal cord lateral hemisection model using conditions identified from in vitro studies. In conclusion, the combination of the multiple channel bridge and gene delivery provided the required physical and chemical guidance cues for spinal cord regeneration [33].

3. Conclusion

The current drug delivery and tissue engineering techniques discussed in this chapter demonstrate that a only a combinatorial approach can provide the desired characteristics required for an efficient repair, regeneration, restoration, reconstruction, and reorganisation of the neural tissue after traumatic CNS injuries. A synergistic therapeutic approach can be designed by incorporating scaffolds with directional cues, bioactives to promote regeneration and repair, neural/progenitor cells for release of growth factors, and functionalized polymers for better neurocompatibility. Most importantly, the design of polymers capable of releasing the drugs, cells and biofactors at a predetermined and controlled rate is essential for the success of these tissue engineering approaches (Table 4). The chapter provides a comprehensive account of recent as well as long established approaches for the delivery of bioactive of neural interest. For further reading, the readers are encouraged to read various enlightening reviews in this area as tabulated in Table 5.

S. No.	Architecture	Biomaterials employed	Bioactive incorporated	Reference
1.	Injectable gel	Hyaluronic Acid-Methyl cellulose (blend)	Nimodipine; Erythropoietin	2-4
2.	Nanoparticles-incorporated multiple channel bridges	PLGA (scaffold); Hydroxyapatite (nanoparticles)	lentiviral vectors encoding NT-3 and BDNF	5

S. No.	Architecture	Biomaterials employed	Bioactive incorporated	Reference
3.	Lipid microtubules-incorporated In situ gelling hydrogels	1,2-bis-(triscosa-10,12-diynoyl)-sn-glycero-3-phosphocholine; Agarose	brain derived neurotrophic factor (BDNF)	6
4.	Photocrosslinked 3D scaffold	Agarose; Sulfosuccinimidyl-6-[4'-azido-2'-nitrophenylamino] hexanoate	Laminin-1	7
5.	Nanoparticles-incorporated injectable gel	PLGA (nanoparticles); agarose gel	Methylprednisolone	9,10
6.	hydrogel-microtube delivery system	Agarose; 1,2-bis-(tricosa-10,12-diynoyl)-sn-glycero-3-phosphocholine microtube	Chondroitinase ABC; Rho GTPase, CA-Rac1 and CA-Cdc42; and BDNF	11,12
7.	3D Scaffolds	PLGA	Schwann cells	13
8.	micro-cylinders embedded hydrogels	1,2-bis(10,12-tricosadiynoyl)-sn-glycero-3-phosphocholine; Agarose	nerve growth factor (NGF)	14
9.	injectable scaffold	Agarose; methylcellulose	-	15
10.	Injectable hydrogel	acrylated poly(lactic acid)-b–poly(ethylene glycol)-b–(poly lactic acid)	NT-3	16
11.	crosslinked hydrogels containing embedded microspheres	hyaluronic acid (HA); poly(lactic-co-glycolic acid) (PLGA)	BDNF and VEGF-loaded	17
12.	scaffolds	Fibrin; heparin; bi-domain peptide (ATIII peptide)	neurotrophin-3 (NT-3)	20
13.	Nerve guidance channels combined with microspheres	poly(hydroxylethylmethacrylate-co-methylmethacrylate); PLGA	Nerve growth factor	24
14.	nanofiber scaffold	Self assembling peptides	RhoA inhibitor	25
15.	Injectable hydrogel	Agarose; carbomer	Chondroitinase ABC (chABC)	29
16.	Self assembling peptide gel	RADA16-1	bone marrow homing motif (BMHP1)	30
17.	microspheres embedded within guidance channels	poly(lactic-co-glycolic acid) (PLGA); Chitosan; fibrin	dibutyryl cyclic-AMP (dbcAMP)	31
18.	disks and multiple channel bridges	poly(lactic-co-glycolic acid) (PLGA)	DNA complexes	33

Table 4. Summary of various bioactive-loaded platforms for spinal cord injury intervention

S. No.	View point discussed in the review	Reference
1.	The current approaches to drug delivery from scaffolds for neural tissue engineering applications and the challenges presented by attempting to replicate the brain, spinal cord, and peripheral nerve tissues were summarized	34
2.	The complex processes of cell guidance occurring within native ECM; strategies to design biomimetic scaffolds able to recapitulate these processes; approaches in controlling the release of the relevant factors; challenges to design novel scaffolds; time and space orchestrated exposure of biomacromolecular moieties	35
3.	Tissue engineering and novel therapeutic approaches to axonal regeneration following spinal cord injury. Axonal growth is supported by inherent properties of the selected polymer, the architecture of the scaffold, permissive microstructures such as pores, grooves or polymer fibres, and surface modifications to provide improved adherence and growth directionality.	36
4.	The state of the art work in electrospinning and its uses in tissue engineering and drug delivery	37
5.	Electrospun fibers mimic the nanoscale properties of native extracellular matrix; the fiber morphology is affected by changing the process parameters	38
6.	Tissue-engineered implant is a biologic-biomaterial combination in which some component of tissue has been combined with a biomaterial to create a device for the restoration or modification of tissue or organ function; Specific growth factors, released from a delivery device or from co-transplanted cells aid in the induction of host paraenchymal cell infiltration and improve engraftment of co-delivered cells for more efficient tissue regeneration; polymeric device development (micropaticles, scaffolds, and encapsulated cells) for therapeutic growth factor delivery in the context of tissue engineering was outlined.	39
7.	The tissue engineering paradigm includes a matrix or scaffold to facilitate tissue growth and provide structural support, cells, and the delivery of bioactive molecules; Injectable materials are designed using processing techniques inherent to both tissue engineering and drug delivery.	40
8.	Basic technology of controlled protein delivery using polymeric materials; techniques under investigation for the efficient administration of proteins in tissue engineering	41
9.	An overview of strategies using natural and artificial substrates to present active biomolecules in the development of vascular structures; the replacement and augmentation of arteries using vascular grafts or stents; the recruitment of microvasculature secondary to an ischemic event or for the purpose of developing perfused, large volume tissue-engineered constructs	42
10.	Polyblend nanofibers and nanostructures can act as proxies of the native tissue, while providing topographical and biochemical cues that promote healing; they are prepared with mixtures of synthetically and naturally derived polymers that can behave cooperatively to demonstrate unique combinations of mechanical, biochemical and structural properties.	43
11.	Synthetic polymers used for tissue growth scaffold fabrication and their applications in both cell and extracellular matrix support and controlling the release of cell growth and differentiation supporting drugs.	44

S. No.	View point discussed in the review	Reference
12.	In the future, engineered tissues could reduce the need for organ replacement, and could greatly accelerate the development of new drugs that may cure patients, eliminating the need for organ transplants altogether.	45
13.	Biodegradable and biocompatible scaffolds have a highly open porous structure and good mechanical strength to provide an optimal microenvironment for cell proliferation, migration, and differentiation, and guidance for cellular in-growth from host tissue; natural and synthetic polymeric scaffolds can be fabricated in the form of a solid foam, nanofibrous matrix, microsphere, or hydrogel; scaffolds can be surface engineered to provide an extracellular matrix mimicking environment for better cell adhesion and tissue in-growth and can be designed to release bioactive molecules, such as growth factors, DNA, or drugs, in a sustained manner	46
14.	To develop electrospun nanofibers as useful nanobiomaterials, surfaces of electrospun nanofibers can be chemically functionalized by plasma treatment, wet chemical method, surface graft polymerization, and co-electrospinning of surface active agents and polymers for achieving sustained delivery through physical adsorption of diverse bioactive molecules such as anti-cancer drugs, enzymes, cytokines, and polysaccharides; surfaces can be chemically modified with immobilizing cell specific bioactive ligands to enhance cell adhesion, proliferation, and differentiation by mimicking morphology and biological functions of ECM.	47
15.	Biomaterials can enable and augment the targeted delivery of drugs or therapeutic proteins to the brain, allow cell or tissue transplants to be effectively delivered to the brain; help to rebuild damaged circuits; promote regeneration; repair damaged neuronal pathways in combination with stem cell therapies; nanotechnology allows greater control over material–cell interactions that induce specific developmental processes and cellular responses including differentiation, migration and outgrowth	48
16.	Application of biomaterials in (i) shunting systems for hydrocephalus, (ii) cortical neural prosthetics, (iii) drug delivery in the CNS, (iv) hydrogel scaffolds for CNS repair, and (v) neural stem cell encapsulation for neurotrauma	49
17.	Recent in vivo studies for the regeneration of injured spinal cord, including stem-cell transplantation, application of neurotrophic factors and suppressor of inhibiting factors, development of biomaterial scaffolds and delivery systems, rehabilitation, and the combinations of these therapies	50
18.	Applications of polymer-based delivery of small molecule drugs, proteins, and DNA specifically relevant to neuroscience research; the fabrication procedures for the polymeric systems and their utility in various experimental models; unique experimental tools with downstream clinical application for the study and treatment of neurologic disease offered by biomaterials	51
19.	Approaches adopted for management of SCI including pharmacologic and gene therapy, cell therapy, and use of different cell-free or cell-seeded bioscaffolds; developments for therapeutic delivery of stem and nonstem cells to the site of injury; application of cell-free/cell-seeded natural and synthetic scaffolds	52

S. No.	View point discussed in the review	Reference
20.	bioengineered strategies for spinal cord repair using tissue engineered scaffolds and drug delivery systems; degradable and non-degradable biomaterials; device design; combination strategies with scaffolds.	53
21.	The merger between the two powerful disciplines—biomaterials engineering and stem cell biology	54
22.	Inclusive survey of biopolymers seeded with Schwann cells (SCs) to be used for axonal regeneration in the nervous system	55
23.	Recent studies that utilize electrospun nanofibers to manipulate biological processes relevant to nervous tissue regeneration, including stem cell differentiation, guidance of neurite extension, and peripheral nerve injury treatments	56
24.	Smart biomaterials are capable to carry and deliver cells and/or drugs in the damaged spinal cord; an overview of a wide range of natural, synthetic, and composite hydrogels	57
25.	Self-assembled materials provide the ability to tailor specific bulk material properties, such as release profiles, at the molecular level via monomer design; an overview of self-assembling molecules, their resultant structures, and their use in therapeutic delivery; current progress in the design of polymer- and peptide-based self-assembled materials.	58

Table 5. Leading review reports incorporating the inherent mechanistic and fabrication details of various neural architectures employed for neural tissue engineering and drug delivery

Author details

Viness Pillay*, Pradeep Kumar, Yahya E. Choonara and Lisa C. du Toit
University of the Witwatersrand, Faculty of Health Sciences,
Department of Pharmacy and Pharmacology, Parktown, Johannesburg, South Africa

Girish Modi
University of the Witwatersrand, Faculty of Health Sciences, Division of Neurosciences,
Department of Neurology, Parktown, Johannesburg, South Africa

Dinesh Naidoo
University of the Witwatersrand, Faculty of Health Sciences, Division of Neurosciences,
Department of Neurosurgery, Parktown, Johannesburg, South Africa

4. References

[1] Chung HJ, Park TG. Surface engineered and drug releasing pre-fabricated scaffolds for tissue engineering. Advanced Drug Delivery Reviews 2007;59: 249–62. http://www.sciencedirect.com/science/article/pii/S0169409X07000270 doi: 10.1016/j.addr.2007.03.015

---

* Corresponding Author

[2] Gupta D, Tator CH, Shoichet MS. Fast-gelling injectable blend of hyaluronan and methylcellulose for intrathecal, localized delivery to the injured spinal cord. Biomaterials 2006;27: 2370–9.
http://www.sciencedirect.com/science/article/pii/S0142961205010410
doi: 10.1016/j.biomaterials.2005.11.015

[3] Wang Y, Lapitsky Y, Kang CE, Shoichet MS. Accelerated release of a sparingly soluble drug from an injectable hyaluronan–methylcellulose hydrogel. Journal of Controlled Release 2009;140: 218–23.
http://www.sciencedirect.com/science/article/pii/S0168365909003289
doi: 10.1016/j.jconrel.2009.05.025

[4] Kang CE, Poon PC, Tator CH, Shoichet MS. A new paradigm for local and sustained release of therapeutic molecules to the injured spinal cord for neuroprotection and tissue repair. Tissue Engineering: Part A 2009;15(3): 595-604.
http://online.liebertpub.com/doi/full/10.1089/ten.tea.2007.0349
doi: 10.1089/ten.tea.2007.0349

[5] Tuinstra HM, Aviles MO, Shin S, Holland SJ, Zelivyanskaya ML, Fast AG, Ko SY, Margul DJ, Bartels AK, Boehler RM, Cummings BJ, Anderson AJ, Shea LD. Multifunctional, multichannel bridges that deliver neurotrophin encoding lentivirus for regeneration following spinal cord injury. Biomaterials 2012;33: 1618-26.
http://www.sciencedirect.com/science/article/pii/S0142961211013408
doi: 10.1016/j.biomaterials.2011.11.002

[6] Jain A, Kim YT, McKeon RJ, Bellamkonda RV. In situ gelling hydrogels for conformal repair of spinal cord defects, and local delivery of BDNF after spinal cord injury. Biomaterials 2006;27: 497–504.
http://www.sciencedirect.com/science/article/pii/S0142961205006216
doi: 10.1016/j.biomaterials.2005.07.008

[7] Dodla MC, Bellamkonda RV. Anisotropic scaffolds facilitate enhanced neurite extension in vitro. Journal of Biomedical Materials Research 2006;78A: 213–21.
http://onlinelibrary.wiley.com/doi/10.1002/jbm.a.30747
doi: 10.1002/jbm.a.30747

[8] Crompton KE, Goud JD, Bellamkonda RV, Gengenbach TR, Finkelstein DI, Horne MK, Forsythe JS. Polylysine-functionalised thermoresponsive chitosan hydrogel for neural tissue engineering. Biomaterials 2007;28(3): 441–9.
http://www.sciencedirect.com/science/article/pii/S0142961206007642
doi: 10.1016/j.biomaterials.2006.08.044

[9] Chvatal SA, Kim YT, Bratt-Leal AM, Lee H, Bellamkonda RV. Spatial distribution and acute anti-inflammatory effects of Methylprednisolone after sustained local delivery to the contused spinal cord. Biomaterials 2008;29: 1967-75.
http://www.sciencedirect.com/science/article/pii/S0142961208000197
doi: 10.1016/j.biomaterials.2008.01.002

[10] Kim YT, Caldwell JM, Bellamkonda RV. Nanoparticle-mediated local delivery of methylprednisolone after spinal cord injury. Biomaterials 2009;30: 2582–90.

http://www.sciencedirect.com/science/article/pii/S0142961209000040
doi: 10.1016/j.biomaterials.2008.12.077

[11] Lee H, McKeon RJ, Bellamkonda RV. Sustained delivery of thermostabilized chABC enhances axonal sprouting and functional recovery after spinal cord injury. PNAS 2010;107(8): 3340–5.
http://www.pnas.org/content/107/8/3340.short
doi: 10.1073/pnas.0905437106

[12] Jain A, McKeon RJ, Brady-Kalnay SM, Bellamkonda RV. Sustained delivery of activated Rho GTPases and BDNF promotes axon growth in CSPG-rich regions following spinal cord injury. PLoS ONE 2011;6(1): e16135.
http://www.plosone.org/article/info%3Adoi%2F10.1371%2Fjournal.pone.0016135
doi: 10.1371/journal.pone.0016135

[13] Moore MJ, Friedman JA, Lewellyn EB, Mantila SM, Krych AJ, Ameenuddin S, Knight AM, Lu L, Currier BL, Spinner RJ, Marsh RW, Windebank AJ, Yaszemski MJ. Multiple-channel scaffolds to promote spinal cord axon regeneration. Biomaterials 2006;27: 419–29.
http://www.sciencedirect.com/science/article/pii/S0142961205007076
doi: 10.1016/j.biomaterials.2005.07.045

[14] Yu X, Dillon GP, Bellamkonda RV. A laminin and nerve growth factor-laden three-dimensional scaffold for enhanced neurite extension. Tissue Engineering 1999;5(4): 291-304.
http://online.liebertpub.com/doi/abs/10.1089/ten.1999.5.291
doi: 10.1089/ten.1999.5.291

[15] Martin BC, Minner EJ, Wiseman SL, Klank RL, Gilbert RJ. Agarose and methylcellulose hydrogel blends for nerve regeneration applications. Journal of Neural Engineering 2008;5: 221–31.
http://iopscience.iop.org/1741-2552/5/2/013/
doi: 10.1088/1741-2560/5/2/013

[16] Piantino J, Burdick JA, Goldberg D, Langer R, Benowitz LI. An injectable, biodegradable hydrogel for trophic factor delivery enhances axonal rewiring and improves performance after spinal cord injury. Experimental Neurology 2006;201: 359–67.
http://www.sciencedirect.com/science/article/pii/S0014488606002731
doi: 10.1016/j.expneurol.2006.04.020

[17] Wang Y, Wei YT, Zu ZH, Ju RK, Guo MY, Wang XM, Xu QY, Cui FZ. Combination of hyaluronic acid hydrogel scaffold and PLGA microspheres for supporting survival of neural stem cells. Pharmaceutical Research 2011;28: 1406–14.
http://www.springerlink.com/content/u721217mn178m517/
doi: 10.1007/s11095-011-0452-3

[18] Lu P, Jones LL, Tuszynski MH. Axon regeneration through scars and into sites of chronic spinal cord injury. Experimental Neurology 2007;203(1): 8–21.
http://www.sciencedirect.com/science/article/pii/S0014488606004365
doi: 10.1016/j.expneurol.2006.07.030

[19] Sakiyama-Elbert SE, Hubbell JA. Development of fibrin derivatives for controlled release of heparin-binding growth factors. Journal of Controlled Release 2000;65(3): 389–402.
http://www.sciencedirect.com/science/article/pii/S0168365999002217
doi: 10.1016/S0168-3659(99)00221-7

[20] Johnson PJ, Parker SR, Sakiyama-Elbert SE. Controlled release of Neurotrophin-3 from fibrin-based tissue engineering scaffolds enhances neural fiber sprouting following subacute spinal cord injury. Biotechnology and Bioengineering 2009;104: 1207–14.
http://onlinelibrary.wiley.com/doi/10.1002/bit.22476
doi: 10.1002/bit.22476

[21] Taylor SJ, Sakiyama-Elbert SE. Effect of controlled delivery of neurotrophin-3 from fibrin on spinal cord injury in a long term model. Journal of Controlled Release 2006;116(2): 204–10.
http://www.sciencedirect.com/science/article/pii/S0168365906003348
doi: 10.1016/j.jconrel.2006.07.005

[22] Taylor SJ, McDonald JW III, Sakiyama-Elbert SE. Controlled release of neurotrophin-3 from fibrin gels for spinal cord injury. Journal of Controlled Release 2004;98(2): 281–94.
http://www.sciencedirect.com/science/article/pii/S0168365904002342
doi: 10.1016/j.jconrel.2004.05.003

[23] Taylor SJ, Rosenzweig ES, McDonald JW III, Sakiyama-Elbert SE. Delivery of neurotrophin-3 from fibrin enhances neuronal fiber sprouting after spinal cord injury. Journal of Controlled Release 2006;113(3): 226–35.
http://www.sciencedirect.com/science/article/pii/S0168365906001957
doi: 10.1016/j.jconrel.2006.05.005

[24] Piotrowicza A, Shoichet MS. Nerve guidance channels as drug delivery vehicles. Biomaterials 2006;27: 2018–27.
http://www.sciencedirect.com/science/article/pii/S0142961205008768
doi: 10.1016/j.biomaterials.2005.09.042

[25] Zhang W, Zhan X, Gao M, Hamilton AD, Liu Z, Jiang Y, Su H, Dai X, He B, Kang X, Zeng Y, Wu W, Guo J. Self-assembling peptide nanofiber scaffold enhanced with RhoA inhibitor CT04 improves axonal regrowth in the transected spinal cord. Journal of Nanomaterials 2012; Article ID 724857.
http://www.hindawi.com/journals/jnm/2012/724857/
doi: 10.1155/2012/724857

[26] Perale G, Veglianese P, Rossi F, Peviani M, Santoro M, Llupi D, Micotti E, Forloni G, Masi M. In situ agar-carbomer polycondensation: A chemical approach to regenerative medicine. Materials Letters 2011;65(11): 1688–92.
http://www.sciencedirect.com/science/article/pii/S0167577X11001522
doi: 10.1016/j.matlet.2011.02.036

[27] Rossi F, Santoro M, Casalini T, Veglianese P, Masi M, Perale G. Characterization and degradation behavior of agar—Carbomer based hydrogels for drug delivery applications: Solute effect. International Journal of Molecular Sciences 2011;12(6):3394–408.

http://www.mdpi.com/1422-0067/12/6/3394
doi: 10.3390/ijms12063394

[28] Santoro M, Marchetti P, Rossi F, Perale G, Castiglione F, Mele A, Masi M. Smart approach to evaluate drug diffusivity in injectable agar-carbomer hydrogels for drug delivery. Journal of Physical Chemistry B 2011;115(11): 2503–10. http://pubs.acs.org/doi/abs/10.1021/jp1111394
doi: 10.1021/jp1111394

[29] Rossi F, Veglianese P, Santoro M, Papa S, Rogora C, Dell'Oro V, Forloni G, Masi M, Perale G. Sustained delivery of chondroitinase ABC from hydrogel system. Journal of Functional Biomaterials 2012;3: 199-208.
http://www.mdpi.com/2079-4983/3/1/199
doi: 10.3390/jfb3010199

[30] Cigognini D, Satta A, Colleoni B, Silva D, Donega M, Antonini S, Gelain F. Evaluation of early and late effects into the acute spinal cord injury of an injectable functionalized self-assembling scaffold. PLoS ONE 2011;6(5): e19782.
http://www.plosone.org/article/info%3Adoi%2F10.1371%2Fjournal.pone.0019782
doi: 10.1371/journal.pone.0019782

[31] Kim H, Zahir T, Tator CH, Shoichet MS. Effects of dibutyryl cyclic-AMP on survival and neuronal differentiation of neural stem/progenitor cells transplanted into spinal cord injured rats. PLoS ONE 2011;6(6): e21744.
http://www.plosone.org/article/info%3Adoi%2F10.1371%2Fjournal.pone.0021744
doi: 10.1371/journal.pone.0021744

[32] De Laporte L, Yang Y, Zelivyanskaya ML, Cummings BJ, Anderson AJ, Shea LD. Plasmid releasing multiple channel bridges for transgene expression after spinal cord injury. Molecular Therapy 2009;17(2): 318–26.
http://www.nature.com/mt/journal/v17/n2/full/mt2008252a.html
doi: 10.1038/mt.2008.252

[33] De Laporte L, Yan AL, Shea LD. Local gene delivery from ECM-coated poly(lactide-co-glycolide) multiple channel bridges after spinal cord injury. Biomaterials 2009;30: 2361–8.
http://www.sciencedirect.com/science/article/pii/S0142961208010272
doi: 10.1016/j.biomaterials.2008.12.051

[34] Willerth SM, Sakiyama-Elbert SE. Approaches to neural tissue engineering using scaffolds for drug delivery. Advanced Drug Delivery Reviews 2007;59: 325–38.
http://www.sciencedirect.com/science/article/pii/S0169409X07000312
doi: 10.1016/j.addr.2007.03.014

[35] Biondi M, Ungaro F, Quaglia F, Netti PA. Controlled drug delivery in tissue engineering. Advanced Drug Delivery Reviews 2008;60: 229–42.
http://www.sciencedirect.com/science/article/pii/S0169409X07002463
doi: 10.1016/j.addr.2007.08.038

[36] Madigan NN, McMahon S, O'Brien T, Yaszemski MJ, Windebank AJ. Current tissue engineering and novel therapeutic approaches to axonal regeneration following spinal cord injury using polymer scaffolds. Respiratory Physiology & Neurobiology 2009;169:

183–99.
http://www.sciencedirect.com/science/article/pii/S1569904809002614
doi: 10.1016/j.resp.2009.08.015

[37] Sill TJ, von Recum HA. Electrospinning: Applications in drug delivery and tissue engineering. Biomaterials 2008;29: 1989-2006.
http://www.sciencedirect.com/science/article/pii/S0142961208000203
doi: 10.1016/j.biomaterials.2008.01.011

[38] Pham QP, Sharma U, Mikos AG. Electrospinning of polymeric nanofibers for tissue engineering applications: A review. Tissue Engineering 2006;12(5): 1197-211.
http://online.liebertpub.com/doi/abs/10.1089/ten.2006.12.1197
doi: 10.1089/ten.2006.12.1197

[39] Babensee JE, McIntire LV, Mikos AG. Growth factor delivery for tissue engineering. Pharmaceutical Research 2000;17(5): 497-504.
http://www.springerlink.com/content/q8157p7k1877p641/
doi: 10.1023/A:1007502828372

[40] Kretlow JD, Klouda L, Mikos AG. Injectable matrices and scaffolds for drug delivery in tissue engineering. Advanced Drug Delivery Reviews 2007;59: 263–73.
http://www.sciencedirect.com/science/article/pii/S0169409X07000282
doi: 10.1016/j.addr.2007.03.013

[41] Baldwin SP, Saltzman WM. Materials for protein delivery in tissue engineering. Advanced Drug Delivery Reviews 1998;33: 71–86.
http://www.sciencedirect.com/science/article/pii/S0169409X98000210
doi: 10.1016/S0169-409X(98)00021-0

[42] Zhang G, Suggs LJ. Matrices and scaffolds for drug delivery in vascular tissue engineering. Advanced Drug Delivery Reviews 2007;59: 360–73.
http://www.sciencedirect.com/science/article/pii/S0169409X07000336
doi: 10.1016/j.addr.2007.03.018

[43] Gunn J, Zhang M. Polyblend nanofibers for biomedical applications: perspectives and challenges. Trends in Biotechnology 2010;28(4): 189-97.
http://www.sciencedirect.com/science/article/pii/S0167779909002388
doi: 10.1016/j.tibtech.2009.12.006

[44] Sokolsky-Papkov M, Agashi K, Olaye A, Shakesheff K, Domb AJ. Polymer carriers for drug delivery in tissue engineering. Advanced Drug Delivery Reviews 2007;59: 187–206.
http://www.sciencedirect.com/science/article/pii/S0169409X07000348
doi: 10.1016/j.addr.2007.04.001

[45] Griffth LG, Naughton G. Tissue engineering - Current challenges and expanding opportunities. Science 2002;295: 1009-14.
http://www.sciencemag.org/content/295/5557/1009.short
doi: 10.1126/science.1069210

[46] Chung HJ, Park TG. Surface engineered and drug releasing pre-fabricated scaffolds for tissue engineering. Advanced Drug Delivery Reviews 2007;59: 249–62.

http://www.sciencedirect.com/science/article/pii/S0169409X07000270
doi: 10.1016/j.addr.2007.03.015

[47] Yoo HS, Kim TG, Park TG. Surface-functionalized electrospun nanofibers for tissue engineering and drug delivery. Advanced Drug Delivery Reviews 2009;61: 1033–42.
http://www.sciencedirect.com/science/article/pii/S0169409X09002324
doi: 10.1016/j.addr.2009.07.007

[48] Orive G, Anitua E, Pedraz JL, Emerich WF. Biomaterials for promoting brain protection, repair and regeneration. Nature Reviews Neuroscience 2009;10: 682-92.
http://www.nature.com/nrn/journal/v10/n9/abs/nrn2685.html
doi: 10.1038/nrn2685

[49] Zhong Y, Bellamkonda RV. Biomaterials for the central nervous system. Journal of Royal Society Interface 2008;5: 957–75.
http://rsif.royalsocietypublishing.org/content/5/26/957
doi: 10.1098/rsif.2008.0071

[50] Hyun JK, Kim HW. Clinical and experimental advances in regeneration of spinal cord injury. Journal of Tissue Engineering 2010; 2010: Article ID 650857.
http://tej.sagepub.com/content/1/1/650857.full.pdf+html
doi: 10.4061/2010/650857

[51] Whittleseya KJ, Shea LD. Delivery systems for small molecule drugs, proteins, and DNA: the neuroscience/biomaterial interface. Experimental Neurology 2004;190: 1–16.
http://www.nature.com/nrn/journal/v10/n9/abs/nrn2685.html
doi:10.1038/nrn2685

[52] Samadikuchaksaraei A. An overview of tissue engineering approaches for management of spinal cord injuries. Journal of NeuroEngineering and Rehabilitation 2007;4: 15.
http://www.jneuroengrehab.com/content/4/1/15
doi:10.1186/1743-0003-4-15

[53] Nomura H, Tator CH, Shoichet MS. Bioengineered strategies for spinal cord repair. Journal of Neurotrauma 2006;23(3/4): 496-507.
http://online.liebertpub.com/doi/abs/10.1089/neu.2006.23.496?2
doi:10.1089/neu.2006.23.496

[54] Chai C, Leong KW. Biomaterials approach to expand and direct differentiation of stem cells. Molecular Therapy 2007;15(3): 467–80.
http://www.nature.com/mt/journal/v15/n3/full/6300084a.html
doi:10.1038/sj.mt.6300084

[55] Tabesh H, Amoabediny Gh, Nik NS, Heydari M, Yosefifard M, Siadat SOR, Mottaghy K. The role of biodegradable engineered scaffolds seeded with Schwann cells for spinal cord regeneration. Neurochemistry International 2009;54: 73–83.
http://www.sciencedirect.com/science/article/pii/S0197018608001861
doi: 10.1016/j.neuint.2008.11.002

[56] Xie J, MacEwan MR, Schwartz AG, Xia Y. Electrospun nanofibers for neural tissue engineering. Nanoscale 2010;2: 35–44.
http://pubs.rsc.org/en/Content/ArticleLanding/2010/NR/b9nr00243j
doi:10.1039/B9NR00243J

[57] Perale G, Rossi F, Sundstrom E, Bacchiega S, Masi M, Forloni G, Veglianese P. Hydrogels in spinal cord injury repair strategies. ACS Chemical Neuroscience 2011;2: 336–45.
http://pubs.acs.org/doi/abs/10.1021/cn200030w
doi:10.1021/cn200030w

[58] Branco MC, Schneider JP. Self-assembling materials for therapeutic delivery. Acta Biomaterialia 2009;5: 817–31.
http://www.sciencedirect.com/science/article/pii/S1742706108002936
doi:10.1016/j.actbio.2008.09.018

Chapter 6

Gene Delivery Systems: Recent Progress in Viral and Non-Viral Therapy

Erdal Cevher, Ali Demir Sezer and Emre Şefik Çağlar

Additional information is available at the end of the chapter

1. Introduction

Thanks to the changes in medicine, pharmacological treatment rapidly progresses into new fields. There is an emphasis on the development of treatment methods to eliminate underlying factors rather than to treat the symptoms of a disease. Therefore, research is increasingly utilizing knowledge from the field of genetics. Genetic mutation and deletion lead to many genetic disorders. Genetic disorders in metabolic pathways, regulation of cell cycle, ligand/receptor function, cell skeleton and extracellular proteins cause serious diseases (Yaron et al., 1997).

Both genetic and acquired diseases may be treated using gene therapy. Genetic diseases are generally caused by deletion or mutation of a single cell. Conversely, in acquired diseases, a single gene cannot be defined as the sole cause of a disease. Gene therapy has increased in prominence, and has shown great potential in treating acquired and genetic diseases (Conwell and Huang, 2005).

Gene delivery systems are categorized as: viral-based, non-viral-based and combined hybrid systems. Viral-mediated gene delivery systems consist of viruses that are modified to be replication-deficient, but which can deliver DNA for expression. Adenoviruses, retroviruses, and lentiviruses are used as viral gene-delivery vectors (Escors and Breckpot, 2010).

Non-viral gene delivery systems were introduced as an alternative to viral-based systems. One of the most important advantages of these systems is improved transfection. Non-viral systems are categorized according to preparation, as physical or chemical types. The most common physical methods are microinjection, electroporation, ultrasound, gene gun, and hydrodynamic applications. In general terms, physical methods refer to delivery of the gene *via* the application of physical force to increase permeability of the cell membrane. In contrast, chemical methods utilize natural or synthetic carriers to deliver genes into cells. In this method, polymers, liposomes, dendrimers, and cationic lipid systems are used as gene delivery systems (Miyazaki et al., 2006; Prokop and Davidson, 2007).

2. Gene therapy

This chapter provides general information on gene delivery systems, how they are used, their relative merits, and selection of the most appropriate methods for new studies on gene therapy.

The drug sector is entering a new era that will enable treatment of the underlying cause rather than the symptoms of a disease. Many human diseases result from mutations or deletions, in genes, which lead to disorders in metabolic pathways, ligand/receptor function, cell cycle regulation, cell skeleton or extra-cellular protein structure and function (Sullivan, 2003). With gene therapy, the disease can be treated by the injection of exogenous nucleic acid sequences designed to target the diseased tissues of the body (Yaron et al., 1997).

Diseases that can be treated by gene therapy are categorized as either genetic or acquired. Genetic diseases are those which are typically caused by the mutation or deletion of a single cell. Conversely, a single gene is not defined as the sole cause of acquired diseases. Although gene therapy was initially used to treat genetic disorders only, it is now used to treat a wide range of diseases such as cancer, peripheral vascular diseases, arthritis, neurodegenerative disorders and AIDS (Mhashilkar et al., 2001). The expression of a single cell, directly delivered to the cells by a gene delivery system can potentially eliminate a disease. Prior to gene therapy studies, there was no alternative treatment for genetic disorders. Today, it is possible to correct genetic mutation with gene therapy studies (Sullivan, 2003).

2.1. Chronology

The term gene therapy was first introduced at the International Congress of Genetics (Yaron et al., 1997). The techniques utilized by Gregor Mendel in the 1850s, which were then developed by Ronald Fischer at the beginning of the twentieth century, formed the turning points in genetics. The work of both Mendel and Fischer laid the foundations of genealogy. The material they studied was later termed as gene by the Danish botanist Wilhelm Johannsen (Yaron et al., 1997). Towards the end of the 1970s, the background of the majority of genetic disorders was understood, and gene therapy came to the fore. The first gene therapy trial in humans was conducted at the beginning of the 1970s, and it was observed that naturally occurring DNA and RNA tumor viruses successfully delivered new genetic information to the genomes of mammal cells (Escors and Breckpot, 2010).

Due to developments in the science of genetics, at the beginning of the twentieth century, it was understood that diseases such as hemophilia were genetic diseases. Similarly, it was found that diseases such as colon cancer, diabetes, and retinoblastoma were also genetic-based diseases. In the 1980s, gene transfer to mammalian cells came to the fore after the development of retroviral vectors (Yaron et al., 1997). In the mid-1980s, gene transfer to mammalian cells became a routine procedure. Retrovirus-based gene therapies brought significant advantages, as they can stably integrate their genomes to host-cell chromosomes. After the 1980s, DNA was defined as a genetic material. Later, it was structurally analyzed and further advances allowed the modification of genetic code. These discoveries on genetic material made cloning possible (Escors and Breckpot, 2010).

In 2006, melanoma was successfully treated for the first time. The treatment used a retroviral formulation of melanoma antigen (MART-1)-specific T-cell receptor (TCR), which encodes α- and β- chains. In recent years, great advances have been made in gene therapy, ranging from somatic cloning and completion of human genome project to the discovery of microRNA-based gene-regulating systems (Escors and Breckpot, 2010).

The use of non-viral gene delivery systems in gene therapy also significantly increased in recent years. Naked plasmid DNA, coated with gold particles was effectively introduced to cells using the non-viral gene gun technique. This technique was first used in plant cells in 1987, and is today commonly used in mammal cells and tissues. One of the most successful current gene therapy techniques is hydrodynamic injection (Willemejane and Mir, 2009).

2.2. Gene delivery systems

Gene delivery systems use various methods to allow uptake of the gene that has been selected to target the cell (Conwell and Huang, 2005). The successful design of a gene delivery system requires complete understanding of the interaction mechanism between the target cell and delivery system. Understanding intercellular traffic and targeting mechanism is the most important factor in designing a more effective gene delivery system. Cell targeting refers to delivery of the therapeutic agent to a specific compartment or organelle of the cell. It is the most commonly used mechanism in endocytosis gene therapy, particularly in cellular uptake of non-viral gene delivery systems (Prokop and Davidson, 2007). After the cellular uptake of the delivery system by endocytosis, cellular release takes place to initiate DNA transcription and translation, and to produce the related protein. A successful gene delivery procedure involves minimizing potential inhibitory inflammatory response while also overcoming certain barriers at each step of the gene delivery procedure, in order to optimize gene activity (Conwell and Huang, 2005).

Viral gene delivery systems consist of viruses that are modified to be replication-deficient which were made unable to replicate by redesigning which can deliver the genes to the cells to provide expression. Adenoviruses, retroviruses, and lentiviruses are used for viral gene delivery. Viral systems have advantages such as constant expression and expression of therapeutic genes (Sullivan, 2003). However, there are some limitations that restrict the use of these systems, which particularly include the use of viruses in production, immunogenicity, toxicity and lack of optimization in large-scale production (Witlox et al., 2007) (Figure 1).

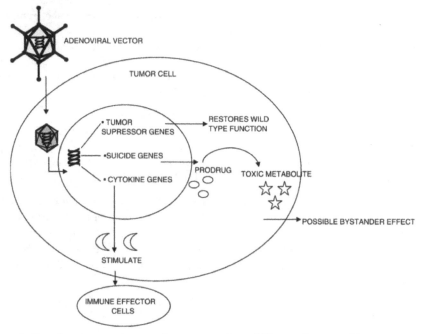

Figure 1. Gene therapy strategies; mutation compensation, suicide gene therapy and immuno-potentiation (Witlox et al., 2007).

Non-viral gene delivery systems were developed as an alternative to viral-based systems. One of the most important advantages of these systems is that they develop transfection. Non-viral gene delivery systems are divided into two categories: physical and chemical. Microinjection, electroporation, gene gun, ultrasound-mediated methods, and hydrodynamic systems are the most widely used physical methods. Physical methods involve the use of physical force to increase the permeability of the cell membrane and allow the gene to enter the cell. The primary advantage of physical methods is that they are easy to use and reliable. However, they also have the disadvantage of causing tissue damage in some applications.

Chemical methods involve the use of carriers prepared from synthetic or natural compounds for gene delivery into the cell, including synthetic and natural polymers, liposomes, dendrimers, synthetic proteins, and cationic lipids. The biggest advantages of these systems are that they are non-immunogenic and generally have low toxicity.

2.2.1. Viral gene delivery systems

Since a large number of viruses have appropriate mechanisms for transfer of genetic material to the target cell, current gene technologies concentrated on the use of viral vectors that provide high transduction effectiveness and advanced level of gene expression. The optimal design of a viral vector depends on the types of virus to be used (Wunderbaldinger et al., 2000).

For safe application of *in vivo* gene therapy, firstly some problems should be eliminated. Therapeutic factors should only be expressed in related cell types, and should not cause any undesired effect in healthy cells (Yaron et al., 1997).

2.2.1.1. Adenoviral systems

Adenoviruses (Ad) were first discovered in 1953 by isolation from human adenoid tissue cultures (Campos and Barry, 2007; Majhen and Ambriovic-Ristov, 2006). They are commonly used as gene vectors (Dinh et al., 2005). C group adenoviruses Ad2 and Ad5 are the most widely studied adenoviruses. The capsid of an adenovirus determines virus tropism. Groups A and C–F first bind to highly-expressed coxsackie virus B-adenovirus receptor, and thus realize their high infectivity in many tissues. In contrast, group B binds to complement-regulatory protein CD46. Adenoviruses are replicated and produce virions, which contain the nucleus of the infected cell (Dinh et al., 2005). These vectors have the ability to be replicated, and purification of the vectors generally involves easier and shorter processes (Armendariz-Borunda et al., 2011).

Adenoviruses are well-characterized, non-integrated, ~26–40 kb in length, relatively large, non-enveloped, linear dsDNA viruses coated with icosahedral particle, with a diameter of ~ 950 Å (excluding elongated fiber proteins) and a molecular weight of approximately 150MDa. They are unreplicated, and infect cells quickly. Adenoviral particles do not contain lipid or membrane; therefore they are stable in solvents such as ether or ethanol. The use of adenoviruses, which are one of the first developed vector systems for gene expression, is a great discovery (Campos and Barry, 2007).

Adenoviruses have important characteristics, which make them indispensable for gene transfer. The most important ones are their well-known molecular biology; delivery capacity of foreign DNA fragments up to 36kb; and ability to transfect DNA into many cell types (Sullivan, 2003).

Adenoviruses are one of the largest and most complex viruses, whose Ad structure was analyzed with cryo-electron microscopy and X-ray diffractometry. An Ad genome of approximately 36kb codes more than forty genomes; however, only 12 of these were demonstrated as the component of the virus particle. As seen in Figure 2 it was reported that crystal structures of single Ad proteins contained fiber knob, shaft, domains, penton base, hexon, and cysteine protease. Ad capsid consists of 252 sub-units called capsomeres, which contain 240 hexonproteins and 12 of the penton base. In addition, the capsid contains pIIIa, pVI, PVIII, and pIX proteins. Each of the 12 capsid corners contains penton bases wrapped by 5 hexons. The penton base serves as a hook for the fiber protein, which projects from the virus like an antenna. Fiber is a homotrimer, where 3 identical polypeptides bind in the same direction, and which contains 3 structurally and functionally different domains: N-terminus, which binds the fiber non-covalently to the penton base; C-terminus, which gives the disc-like knob form, which is responsible for binding to the receptor; and the rod-like shaft, which varies in length according to the serotype of the virus (Medina-Kauwe LK. 2003; Majhen and Ambriovic-Ristov, 2006).

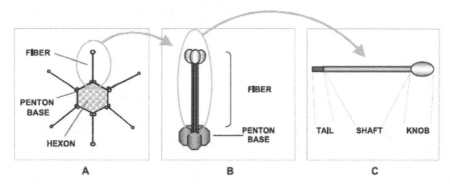

Figure 2. Schematic of the adenovirus capsid. (A) Whole capsid identifying fiber, penton base, and hexon. (B) Enlargement of circled region in (A), showing homotrimeric fiber bound to homopentameric penton base. (C) Fiber monomer, identifying tail, shaft, and knob domains. Pictures are not drawn to scale (Medina-Kauwe LK. 2003).

A viral genome is in a condensed state inside cell nucleus, together with protein V, VII and X, and the 5′ terminus of the AdDNA is covalently linked to a terminal protein (TP). The terminal protein (TP) functions as the initiation primer in viral DNA replication. An Ad genome consists of 5 early (E1A, E1B, E2, E3 and E4), 4 interim (IVa2, IX, VAI, VAII) and one late transcriptional unit. E1A is the first viral transcriptional unit, which will be expressed after entering the cell. E1A proteins activate other *trans*early transcription units, which will create an optimum medium for virus replication by causing the products to enter in S phase of the cell E1B proteins bind to p53, Bak, and Bax proteins, and allows the infected cell survive by inhibiting p53 dependent apoptosis. The E2A unit encodes the proteins that function in viral genome replication, including DNA polymerase, prethermal protein, and single-stranded DNA-binding protein. While the E4 transcription unit encodes the proteins that affect cell cycle control and transformation, E3 protein disrupts the immune response of the host and ensures the continuation of the infected cell (Majhen and Ambriovic-Ristov, 2006).

The nucleus is surrounded by an icosahedral capsid with a symmetrical structure, formed by the non-covalent interactions between 7 proteins (II, III, IIIa, IV, VI, VIII, and IX) (Smith et al., 2010). Adenoviral structural proteins are responsible for the stabilization of genome and encapsidation of the nucleoprotein nucleus. The icosahedral capsid consists of seven peptides:trimerichexons, which are found in complex form with three minor capsid polyproteins (VI, VIII and IX), which provides stabilization (II); pentonbase (III); receptor binding fiber (IV) and penton-bound protein which serves as a bridge between protein and the hexon base (III). The fiber consists of 3 domains which are tail in N-terminus, rod-like shaft and globular knob in C-terminus (Couglan et al., 2010). Adenoviruses enter target cells *via* receptor-mediated endocytosis. Instead of combining its own DNA with the genomes of the host cell, the adenovirus, remains as an episome within the infected cell. This provides high efficiency (10); however, it should not be ignored, since it will restrict the longevity of expressed trans genes; in other words, protein expression will quickly cease (Yaron et al., 1997; Muzzonigro et al., 1999).

Penton and fiber proteins of virus capsid interact with the coxsackievirus-adenovirus receptor cell surface protein to provide cell binding. These proteins are then localized in clathrin-coated pits through NPXY motive of β_3 and β_5 integrin sub units of the cell. Dinamine, which is systolic GTPase, mediates cellular uptake of the virus into the cell via endocytosis by providing construction and development of clathrin-coated pits. Viral capsid proteins dissociate prior to endocytosis, and the pH value of the viral endosome decreases due to proton pumps. At pH 6.0, the virus has the ability to detach from the vesicle and enter the cytosol. Capsid proteins of the virus move towards the nucleus through microtubules and fragment in the following stages. Although a considerable part of the capsid proteins remain in the periphery of the nucleus, viral DNA crosses *via* nuclear pores (Ziello et al., 2010).

For successful delivery of DNA to the nucleus, viruses must facilitate cell-specific binding, endocytosis internalization, propagation from endocytic vesicles to cytosol, delivery into cytoplasm, translocation from one terminus of the nuclear envelope to other, and finally expression of the delivered gene (Dinh et al., 2005).

Direct injection or bolus delivery through inhalation is the easiest form of viral delivery. However, since the virus will spread from the injection area, a high dose is required to achieve therapeutic effectiveness. The spread of the virus from the injection site limits the regional effectiveness and immune response. Adenoviral vectors can be targeted *via* selective modification of coat proteins. There is a relatively high level of protein expression following the transduction, equal to approximately 35% of total cellular protein (Zhang et al., 2009).

Adenoviruses have many natural properties that enable them to be used as a vector for on colitic, vaccine, or gene therapy. Non-enveloped viruses can be kept in lyophilized form in a stable state inside a flacon tube or capsule; they can be transported without cold chain; by mediating in high transduction effectiveness in dividing and non-dividing cells, they can form 104 virus particles per infected cell (Khare et al., 2011). Adenoviruses achieve suitable transduction through a high level of expression and become beneficial in *in vivo* conditions (Muzzonigro et al., 1999).

Adenoviruses have been one of the most promising methods for high effectiveness in *in vivo* gene therapy. For example, following systemic vector delivery, transduction levels of hepatocytes were observed by adenoviral systems. These are some of the most effective vectors for gene delivery to various organs; however, they have very significant disadvantages. Some target cells have low ratios of appropriate primary and/or secondary adenoviral receptors, and this requires a high dose of vector application to cause target-cell cytotoxicity. Additionally, non-discriminating tropism of the virus can also lead to transduction to untargeted cells (Reynolds et al., 1999). The most serious problem in the use of Ad vectors is their tendency to cause strong immune and inflammatory responses at high doses (Navarro et al., 2008).

2.2.1.2. Retroviral systems

Retroviruses are diploid, single-stranded, circular-enveloped RNA viruses of the family Retroviridae, with a genome of 7–11 kb, and a diameter of approximately 80–120 nm (Osten et al., 2007; Escors and Brecpot, 2010). The Retroviridae family is divided into two sub-families: Orthoretrovirinae and Spumaretrovirinae species (Osten et al., 2007). Retroviruses cause diseases such as AIDS, leukemia, and cancer; however, their use as a vector in gene therapy brought new developments in treatment (Pages and Danos, 2003).

The ability of retrovirus-based gene delivery vectors to carry foreign genetic material was first realized in the early 1980s (El-Aneed, 2004; Escors and Brecpot, 2010). Retroviruses are viruses that integrate with host genome to produce viral proteins (gag, pol, env) that are extracted during gene delivery (El-Aneed, 2004). Retroviral vectors have the capacity to delivery DNA up to 8 kb (Navarro et al., 2008). The most commonly used retroviruses are the Moloney murine leukemia virus species, which have the capacity to deliver exogenous genetic material up to approximately 9 kb (Muzzonigro et al., 1999).

A virion nucleus consists of circular or triangular gag-encoded capsid proteins. They are coated with gag-encoded nucleocapsid protein. The nucleus contains pol-encoded enzymes, reverse transcriptase, and integrase. Retrovirus genomes have various characteristics. For example, these viruses are diploid in the real sense, and their genomes are produced by cellular transcriptional mechanism. In addition, these viruses require cellular (tRNA) for replication (Luban, 2000). The genome of these (+) sense RNA viruses is not directly processed as mRNA immediately after infection Considering the structure of the genome, retroviruses are categorized as either simple or complex forms. Simple and complex retroviruses encode gag (group-specific antigen), pro (protease), and pol (polymerase) genes; complex retroviruses also encode a large number of additional genes. Retroviruses were the first viruses to be modified for gene delivery, and have also been used in the majority of clinical trials of gene therapy (Hu and Pathak, 2000).

Most of retroviral vectors used in clinical studies are based on the Moloney murine leukemia virus (MMLV). MMLV is a well-studied and characterized virus; its genome encodes three polyproteins that are required in trans form for replication and packaging: gag, pol and env (Escors and Brecpot, 2010).

An ideal retroviral vector for gene delivery should be cell-specific, regulated, and safe. Effectiveness of delivery is important, as it will also determine the effectiveness of therapy (Hu and Pathak, 2000). Retroviruses have a lipid envelope. In order to enter a host cell, they use the interactions between cellular receptors and virally encoded proteins, which are embedded in the membrane (Hu and Pathak, 2000). Combination of chimeric envelope protein with viral particles allows the retrovirus to bind receptor-positive target cells (Yi et al., 2011). SU in the virion surface binds to CD, which is a cell-surface protein expressed by some T-cells and is found in macrophages. Binding to CD4 induces some changes in the envelope protein (SU) of the domain of epidermal growth factor (EGF), which allows for interaction with chemokine receptors (CKR). CKRs are a family of cell-surface-G-proteins functioning as receptors to stain molecules called chemokines.

Infusion of viral and cellular membranes starts the internalization of the viral nucleus (Yi et al., 2011); the viral envelope combines with the cell membrane. Envelope glycoprotein (Env) of retroviruses is responsible for determining tropism. Binding of Env to cellular receptor and fusion of viral and cellular membranes are the first stages of infection. Trials that targeted retroviruses by adding single-stranded antibodies or Env cell-binding ligands showed limited success. The addition of such large ligands to Env protein prevents Env from binding to the virion (Bupp and Roth, 2002). Env protein takes a particle-coated structure and releases the viral nucleus into the cytoplasm. Single-stranded DNA gets reversely transcripted to double-stranded DNA in the nucleus (Osten et al., 2007; Karlsson et al., 1987). Viral RNA is reverse transcribed to a DNA copy using virally-encoded reverse-transcriptase enzyme in the virion (Hu and Pathak, 2000). Retroviruses follow a different replication cycle through transformation of single-stranded RNAs into double-stranded DNA in the infected cell. Viral DNA synthesis takes place in cytoplasm by virion-dependent DNA polymerase, which is termed reverse transcriptase. Viral DNA enters the nucleus, where takes the ring form for the first time, and serves as a draft for RNA synthesis (Olsen and Swanstorm, 1985). The first DNA product is a linear double layer molecule, which forms during DNA synthesis. Within the nucleus, some linear DNA is turned into many different forms of ring DNA; these mainly contain two copies of LTR units in tandem, or a single copy of LTR unit (Olsen and Swanstorm, 1985). The end of each LTR unit creates short, deficient repetitions; this represents the strand domain required for this integration (Olsen and Swanstorm, 1985), and is delivered to the nucleus. This delivery takes place through cell division for oncoretroviruses, and through active transport for lentiviruses. Here, lentiviruses are observed to be more advantageous than oncoretroviruses, as they have the ability to deliver genes to non-dividing cells. When viral DNA enters the nucleus, it integrates with the DNA of the host cell (provirus). Retroviruses introduce their genetic material to the host cell genome in a stabile manner during mitotic division. Since these types of retroviruses only transfer genes to dividing cells, many procedures that utilize retroviruses are applied *ex vivo*. However, more recent lentiviral-based retroviral vectors reduce these restrictions (Muzzonigro et al., 1999). Most retroviruses infect cells that can be actively divided during mitotic division. This property protects normal tissue, and although it naturally targets the tumor, all tumors contain non-dividing cells in G0, which is the resting phase of the tumor cell cycle (Hu and Pathak, 2000; Kitamura et al., 2003; El-Aneed, 2004) (Figure 3).

Infected cells are then transcribed and spliced. Full-length viral RNA (which is the RNA that encodes all proteins) is delivered to cytoplasm and translated; other cellular procedures are modification and delivery of RNA from the nucleus (Hu and Pathak, 2000). Spliced full-length viral RNA is packaged into viral particles. Retroviruses are RNA viruses that are replicated over integrated DNA intermediate products. Retroviral particles surround two copies of full-length viral RNA, containing all of the genetic information required for virus replication, with capsid (Hu and Pathak, 2000). Virologic and genetic studies indicated that specific packaging of retroviral genomic RNA was carried out through the interaction with the nucleocapsid (NC) domain of Gag polyprotein. Retroviral NC domains are generally very simple, and contain one or two zinc knob motifs consisting of C-C-H-C sequences. Zinc knobs form metal-coordinated reverse turn, stabilized by NH-S hydrogen bonds. Most retroviral zinc knobs contain a hydrophobic cut on the surface of the mini-globular domain,

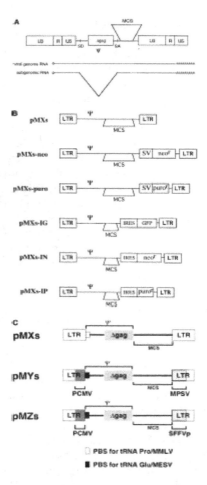

Figure 3. Structures of retrovirus vectors. **(A)** Basic structure of retrovirus vectors and two transcripts from the vector. In the replication competent MMLV, the Gag-Pol and the Env proteins are translated from the genomic RNA and the subgenomic RNA, respectively. The subgenomic RNA is a spliced form RNA, and the splicing occurs from the splice donor site (SD) to the splice acceptor site (SA). Both 5´ and 3´ LTRs consist of U3, R, and U5 regions. Ψ = packaging signal; Δgag = truncated *gag* sequence. **(B)** Structures of versatile pMXs-derived vectors. LTR = long terminal repeat; Ψ = packaging signal; MCS = multi-cloning site; IRES = internal ribosomal entry site; GFP = green fluorescent protein' neor = neomycin-resistant gene; puror = puromycin-resistant gene. (C) Structures of pMXs, pMYs, and pMZs vectors. The 5´ LTR, primer binding site (PBS), and the extended packaging signal of pMXs are derived from the MFG vector. PBS used in pMYs and pMZs are derived from MESV (murine embryonic stem cell virus) and binds tRNA-glu instead of tRNA-pro. MCS is designed for cDNA library construction and is preceded by triple stop codons (not shown). White box = MMLV LTR; gray box = PCMV LTR; hatched box = MPSV LTR or SFFVp LTR. MCS = multi-cloning site (Kitamura et al., 2003).

recognizing the specific structure of RNA or DNA. Base N- and C- terminal tails of nucleocapsid domains are conformationally indurable (Miyazaki et al., 2011). Retroviral genome packaging is generally localized between the binding donor (SD) region and the gag start codon in the 5′ head region. It should be noted that the packaging sign generally coincides with the dimerization region, which indicates that packaging combines with genome dimerization (Miyazaki et al., 2011). Inhibition of genome dimerization through addition or deletion of mutations at dimer initiation sites (DIS) causes a significant decrease in genome packaging. Studies of mutant viruses containing two retroviral genomes showed that these were non-covalently dimerized in progen viruses. 5′ untranslated region (UTR) packages monomeric genome, which indicates that the genome packaging procedure occurs *via* the interaction of two 5′ UTR (Miyazaki et al., 2011). Virion maturation occurs by the budding of the particle from the cell (Escors and Brecpot, 2010). The translational mechanism of the host synthesizes and modifies viral proteins. Newly synthesized viral proteins and full-length RNAs combine to produce a new virus form, which will be budding from the host cell (Hu and Pathak, 2000).

A retrovirus infects the target cell by providing interaction between viral envelope protein and cell surface receptor on the target cell. The virus then internalizes to the place where its single-stranded RNA turns into double-stranded DNA. Double-stranded DNA is delivered to the nucleus and integrated to the host cell genome there. Many types of retrovirus types require degradation of mitosis and then the nuclear envelope for the arrival of a viral genome within the nucleus (Robbins and Ghivizzani, 1998).

Stable binding of viral DNA to the host genome is advantageous because it will provide long-term expression of transgenes required for therapeutic effect. However, one of the disadvantages of current retroviral transfer systems is that they are not specific to types of target cells (Yi et al., 2011).

One of the most important properties of retroviruses is that they can integrate a reverse transcribed genome to the host cell chromosome (Miyazaki et al., 2011).

Unlike adenoviral vectors, retroviral vectors realize transfection through transgene integration to the target cell genome. However, transgene expression ceases within a few days or weeks. Retroviral vectors reveal gene transfer that is unsuitable for many cells in *in vivo* conditions, and this partly stems from rapid inactivation of the human complement system. This silencing is not well characterized; however, it appears as a result of methylation in DNA or promoter regions, or participation of splice region to condensed chromatin (Reynolds et al., 1999; Navarro et al., 2008).

The ability of retroviruses to enter their genomes to host DNA enables them to make stable modifications to the life cycle of the host cell. This stability is greater than viruses such as adenovirus, herpes simplex virus (HSV), and papilloma virus, which remain episomal (Robbins and Ghivizzani, 1998).

2.2.1.3. Lentiviral systems

In recent years, studies mainly concentrated on the use lentiviral vectors. Lentivirals are viral systems without small, retrovirus-like viral proteins and no capacity for replication;

they provide gene delivery to non-dividing cells. This characteristic property is an advantage for various gene therapy applications used in targeting in post-mitotic and highly differentiated cells. The most important advantage of lentiviruses compared with other retroviruses is their ability for gene transfer to non-dividing cells (Escors and Brecpot, 2010; Yi et al., 2011; Matrai et al., 2009; Freed, 1997). This characteristic is believed to be related to the pathogenic characteristics of lentiviruses, which infect terminally differentiated cells of monocyte/macrophage lineage (Freed, 1997). For this reason, lentiviral vectors can be used for transgene expression to neuron cells (Yi et al., 2011).

Genome of lentiviruses have a more complicated structure; they contain accessory genes which regulate viral gene expression, control combination of infectious particles, modulate viral replication in infected cells, and are associated with the continuance of infection (Howarth et al., 2010). In other words, the fact that it contains regulatory and accessory genes apart from gag, pol and env, requires lentiviruses to adopt a more complex form (Osten et al., 2007). For example, HIV-1 is one of the most widely used lentiviral vectors, and contains six accessory genes (tat, rev, vif, vpr, nef, vpu) (Osten et al., 2007; Yi et al., 2011). These proteins are involved in all steps of cell cycles, which are termed: budding, maturation, and integration. In addition to helping combination of virions, these proteins ensure nuclear export and transcription ratio of RNA (Yi et al., 2011).

HIV infects CD4-positive T lymphocytes and macrophages (CD4 antigen acts as a primer surface receptor for HIV-1), and causes chronic immune deficiency, known as acquired immune disorder syndrome (AIDS). HIV-1 genome additionally contains 2 regulatory genes (*tat* and *rev*), and 4 accessory genes (*vpr, vpu, vif, nef*). The lenti viral genome is 9.2 kb in length. *Tat* protein increases transcriptional activity in 5' LTR of integrated provirus from promoter regions. Rev protein transports non-spliced HUV mRNA from the nucleus. In general, accessory proteins increase virulence against the host organism. Development of HIV-1-based vectors was first achieved by utilizing the abilities of lentiviral vectors of infecting post-mitotic cells. The design of other retrovirus-based vectors, such as self-inactivating MoMLV vectors, can be directly transferred to lentiviral vectors. In the most recent generations of HIV-1-based vectors, all accessory genes and the regulatory tat gene are deleted (Osten et al., 2007). In the self-inactivating (SIN) expression vector, the U3 promoter region is deleted from the 3'LTR. This region was copied to the 5' end of dsDNA during reverse-transcription. Therefore, SIN modification results in transcriptional inactivation of the integrated provirus, which allows for the restriction of the likelihood of recombination with latent retroviral sequences and mobilization of latent retroviral sequences in the host cell genome (Osten et al., 2007).

Tropism of lentiviral vectors depends on the type of envelope protein used for viral production (Escors and Brecpot, 2010). The use of heterologous Env proteins is called pseudo typing. The most widely used Env protein is "vesicular stomatitis virus glycoprotein (VSV-G)". This protein permits the virus high titration values *via* ultracentrifugation and a wide tropism (VSV-G binds to suitable phospholipid component of plasma membrane) (Osten et al., 2007).

Lentiviral vectors do not require degradation of the nuclear membrane for integration. Lentiviruses that are encoded with the Gag matrix protein integrase enzyme and vpr protein interact with the nuclear import mechanism of the target cell and manage active transport of pre-integration complex *via* nucleopores. This characteristic enables transfection to non-dividing cells and, in conclusion, "complex retroviruses" become suitable for use as gene transfer vectors, particularly for post-mitotic cells like neurons (Howarth et al., 2010). Receptors have been defined for many retroviruses. The best-characterized example is CD4 molecule, which serves as a receptor for lentiviruses including HIV (Freed, 1997).

Frequently, pseudotype lentiviral vectors are formed by "vesicular stomatitis virus" envelope (VSV-G). VSV-G is a glycoprotein that interacts with the phospholipid component of a number of receptors or cell membrane. VSV-G offers large host-cell range and high vector particle stability, which are attractive characteristics for *ex vivo* gene modification. However, restriction of infection to specific cells, which is called transduction altargeting, is effective and reliable and critical in the case of *in vivo* gene delivery. In addition, it is the key to increase therapeutic effectiveness, reduce adverse effects, and reducing the required amount of the vector. Two methods can be used to achieve this: (a) benefiting from natural characteristics of existing viral proteins, (b) using gene engineering to continue, stop or increase the original tropism of the vector (Escors and Brecpot, 2010).

Recently-developed lentiviral gene transfer systems have many characteristics of retroviral systems. A viral genome integrates with host chromosomes, and genes that are desired to remain permanently are placed (Yi et al., 2011).

2.2.2. Non-viral gene delivery systems

The basic concept underlying gene therapy is that it develops gene expression to specific cells in order to treat human diseases or for transfer of genetic material to inhibit the production of a target protein (He et al., 2010).

In theory, viral carriers can achieve rapid transfection of foreign material spliced to viral genome with high transfection ratio. However, many studies that used viral vectors reported unsatisfactory results, due to the immunologic and oncogenic adverse effects of these vectors. On the other hand, non-viral vectors have many advantages, such as easy of fabrication, cell/tissue targeting, and low immune response. The biggest disadvantage of non-viral vectors in clinical use is low transfection efficiency (He et al., 2010). Therefore, the most important points that should be taken into account in gene therapy are the introduction of the gene into the cell and increasing transfection efficiency. Using transfection, cells are induced for the production of chemicals used in pharmacological arrangements like hormone replacement or specific protein production (Godbey and Mikos, 2001). Naked DNA molecules cannot effectively enter to the cell due to their hydrophilic structures and large size resulting from negatively-charged phosphate groups. In addition, they are easily fragmented by nuclease enzymes. Therefore, the biggest difficulty in gene therapy is the development of physical methods to ensure gene transfer to target cells of the gene delivery vectors and delivered gene (Al-Dosari and Gao, 2009).

As seen in Figure 4, natural and synthetic polymers are used to prepare non-viral gene delivery systems. Compared to viral delivery systems, non-viral carriers are less toxic and immunogenic. Another advantage of non-viral vectors is ease-of-production (DeLaporte et al., 2006). Much of the previous research found that non-viral systems were less effective than viral systems. However, in gene therapy conducted with physical methods, the effectiveness of gene transfection and therapy increased, and the duration of gene expression was extended significantly in clinical terms (Al-Dosari and Gao, 2009).

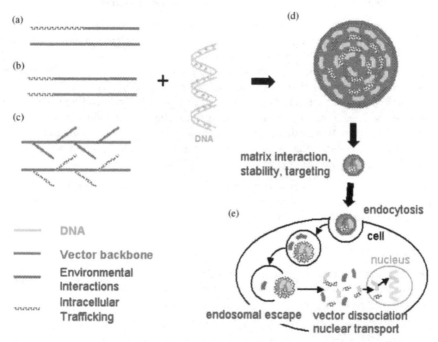

Figure 4. Modular design of non-viral vectors schematic. Modules associated with vector design are: vector backbone (grey), functional groups for regulating environmental interactions (purple), and intracellular trafficking (red). The vector backbone, typically containing polymers, lipids, or polysaccharides, is designed for DNA binding and complexation, which can protect against nuclease degradation, create a small, less negatively charged particle that can be internalized by cells, and facilitate some intracellular trafficking. The function of the vector backbone is being augmented by the attachment of groups that address the extracellular and intracellular barriers. The environmental functional groups can serve to limit interactions with serum components, promote specific cell binding or tissue targeting, or facilitate interactions with the extracellular matrix or biomaterials. The intracellular functional groups aim to enhance nuclear accumulation of the DNA either by facilitating endosomal escape, movement along the cytoskeleton, or nuclear pore trafficking. The individual modules can be assembled in different ways (a – c) for complexation with DNA (green), which may affect the structure and function of the resulting non-viral vector. (d) Schematic illustrating the distribution of the modules and DNA throughout the vector cross section, with the desired organization of functional groups regulating the environmental interactions presented primarily on the exterior and the groups for intracellular trafficking protected within the vector interior for activity following internalization. (e) Vectors are internalized by endocytosis and must subsequently escape the endosome for transport to the nucleus. Additionally, the modular components must dissociate from the DNA to allow for transcription (DeLaporte et al., 2006).

A number of barriers need to be overcome in order to increase the effectiveness of non-viral vectors in humans. These barriers are classified as production/formulation/storage; extracellular barriers; and intracellular barriers (Davis, 2002). Anatomic barriers are extracellular matrixes coating the cells, which prevent direct transport of macromolecules to target cells through epithelium and endothelial cell sequences. Phagocytes like Kupffer cells in the liver and residential macrophages in the spleen are responsible for theclearance of DNA-loaded colloidal particles in blood circulation. Similarly, nucleases found in blood and extracellular matrix cause free and unprotected nucleic acids to be rapidly inactivated following systemic application. The most critical barrier to effective DNA transfection was regarded as the transition of plasma membrane. Typically, naked nucleic acids cannot cross cell membrane by cellular uptake mechanisms such as endocytosis, pinocytosis, and phagocytosis without application of physical methods or being loaded to a carrier (Al-Dosari and Gao, 2009). There is a substantial body of research on developing effective physical, chemical, and biological systems to deliver transgenes into the cell to provide appropriate expression (Gao et al., 2007). Physical approaches, including electroporation, gene gun, ultrasound, and hydrodynamic delivery are based on the application of a force to increase the permeability of the cell membrane and promote intracellular gene transfer. In chemical applications, synthetic or natural carriers are used to transport transgenes to the cells. An ideal gene delivery system should meet 3 criteria: The carriers should protect the transgene from nuclease enzymes inside intracellular matrixes; should transport the transgene from plasma membrane to the target cell nucleus; and should not cause any toxic effect (Gao et al., 2007).

Two of the most important advantages of synthetic carriers are that they do not display immunogenicity, and large-scale production is easy. Furthermore, the size of the gene to be delivered does not reduce efficiency of these systems. Even mammalian artificial chromosomes of 60 megabase were successfully transfected by these types of carriers (Schatzlein, 2003).

Non-viral vectors can trigger an inflammatory response, since they do not provide a specific recognition; they are much less dangerous than viral vectors in terms of antigen specific immune response. However, although non-viral vectors seem to be more suitable, there are some important points to be contemplated in vector design. Non-viral vectors should be designed according to specific cell targeting; cellular uptake and cellular release should be optimized; and potential immune response should be minimized (Conwell and Huang, 2005; Mrsny, 2005).

2.2.2.1. Physical methods

Gene Gun

Delivery with gene gun method is also termed ballistic DNA delivery or DNA-coated particle bombardment, and was first used for gene transfer to plants in 1987 (Al-Dosari and Gao, 2009; Lin et al., 2000). This method is based on the principle of delivery of DNA-coated heavy metal particles by crossing them from target tissue at a certain speed. The particles achieve sufficient speed due to a pressurized inert gas (generally helium). Generally, gold, tungsten or silver microparticles were used as the gene carrier (Mhashilkar et al., 2001; Al-

Dosari and Gao, 2009; Miyazaki et al., 2006). Momentum allows penetration of these particles to a few millimeters of the tissue and then cellular DNA release (Gao et al., 2007). These particles typically have a diameter of 1μm. Due to its small size, the particle easily penetrates the cell membrane and can transport DNA into the cell. At this point, DNA separates from the carrier particle and can be expressed (Lin et al., 2000).

Gas pressure, particle size and dose frequency are critical factors in determining the degree of tissue damage and penetration effectiveness of the application (Al-Dosari and Gao, 2009).

Gene-gun-based gene transfer is a widely tested method for intramuscular, intradermal and intratumoral genetic immunization (Miyazaki et al., 2006). Numerous animal tests and clinical trials indicated that this method caused a greater immune response than microinjection, even in low doses (Al-Dosari and Gao).

The advantages of gene gun over other *in vivo* gene delivery systems are as follows: [1] It does not use toxic chemicals or complex biological systems, [2] delivery is achieved without the need for a receptor, [3] DNA fragments of various sizes, including large ones, are transported, [4] there is no need to introduce foreign DNA or protein, [5] it has high repeatability, [6] production of heavy metal particles is easy (Lin et al., 2000). However, in this method, gene expression is short-term and low (Mhashilkar et al., 2001).

Electroporation

The future of gene therapy requires the advancement of effective and non-toxic polynucleotide gene delivery mechanisms. Electroporation includes controlled electric application to increase cell permeability. Electroporation was first developed in 1960s, with studies on the degradation of cell membrane with electric induction. Neumann et al., first reported transfection of eukaryotic culture cells through electroporation in 1982. In many subsequent studies, transfection was performed on animal and plant cells *via* electroporation (Al-Dosari and Gao, 2009; Somiari et al., 2000).

Electroporation introduces foreign genes into the cell by electric pulses. In this method, pores are formed on the membrane surface to enable the DNA to enter the cell. Pore formation occurs very rapidly, in approximately 10 nanoseconds. The size of the electric pore is estimated to be smaller than 10 nm radius. If the molecule is smaller than the pore size (as in oligonucleotides and chemical compounds), it can be transferred to the cell cytosol through diffusion (Somiari et al., 2000; Miyazaki et al., 2006). In addition to passive diffusion, loaded molecules and ions can be transported from the membrane *via* electrophoretic and electro-osmotic means *via* the effect of electric regions. The pores close following cellular uptake of DNA. In recent years, *in vivo* electroporation became common in nucleic acid vaccines and improving non-viral gene therapy. There are critical steps defined for transportation *via in vivo* gene delivery with electroporation. The first step is fusing together, attachment or proximity between the cell membrane and nucleic acid. The second step is adding nucleic acid to the membrane, which is immediately followed by the third step, involving the delivery of nucleic acid from the membrane. The delivery procedure results in decreased pore size and permeability (Somiari et al., 200).

In vivo electroporation technique is a generally reliable method that is more efficient than other non-viral systems. When the parameters are optimized, this technique is equally effective as viral vectors. In addition to local injection and electroporation, it was previously shown that *in vivo* electroporation can be applied in localized form after the injection of plasmid DNA (Al-Dosari and Gao, 2009).

There are some difficulties in *in vivo* applications of electroporation. There is an effectiveness region of approximately 1 cm between the electrodes, and this makes transfection of the cells in large regions of the tissues difficult. It is difficult to use in internal organs, and surgery is required to implant electrodes. High temperature due to high voltage application can cause irreversible tissue damage. The application of high voltage to cells can affect the stability of genomic DNA (Al-Dosari and Gao, 2009; Gao et al., 2007).

Ultrasound

Ultrasound has many clinical advantages as a gene delivery system, due its easy and reliable procedure (Pitt et al., 2004; Ferrara, 2010). In recent years, it was found that microbubbles applied by ultrasound increased gene expression. Microbubbles or ultrasound contrast agents decrease cavitation threshold with ultrasound energy. In many applications, perfluoropropane-loaded albumin microbubbles (Mallinckrodt, San Diego, USA) were used. The microbubbles were modified with plasmid DNA before the injection and then ultrasound was applied (Niidome and Huang, 2002).

Ultrasound has been used for therapeutic purposes for more than a half century, even before the use of ultrasound for diagnosis and imaging purposes. In diagnostic use, low-intensity ultrasound is used to prevent energy accumulation in tissue causing biological effects. Conversely, therapeutic applications are based on the principle of intensification of ultrasound energy within the tissue (Frenkel, 2008).

After the discovery of the applicability of ultrasound to gene therapy at the cellular and tissue level, this was taken one step further with physical methods. Reporter gene expression, where naked DNA is used, advanced for10 times thanks to this discovery. The transfection efficiency of this system is based on frequency, time of ultrasound treatment, the plasmid DNA mount used, etc. In conclusion, size and local concentration of DNA plays an important role in the effectiveness of transfection (Gao et al., 2007).

Hydrodynamic therapy

Hydrodynamic gene delivery is based on the principle of understanding the characteristics and structure of capillaries, an understanding of the dynamic characteristics of the fluids passing through blood veins (Suda and Liu, 2007). Hydrodynamic gene delivery uses the hydrodynamic pressure created by the injection of the large volume of DNA solution with blood pressure inside veins (Suda and Liu, 2007), and thus the permeability of the capillary endothelium increases and pores form in the plasma membrane encircling parenchyma cells (Gao et al., 2007; Suda and Liu, 2007). DNA or other related molecules can reach the cell from these pores. Membrane pores are later closed, and these molecules are retained within the cell. In hydrodynamic gene therapy, the principle reason for targeting parenchyma cells is that capillary endothelium and parenchyma cells are closely related, and when the endothelial barrier is breached, this allows DNA to easily reach parenchyma cells. In addition, the capillary's thin wall structure has a stretchable and easily fragmented structure (Suda and Liu, 2007). The effectiveness of hydrodynamic procedure depends on capillary structure, the structure of the cells encircling capillaries, and the hydrodynamic force applied (Gao et al., 2007; Suda and Liu, 2007).

2.2.2.2. Chemical methods

Polymers

Polymers are long-chained structures composed of small spliced molecules called monomers. Polymers that are composed of a repeated monomer are called homopolymers, while those composed of two monomers are called copolymers. Natural and synthetic polymers are used in drug delivery systems. Biodegradable and non-biodegradable polymers are used according to the type of controlled release mechanism. Biodegradable polymers are non-water soluble, and undergo chemical or physical change in biologic environments (Tuncay and Calis, 1999). Polyamides, dextran, and chitosan are examples of biodegradable polymers. On the other hand, non-biodegradable polymers are not degraded in biological environments; hydrophilic polymers are hydrogels, which are non-water soluble and swell in water, while hydrophobic polymers are non-water soluble and do not swell. Examples of hydrophilic hydrogel polymers include polyvinylalcohol, polyvinylacetate, polyethyleneglycol, polyacrylic acid, polyhydroxyethyl methacrylate, and polymethacrylic acid. Examples of hydrophobic polymers include silicones, and polyethylene vinyl acetate. Polymers such as ethyl cellulose (EC), hydroxypropyl methyl cellulose (HPMC), cellulose acetate phthalate (CAP), and eudragit derivatives are commonly used in controlled release systems (Tuncay and Calis, 1999).

Selection and design of a polymer is difficult due to structural differences; achieving the desired chemical, mechanical, and biological functions requires understanding of the characteristics and surface of a polymer. For polymer selection, in addition to its physicochemical characteristics, characterization of extensive biochemical characteristics and preclinical tests are required to demonstrate its reliability (Pillai and Panchagnula, 2001).

The physical properties of a polymer carrier, such as hydrophilicity, surface charge, permeability and diffusibility, biocompatibility with tissue and blood (Pillai and Panchagnula, 2001).

For successful delivery, polymers should package DNA in small sizes. Thus, extracellular and intracellular stability of DNA is increased; cellular uptake by endocytosisis enabled; and, by transporting it to the nucleus, the active form of DNA can be released within the nucleus (Mrsny, 2005).

Polymeric gene transporters deliver genetic material through electrostatic interactions with nano-sized polyplexes for gene therapy (Kim et al., 2011).

A synthetic gene delivery system: [1] should protect the negatively-charged phosphate DNA skeleton against anionic cell surface from load repulsion, [2] should be condensed to suitable length intervals of DNA with a macromolecular structure for cellular internalization (condensing at nanometer size for receptor compatible endocytosis or condensing at micrometer size for phagocytosis); and [3] should protect DNA from all extracellular and intracellular nuclease degradations. To meet this need, researchers concentrated on three strategies: electrostatic interaction, encapsulation, and adsorption (Wong et al., 2007).

Electrostatic interaction

The majority of polymeric vectors presently in use form complexes with negatively charged DNA by electrostatic interaction. All polymers have amino groups. At adequate nitrogen–phosphate ratio, the polymer and the DNA form nanocomplexes, which allows both cellular DNA uptake and also protects the DNA from nuclease enzyme (Wong et al., 2007).

Encapsulation

An alternative to electrostatic condensation of DNA is encapsulation of DNA with a biodegradable polymer. Polymers that have an ester linkage in their structures (like polyesters) are hydrolytically degraded to short oligomeric and monomeric compounds, which are more easily discharged from the body. Furthermore, the degradation mechanism and DNA release can be controlled by changing the physicochemical characteristics and composition of the polymer. DNA is protected from enzymatic degradation by encapsulation (Wong et al., 2007) (Figure 5).

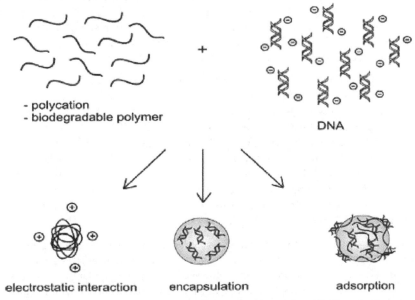

Figure 5. Gene packaging—The three main strategies employed to package DNA are *via* (1) electrostatic interaction, (2) encapsulation within or (3) adsorption onto biodegradable nano- or microspheres (Wong et al., 2007).

Adsorption

Alternative DNA packaging methods, such as adsorption techniques, were developed to overcome the limitations of encapsulation methods. DNA adsorption represents the combination of the above mention two models. In this method, DNA is conjugated to the surface of biodegradable cationic particles, or is electrostatically adsorbed due its negative charge. This method prevents the DNA from being exposed to heavy encapsulation conditions, and also increases rapid release DNA (Wong et al., 2007).

Adsorption methods attracted much research interest, as it does not cause immunogenicity, does not require the integration of exogenous genes to host chromosomes, is a simple and cheap method, and is suitable for effective gene delivery. However, low transfection efficiency, some cytotoxic effects, and *in vivo* instabilities are still significant restricting factors in gene therapy. One of the strategies to solve these problems is the synthesis of biologically degradable polymers (Kim et al., 2011).

Liposomes

Liposomes are colloidal drug delivery systems. They are biologic membrane-like sacs in sphere form, formed by one or more lipid layers, and include an aqueous phase. The phospholipid phase consists of principle components like aqueous phase and cholesterol. Liposomes are classified according to the number of layers they contain. The advantages of liposomes include effectiveness at small doses, extended dosing interval, and ideal transport for active substances with a short half-life. Cellular uptake mechanism of active substances in liposomes can be categorized as endocytosis, combination by melting, and adsorption. Liposomes are used for application of carcinogenic, antifungal, antiparasitic, antiviral, and anti-inflammatory drugs, hormones, DNAs, and cosmetics (Bogdansky, 1990).

Cationic lipids, which are used for the entrance of plasmid DNAs in the cell, have been studied for more than 20 years. During this period, many cationic liposome formulations were developed, and were tested as nucleic acid transported in animals and human with phase I and phase II studies. When compared to other gene delivery systems such as viral vectors and transfection agents, cationic liposome delivery systems are more easily formulated and cause no biological damage like viral vectors (Dass and Choong, 2006). Critical parameters that determine the behavior of liposomes in *in vitro* and *in vivo* conditions include size, number of layers, and surface charge. Unilamellar or mutilamellar vesicles can be produced depending on the preparation method; the diameter of these vesicle ranges from 25 nm to 50 μm (Bogdansky, 1990).

Liposomes are divided into three categories according to their charges: cationic, anionic, or neutral. Compared to viral vectors, liposome delivery systems are non-pathogenic and non-immunogenic, with easy of preparation. However, the most important disadvantage of liposomes is short gene expression time and low transgene expression level. Since liposomes are generally non-toxic and non-immunogenic structures, they are considered reliable carriers for gene therapy. Liposome-based gene delivery was first reported by Felgner (1987). In the 1990s, liposomes were used in numerous cationic lipid gene therapy tests.

Liposomes are not as effective as viral vectors in *in vivo* gene delivery, and it is generally difficult for them to transfect targeted gene to selected cells (Miyazaki et al., 2006).

Dendrimers

Dendrimers were first defined in the late 1970s and early 1980s. Dendrimers consist of symmetrical branches projecting from a central core (Dufes et al., 2005; Genc, 2008; Bulut and Akar, 2012). Dendrimers are 10–200 Angstrom in diameter; they are repeating, branched, large spherical molecules, and have functional groups on their surface that can be used as a building block to connect many biological materials (Ward and Baker, 2008). These functional groups determine the variability of dendrimers, whereas branching provides the growth of the structure (Dufes et al., 2005; Bulut and Akar, 2012). As seen in Figure 6, the most important advantages of dendrimers are conjugation of a large number of different molecules on the dendrimer surface, and the conjugation of molecules that will be used for diagnosis and treatment (Ward and Baker, 2008; Dufes et al., 2005).

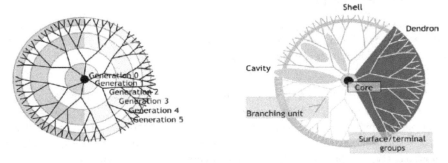

Figure 6. Dendrimer structure. The stepwise synthesis of dendrimers means that they have a well defined hierarchical structure. This hypothetical dendrimer is based on a core with three covalent root attachment points but other common cores have di- or tetracovalent cores. The valency of the core dictates the number of linked dendrons and the overall symmetry of the molecule. The dendrons are synthesised by covalent coupling of the branch units. For each additional layer or *generation* that is being added to the structure the reaction sequence is repeated. In this case the units have two new branching points at which additional units can be attached. (The generation count is not always consistent: normally *generation* 0 refers to the core while sometimes it is used to describe the dendrimer after the first reaction cycle.) The number of branching points, branching angles, and the length of the branching units determine to what extent each generation increases molecular volume vs. surface area. For the higher generations the density of the terminal groups reaches a point where for steric reasons no groups can be added (starburst effect). Dendrimers of higher generation also have a typical molecular density profile under favourable conditions; the high peripheral molecular density establishes a steric outer shell and the lower density at the centre creates cavities which can accommodate guest molecules. (Dufes et al., 2005).

The degree of polymerization of dendrimers is represented by the number of generations (G) of repeated branching cycles during synthesis. Generation number can be easily identified by calculating number of branching points from the core to the outer surface.

The number of branching points increases proportional to dendrimer growth. For example, a dendrimer with no connection points is termed zero generation (G-0) (Bulut and Akar, 2012).

Equal layer groups of dendrimers with an equal number of layers are highly suitable for use in drug delivery due to their perfect encapsulation characteristics and highly controllable chemical behaviors. Drugs can be encapsulated in a dendrimer or can electrostatically or covalently connect to functional groups on the surface (Ward and Baker, 2008; Bulut and Akar, 2012). On the other hand, targeted drug delivery can be achieved by covalent conjugation of the targeting agent to functional groups of dendrimers (Ward and Baker, 2008).

Although the toxicity of dendrimers that form complexes with DNA generally decreases, toxicity and cellular effects of free dendrimers should be taken into account (Dufes et al., 2005).

Cationic lipid compatible systems

Felgner et al. pioneered cationic lipid-based gene transfer (Felgner et al., 1987; Al-Dosari and Gao, 2009). Today, hundreds of lipids have been developed and tested for gene transfer. Lipid-based systems consist of a positively-charged hydrophilic head and hydrophobic tail structure.

Most common hydrophilic head groups are primary, secondary, tertiary amines, or quaternary amine salts. These positively charged sections connect to negatively charged phosphate groups in nucleic acid. The hydrophobic tail consists of aliphatic chain, cholesterol, or steroid rings. The connection region between hydrophilic and hydrophobic sections consists of the bonds that affect biodegradability ratio, such as ether, ester, carbamate, or amid (Al-Dosari and Gao, 2009; Uyechi-O'Brian and Szoka, 2003).

Each lipid has a different sized head group and hydrocarbon tail length, and these characteristics have a significant impact on the formation of DNA–lipid complexes and intake by the cell (Balasz and Godbey, 2010). The transfection effectiveness of cationic lipids varies according to the structure of the lipid and the charge ratio used to form the DNA–lipid complex. Compared to negatively-charged DNA, a positively-charged lipid spontaneously forms structures called lipoplexes. In lipoplex structure, the DNA molecule is encircled by positively-charged lipids, which protect it from extracellular and intracellular nucleases. In addition, due to their positive charges, lipoplexes electrostatically interact with the cell membrane and thus cellular uptake is achieved (Al-Dosari and Gao, 2009; Uyechi-O'Brian and Szoka, 2003).

Cationic lipids such as N-[1-(2,3-dioliloksi)propyl]-N,N,N-trimethlammoniumchloride (DOTMA), [1,2-bis(oliloxy)-3-(trimethlamonnium) propane] (DOTAP), 3β[N-(N_,N_-dimethlaminoethane)-carbamile] cholesterol (DCChol) and dioctadecylamidolysisspermine are used to prepare lipid carriers (Balasz and Godbey, 2010).

The aim of cationic lipid-based gene therapy is to transport plasmid DNA to the cell and thus to achieve the desired protein/peptide transcription and translation. DNA–lipid complex is internalized into the cell through the vesicular path, which is followed by the release of cell cytoplasm of DNA from the lipoplex. Some fractions of the released DNA are transported to the nucleus (Uyechi-O'Brian and Szoka, 2003). Strong DNA–cationic lipid complexes alone are insufficient for gene transfer; however, DNA release before or after transport to the nucleus is critically important (Khalid et al., 2008). Lipid–cationic lipid ratio, cationic lipid–DNA ratio and DNA mount presented to the cell are important parameters that significantly influence transfection efficiency (Hofland et al., 1996).

Although gene expression is provided by cationic lipids, for clinical benefit, the effectiveness, expression time and degree of gene transfer were not found to be adequate. The most significant disadvantages of cationic lipids are structural instability and heterogeneity, inactivation in blood, low effectiveness, and weak targetability when compared to other systems (Navarro et al., 2008).

Cationic lipid-based transfection systems are easy to prepare and reliable; they also have low immunogenicity, and there is no need to classify the size of DNA which will be transported (Mortimer et al., 1999). Many cationic lipid-DNA based systems are effectively taken up by endocytosis; however, the mechanism of DNA release from endosome and translocation to the nucleus are not well known (Mortimer et al., 1999).

2.3. The use of gene delivery systems in treatment

2.3.1. Cancer

Any change in the structure of genes that cause diseases is called mutation. In a mutated cell, variations occur in the sequence of nucleotides. As a result, chemical substances that are produced under the control of the gene have abnormal structure and function. If the gene is associated with the growth, differentiation, or division of cells, then the mutation might cause cancer (Wang et al., 2012). There are two main groups of genes responsible for formation of cancer. These are oncogenes and tumor suppressor genes. Oncogenes are mutated versions of normal genes that are responsible for controlling cell growth. After mutation, they compel the cell to become a cancer cell. There are more than 100 known oncogenes, most of which were identified in human tumors. The "ras gene" is the most widely known and most commonly studied of these genes. After mutation, the ras gene initiates division and cancer formation in cells with the "ras protein" it forms (Luo et al., 2012).

Tumor suppressor genes normally inhibit cell division and tumor development in cells. The mutated forms of these genes cannot inhibit cell division, and instead cause tumor formation. Among these genes, the RB and P53 genes are the most widely known. These genes show their effect with p-RB protein and P53 protein, which are produced under their control. Normally, these proteins inhibit DNA replication and cell division, and regulate apoptosis. If the created genes are mutated, these proteins lose their activity and uncontrolled cell division occurs, which results in cancer development. It was indicated that RB protein was inactive in approximately 40% of human cancers. Similarly, it was found that P53 gene had an abnormal structure in 50% of all tumors (Morandell & Yaffe, 2012).

Gene therapy is based on the principle of replacing damaged genes in diseased cells with corresponding healthy genes that were prepared outside the body. This approach is the most difficult type of gene therapy. Successful treatment involves healthy genes, which are prepared out side the body, targeting specific cells in the body *via* certain transporters (carriers). Current technology has simplified the process of preparing healthy genes. However, the subsequent process of targeting cells remains imperfect (Lagisetty & Morgan, 2012).

In addition to the correction of defective genes, gene therapy includes other treatment principles. In a different method, cancer patients were injected "cytosinedeaminase" enzyme, which is not normally produced in humans, *via* viral carriers,thereby allowing this enzyme to be synthesized in tumor cells (Logue & Morrison, 2012). The drug 5-FC is injected at high doses with no adverse effects; this is converted to 5-FU in tumor cells by cytosine deaminase enzyme. Using this method, effective levels of drug activation are achieved without damaging healthy cells.

In a similar method, carrier viruses injected with "thymidinekinase enzyme gene" found in the herpes simplex viruses reach cancer cells and produce thymidine kinase enzyme in these cells. This enzyme enables the drug ganciclovir, which has no adverse effects on normal body cells, to be active in tumor cells and destroy cancer cells (Etienne-Grimaldi et al., 2012)

Another treatment approach involves inhibition of oncogene proteins that were mentioned above. Oncogenes cause cancer formation *via* the proteins they control. If the production of these proteins is inhibited, their cancer-causing effects will be reduced. One example is the farnesyltransferase enzyme, which plays a role in the formation stages of RB protein. It was reported that new tumor formation was inhibited in patients who were injected with drugs that inhibited the function of this enzyme (Logue & Morrison, 2012). Cancer treatment is the most studied application of gene therapy. A large number of genetic changes occur by the transformation of a normal cell to a neoplastic cell (El-Aneed, 2004).

Tumor suppressor genes eliminate cancer cells through apoptosis, whereas oncogenes accelerate proliferation. For this reason, apoptotic genes and anti-oncogenes are frequently used in cancer treatment. In addition to oncogenes and tumor suppressor genes, chemotherapy and gene therapy were combined *via* a 'suicide gene' strategy. A suicide gene encodes an enzyme that does not belong to mammals, and this enzyme converts non-toxic product into active cytotoxic metabolite in cancer cells. Tumor suppressor genes, anti-oncogenes, and suicide genes target cancer cells at the molecular level. Generally the genes that encode cytokine revive immune response to cancer cells (Wang et al., 2012).

Transformation of a normal cell to a neoplastic cell occurs by multi-mutationary changes of the cells at the genetic level. Due to the complicated nature of cancer, cancer gene therapy involves many therapeutic strategies. These strategies can be analyzed according to two categories: immunogenic and molecular (El-Aneed, 2004).

2.3.2. Immunologic approach

The human immune system has two pathways to respond to foreign antigens. The first pathway includes antibodies secreted by B cells following activation of membrane immunoglobulin via (B cell receptor)-antigen connection. Antibodies are water-soluble proteins that move within the circulatory system to reach the target antigens. T cells, the second immune pathway, directly interact with antibodies without secreting antibody. T cells can produce multiple immune reactions, including cytotoxic effects (Lagisetty & Morgan et al., 2012).

Cancer cells are immunogenic in nature with their cancer antigens, which are intracellular molecules. Therefore, cellular immunity (T-cell mediated), is more important than humoral immunity (B-cell mediated) (Restifo et al., 2012). Normal immune response is not sufficient to eliminate tumor cells. The ability of cancer cells evade immune-system responses is associated with secretion of immunosuppressive factors, down-regulation of antigen expression or MHC (major histocompatibility complex) molecules, and co-stimulation deficiency. One of the common genetic immunotherapy strategies includes transfer of immune-stimulating molecular genes like cytokines. Immune response is created by the activation of interleukin-12 production by tumor cells with numerous components of immune system, particularly including cytotoxic T lymphocytes and natural killer cells (McDonald et al., 2012).

Another immunologic approach involves *in vitro* manipulation of the antigen-presenting cells to produce active tumor antigens. Dendritic cells are the strongest antigen-presenting cells (El-Aneed, 2004). Application of antigen-encoding genes *via* direct vaccination might induce the desired immune response to cancer cells. When injected subcutaneously or intramuscularly, DNA enters local cells like fibroblast and myocytes, and antigen is subsequently produced and secreted. Antigen-presenting cells move towards lymphoid organs where new antigens will be caught and the desired immune response will be initiated (El-Aneed, 2004). Another method to increase the specificity of chemotherapy might be enzyme-encoding enzyme-activate prodrug therapy, which converts non-toxic products into specific and toxic metabolites (Altaner, 2008). This approach is known by many different names, including enzyme prodrug therapy in gene management; suicide gene therapy or enzyme prodrug therapy in virus management; and gene prodrug activation therapy (Scheier et al., 2012). All of these expressions define the same two-step treatment process. The first step involves the targeting and transport of the foreign enzyme to the tumor *via* various pathways. In the second step, non-toxic prodrug is applied and converted to active systolic metabolite. In *in vivo* approaches, expression of foreign genes does not occur in each cell of the target tumor. As a result, the active drug can enter the transduced cell and cell deaths take place, including the cells which do not express enzyme. This procedure is also termed the bystander effect or neighbor cell death effect. In addition, dead cells can induce host immune response due to T cells and NK cells. This therapeutically beneficial effect is known as the slight bystander effect. To increase the effectiveness of enzyme-activated product therapy, therapeutic genes in the vector should be expressed at a sufficiently high ratio to achieve effective prodrug transformation; it should remain as active as possible in order to support the killing mechanisms of the produced systolic metabolite, and the suicide gene should be specifically targeted only to the tumor. These arrangements will also reduce adverse effects (Altaner, 2008).

2.3.3. Cardiovascular disorders

Recombinant adenovirus is one of the most practical vectors for localized gene therapy. In addition, these vectors allow for tissue-specific delivery, and are suitable for re-targeting. Bispecific antibodies were used to coat adenovirus particles by connecting the antibody ligand on the cell receptor surface. Genetic modifications also include gene modifications for some viral coat proteins to change tropisms of adenoviruses (Ji et al., 2012).

Antiviral vectors are the most recently developed vectors; they are HIV-based and generally used for HIV treatment. These vectors have the ability to transfect non-dividing and dividing cells. The effectiveness and reliability of these cells are currently being analyzed (Kozarsky, 2001).

2.3.3.1. Angiogenesis

One exciting recent development is that blood circulation can be provided to ischemic tissues. The development of new blood veins was observed in the region of endothelial growth factor (VEGF) expression (Katz et al., 2012). Gene transfer has advantages for protein therapy, and the use of permanent VEGF is preferred. This method can be fulfilled by a single injection of gene-transfer vector; however, transgene expression of VEGF should last for a limited period, because long-term unregulated VEGF expression might cause abnormal angiogenesis. Therefore, rapid gene expression obtained from adenoviral and plasmid vectors are among the ideal vectors for local delivery of VEGF gene by direct injection (Kozarsky, 2001; Katz et al., 2012).

2.3.3.2. Cardiac failure

Treatment of cardiac failure by gene therapy is still limited, due to the need to determine suitable transgenes and develop effective gene delivery methods to the myocardium. Genes can be directly transported to the heart. However, if these genes have to be transported to larger regions, as in the case of cardiac failure, this method is not regarded as successful. Another method involves transporting gene delivery vectors to coronary veins *via* a catheter; however, some catheter materials inactivate recombinant adenovirus (Kozarsky, 2001; Kairouz et al., 2012).

2.4. Pulmonary disorders

According to some authors, lungs are ideal organs for gene therapy. However, cystic fibrosis and α_1-antitripsin deficiency are the only common disorders with known genetic background for which existing treatments are not curative. Although cystic fibrosis is the first target for pulmonary gene therapy, this method is used to treat many acquired diseases, mainly cancer (Davies et al., 2003).

After the discovery of CTFR in 1989, considerable new progress was made to improve gene transfer system for somatic gene therapy of cystic fibrosis. Cystic fibrosis affects approximately1 in 2500 newborns, which makes it the most common recessive genetic lethal disorder (Davies et al., 2003). Even a copy of a single normal SF gene is sufficient for normal function (Klink et al., 2004). Therefore, somatic gene therapy is relatively straightforward. The only requirement is to provide a cell affected by a gene which makes CFTR protein expression (94). CFTR is cAMP-regulated chloride channel in epithelium cells. Dysfunction of CFTR arises from production deficiency, problems in transport of apical membrane of the cell to the effective region, or due to functional defects (Davies et al., 2003). Air tract epithelium is the most important target among lung diseases that cause mortality and morbidity. In order to address this aim, many gene delivery systems were developed and their effectiveness *in vitro* and *in vivo* was analyzed.

The use of adenoviral vectors gave rise to safety concerns due to low transduction effectiveness and increasing inflammation in human lungs. Tests with cationic liposomes showed low toxicity and effectiveness (Klink et al., 2004).

Some individuals have to be overcome to perform gene therapy. Mucociliary clearance is the primary one of these individuals. Air tract secretions and the mucociliary clearance system act as significant barriers to exogenous gene transfer. The epithelia of a healthy respiratory system create a thin mucus layer required for normal cilia function; however, this layer inhibits gene transfer by cationic liposomes (Davies et al., 2003).

Similarly, a potential gene transfer agent has to overcome the barrier formed by secretions in order to enter the cell. The glycocalyx structure and endocytosis ratio of a cell were defined as the factors that restrict the effectiveness of gene transfer. A number of intracellular process, including endosomal system, cytoplasmic delivery, and the entrance to the nucleus serve as barriers to successful gene transfer. Similarly, host immune response causes problems in the application of gene transfer agents to lungs (Davies et al., 2003).

Adenovirus/CFTR was applied to the nasal epithelia of three patients to treat cystic fibrosis. No viral replication was observed, but mild inflammation was reported. PD returned to normal baseline values in all three patients (Davies et al., 2003). However, one of the problems of this vector system is that low expression levels of viral gene wastes leads to cytotoxic T-cell response that targets vector-containing cells. The fact that adenoviruses are generally air tract pathogens is a both advantageous and disadvantageous. Many potential receivers have circulating antibodies that reduce vector effectiveness and T-cell response. Most importantly, systemic application of adenoviral vectors causes acute and potentially life-threating inflammation responses due to activation of antigen-presenting cells (Klink et al., 2004). On the other hand, when compared to other gene delivery systems, lentiviral vectors are advantageous. Lentiviral vectors are integratable retrovirus derivatives with a high cloning capacity. When suitable regular sequences such as LCS (locus control sections) are used, stable and cell-specific expression can be achieved. When envelope proteins of pseudo-written lentiviral vectors are applied to apical surface with vesicular stomatitis virus, it is not possible to effectively transduce polarized air tract epithelia. Retroviral vectors, pseudo-written with apical membrane-connecting envelope proteins, are used to overcome this problem (Klink et al., 2004).

The first clinical trial of liposome-compatible CFTR gene transfer was reported in 1995. This method involves direct application of DC-Chol/DOPE/CFTR to the nasal epithelia of SF patients. No adverse clinical effects were observed, and nasal biopsy analyses showed no histologic change. Specific mRNA and plasmid DNA were found in five out of eight patients who received CFTR gene vector (Klink et al., 2004).

3. Conclusion

Current gene delivery systems are divided into three categories: viral-based, non-viral based, and combined hybrid systems. Viral gene delivery systems consist of viruses that are modified to be replication-deficient which can deliver genes to the target cells to provide expression. Although viral systems have many advantages, such as long-term expression, and the effectiveness and expression of therapeutic genes, they also have various disadvantages. These disadvantages include risks due to working with viruses, optimization problems when producing large batches, and problems of immunogenicity and toxicity. To date, adenoviruses, retroviruses, and lentiviruses have been used as viral gene carrier vectors. Non-viral systems include physical and chemical methods. In its broadest sense, this refers to delivery of the gene into the cell by applying a physical force in order to increase the permeability of the cell membrane. The most common physical methods are microinjection, electroporation, ultrasound, gene gun, and hydrodynamic delivery. Chemical methods use natural and synthetic compounds are to deliver the gene into the cell. The gene delivery system generally includes polymers, liposomes, dendrimers, and cationic lipids. Non-viral vectors have many advantages, such as easy of synthesis, effective targeting of cell/tissue, low immune response, and potential to use plasmid at desired molecular weight. The biggest disadvantage of non-viral vectors in clinical use is low transfection efficiency. A large number of viral and non-viral gene delivery systems have been developed. Both systems have many advantages and disadvantages. Hybrid systems were developed to combine the advantageous parts of both the individual systems, while minimizing their respective disadvantages, thereby producing a gene therapy with higher effectiveness and low toxicity. The biggest advantage of hybrid systems is that they are less toxic than viral systems, and are not as low-efficient as non-viral systems.

Author details

Erdal Cevher * and Emre Şefik Çağlar
Department of Pharmaceutical Technology, Faculty of Pharmacy, Istanbul University, Beyazıt, Istanbul, Turkey

Ali Demir Sezer
Department of Pharmaceutical Biotechnology, Faculty of Pharmacy, Marmara University, Haydarpaşa, Istanbul, Turkey

4. References

Al-Dosari MS, Gao X. (2009). Nonviral Gene Delivery: Principles, Limitations, and Recent Progress. *American Association of Pharmaceutical Scientist Journal*; 11; 671-681.

Altaner C (2008). Prodrug cancer gene therapy. *Cancer Letters*; 270; 191–201.

Armendáriz-Borunda J, Bastidas-Ramírez BE, Sandoval-Rodríguez A, González-Cuevas J, Gómez-Meda B, García-Bañuelos J. (2011). Production of first generation adenoviral vectors for preclinical protocols: Amplification, purification and functional titration. *Journal of Bioscience and Bioengineering*; 112; 415–421.

Balazs DA, Godbey WT. (2010). Liposomes for Use in Gene Delivery. *Journal of Drug Delivery*; 2011; 1-12.

Bogdansky S. (1990). In Chasin M, Langer R(ed). Natural Polymers as Drug Delivery Systems. *Biodagradable Polymers as Drug Delivery Systems*. Marcel Dekker Inc, ABD. pp: 231-261.

Bulut MO, Akar E. (2012). Dendrimerlerin Önemi Ve Kullanım Alanları. Süleyman Demirel Üniversitesi Teknik Bilimler Dergisi: 1; 5-11.

Bupp K, Roth MJ. (2002). Altering Retroviral Tropism Using a Random-Display Envelope Library. *Molecular Therapy*; 5; 329-335.

Campos SK, Barry MA. (2007). Current Advances and Future Challenges in Adenoviral Vector Biology and Targeting. *Current Gene Therapy*: 7; 189-204.

Conwell CC, Huang L, In K. Taira, K. Kataoka, T. Niidome (ed). (2005). Recent Progress in Non-viral Gene Delivery. *Non-viral Gene Therapy Gene Design and Delivery*. Springer-Verlag Tokyo. Japan; pp: 3-11.

Coughlan L, Alba R, Parker A, Bradshaw AC, McNeish IA, Nicklin SA Baker AH. (2010). Tropism-Modification Strategies for Targeted Gene Delivery Using Adenoviral Vectors. *Viruses*: 2; 2290-2355.

Dass CR, Choong PFM. (2006). Selective gene delivery for cancer therapy using cationic liposomes: *In vivo* proof of applicability. *Journal of Controlled Release*; 113; 155–163.

Davies JC, Geddes DM, Alton EWFW. (2003). Pulmonary Gene Therapy. *Pharmaceutical Gene Delivery Systems*. Eastern Hemisphere Distribution, ABD. Chapter 14.

---

* Corresponding Author

Davis ME. (2002). Non-viral gene delivery systems. *Current Opinion in Biotechnology*: 13: 128–131

Dinh AT, Theofanous T, Mitragotri S. (2005). A Model for Intracellular Trafficking of Adenoviral Vectors. *Biophysical Journal*; 89; 1574–1588.

Dufes C, Uchegbu IF, Schatzlein AG. (2005). Dendrimers in gene delivery. *Advanced Drug Delivery Reviews*; 57; 2177– 2202.

El-Aneed A. (2004). An overview of current delivery systems in cancer gene therapy. *Journal of Controlled Release*; 94; 1– 14.

Escors D, Brecpot K. (2010). Lentiviral vectors in gene therapy: their current status and future potential. *Archivum Immunologiae et Therapia Experimentalis*;58;107–119.

Etienne-Grimaldi MC, Bennouna J, Formento JL, Douillard JY, Francoual M, Hennebelle I, Chatelut E, Francois E, Faroux R, El Hannani C, Jacob JH, Milano G. (2012). Multifactorial pharmacogenetic analysis in colorectal cancer patients receiving 5-fluorouracil-based therapy together with cetuximab-irinotecan. *British Journal of Clinical Pharmacology*; 73; 776-785.

Felgner PL, Gadek TR, Holm M, Roman R, Chan HW, Wenz M, orthrop JP, Ringold GM, Danielsen M. (1987) Lipofection: a highly efficient, lipid-mediated DNA-transfection procedure. *Proceedings of the National Academy of Sciences of U.S.A*; 84; 7413–7417.

Ferrara KW. (2010). Driving delivery vehicles with ultrasound. *Advanced Drug Delivery Reviews*; 60: 1097–1102.

Freed EO. (1997). Retroviruses. *Encyclopedia of Cancer*:4; 167-172

Frenkel V. (2008). Ultrasound mediated delivery of drugs and genes to solid tumors *Advanced Drug Delivery Reviews*; 60: 1193–1208

Gao X, Kim KS, Liu D. (2007). Nonviral Gene Delivery: What We Know and What Is Next. *American Association of Pharmaceutical Scientist Journal*; 9: 92-104.

Genç R. (2008). Dendrimerler: Yeni Nesil Polimerik Ağaçlar. *Katalizör*: 1; 24-28.

Godbey WT, Mikos AG. (2001). Recent progress in gene delivery using non-viral transfer Complexes. *Journal of Controlled Release*: 72; 115–125.

Gönen Korkmaz C. (2008). Gen Transferi-Transfeksiyon: Prostat Kanseri STAMP2 Stabil Hücre Hattının Oluşturulması. *DEÜ Tıp Fakültesi Dergisi*; 22: 39 – 45.

He CH, Tabata Y, Gao JQ. (2010). Non-viral gene delivery carrier and its three-dimensional transfection system. *International Journal of Pharmaceutics*:386; 232–242.

Hofland HEJ, Shephard L, Sullivan SM. (1996). Formation of stable cationic lipid/DNA complexes for gene transfer. *Proceedings of the National Academy of Sciences*; 93: 7305-7309.

Howarth JL, Lee YB, Uney JB, (2010). Using Viral Vectors as Gene Transfer Tools. *Cell Biology Toxicology*; 26; 1-20.

Hu WS, Pathak VK (2000). Design of Retroviral Vectors and Helper Cells for Gene Therapy. *Pharmacological Rewievs*; 52; 494-507.

Smith JG, Wiethoff CM, Phoebe LS, Nemerow GR. (2010). Adenovirus. *Current Topics in Microbiology and Immunology:* 343; 195-224.

Ji J, Ji SY, Yang JA, He X, Yang XH, Ling WP, Chen XL. (2012). Ultrasound-targeted transfection of tissue-type plasminogen activator gene carried by albumin nanoparticles to dog myocardium to prevent thrombosis after heart mechanical valve replacement. *International Journal of Nanomedicine;*7;2911-2919.

Karlsson S, Papayannopoulou T, Schweiger S (1987). Retroviral-mediated transfer of genomic globin genes leads to regulated production of RNA and protein. *Proceedings of the National Academy of Sciences;* 84; 2411-2415.

Katz MG, Fargnoli AS, Pritchette LA, Bridges CR. (2012). Gene delivery technologies for cardiac applications. *Gene Therapy;*19;656-669.

Kairouz V, Lipskaia L, Hajjar RJ, Chemaly ER. (2012). Molecular targets in heart failure gene therapy: current controversies and translational perspectives. *Annals of the New York Academy of Sciences;* 1254; 42-50.

Khalid S, Bond JB, Holyoake J, Hawtin RW, Sansom MSP (2008). DNA and lipid bilayers: self-assembly and insertion. *Journal of the Royal Society Interface;* 5; 241–250.

Khare R, Chen CY, Weaver EA, Barry MA. (2011). Advances and Future Challenges in Adenoviral Vector Pharmacology and Targeting. *Current Gene Therapy:* 11; 241-258.

Kim T, Rothmund T, Kissel T, Kim SW. (2011). Bioreducible polymers with cell penetrating and endosome buffering functionality for gene delivery systems. *Journal of Controlled Release:* 152; 110–119.

Kitamura T, Koshino Y, Shibata F, Oki T, Nakajima H, Nosaka T, Kumagai H. (2003). Retrovirus-mediated gene transfer and expression cloning: powerful tools in functional genomics. *Experimental Hematology;* 31;1007-1014.

Klink D, Schindelhauer D, Laner A, Tucker T, Bebok Z, Schwiebert EM, Boyd AC, Scholte BJ. (2004). Gene delivery systems—gene therapy vectors for cystic fibrosis. *Journal of Cystic Fibrosis;* 3; 203– 212.

Kozarsky KF (2001). Gene Therapy for Cardiovascular Disease. *Current Opinion in Pharmacology* 2001; 1; 197–202.

Lagisetty KH, Morgan RA. (2012). Cancer therapy with genetically-modified T cells for the treatment of melanoma. *Journal of Gene Medicine;* 14; 400-404.

Lin MTS, Pulkininen L, Uitto J, Yoon K. (2000). The Gene Gun: Current Applicationsin Cutaneous GeneTherapy. *International Journal of Dermatology;* 39; 161-170.

Logue JS, Morrison DK. (2012). Complexity in the signaling network: insights from the use of targeted inhibitors in cancer therapy. *Genes & Development;* 26; 641-650.

Luo Y, Kofod-Olsen E, Christensen R, Sørensen CB, Bolund L. (2012). Targeted genome editing by recombinant adeno-associated virus (rAAV) vectors for generating genetically modified pigs. *Journal of Genetics and Genomics;* 39; 269-274.

Majhen D, Ambriovic-Ristov A. (2006). Adenoviral vectors-How to use them in cancer gene therapy? *Virus Research;*119; 121–133.

Mátrai J, Chuah MKL, Vanden Driessche T. (2009). Recent Advances in Lentiviral Vector Development and Applications. *Molecular Therapy*; 18: 477–490.

McDonald PC, Winum JY, Supuran CT, Dedhar S. (2012). Recent developments in targeting carbonic anhydrase IX for cancer therapeutics. *Oncotarget*; 3, 84-97.

Medina-Kauwe LK. (2003). Endocytosis of adenovirus and adenovirus capsid proteins. *Advanced Drug Delivery Reviews*; 55;1485-1496.

Mhashilkar A, Chada S, Roth JA, Ramesh R. (2001). Gene therapy; Therapeutic approaches and implications. *Biotechnology Advances*; 19; 279-297.

Miyazaki M, Obata Y, Abe K, Furusu A, Koji T, Tabata Y,Kohno S. (2006). Technological Advances in Peritoneal Dialysis Research: Gene Transfer Using Nonviral Delivery Systems. *Peritoneal Dialysis International*; 26; 633–640.

Miyazaki Y, Miyake A, Nomaguchi A, Adachi A. (2011). Structural dynamics of retroviral genome and the packaging. *Frontiers in Microbiology*; 2; 2-9.

Mortimer I, Tam P, MacLachlan I, Graham RW, Saravolac EG, Joshi PB. (1999). Cationic lipid-mediated transfection of cells in culture requires mitotic activity. *Gene Therapy*; 6; 403–411.

Mrsny R. (2005). In Amiji MM (ed). Tissue-and Cell-Specific Targeting for the Delivery of Genetic Information. *Polimeric Gene Delivery*. CRC PRESS, USA. pp: 1-30.

Muzzonigro TS, Ghivizzani SC, Robbins PD, Evans CH. 1999. The Role of Gene Therapy: Fact or Fiction? *Clinics in Sports Medicine*; 18; 223-237.

Navarro J, Risco, Toschi M,Schattman G. (2008). Gene Therapy and Intracytoplasmatic Sperm Injection (ICSI) – A Review. *Placenta*; 29; S193–S199.

Niidome T, Huang L. (2002). Gene Therapy Progress and Prospects: Nonviral vectors. *Gene Therapy*; 9; 1647–1652.

Olsen JC, Swanstorm R. (1985). A New Pathway in the Generation of Defective Retrovirus DNA. *Journal of Virology*; 56; 779-789.

Osten P, Grinevich V, Cetin A. (2007). Viral Vectors: A Wide Range of Choices and High Level Services. *HEP*; 178; 177-202.

Pages JC, Danos O. (2003). In Rolland A, Sullivan SM. Retrovectors Go Forward. *Pharmaceutical Gene Delivery Systems*. Eastern Hemisphere Distribution, USA. Chapter 9.

Pillai O, Panchagnula R. (2001). Polymers in drug delivery. *Current Opinion in Chemical Biology*; 5: 447–451.

Pitt WG, Husseini GA, Staples BJ. (2004). Ultrasonic Drug Delivery – A General Review. *Expert Opinion on Drug Delivery*; 1; 37–56.

Prokop A, Davidson JM. (2007). In Lanza R, Langer R, Vacanti J (ed). Gene Delivery into Cells and Tissues. *Princeples of Tissue Engineering*. Elsevier Academic Press, ABD; pp: 493-515.

Restifo NP, Dudley ME, Rosenberg SA. (2012). Adoptive immunotherapy for cancer: harnessing the T cell response. *Nature Reviews Immunology*; 12; 269-281.

Reynolds PN, Feng M, Curiel DT. (1999). Chimeric viral vectors – the best of both worlds? *Molecular Medicine Today*; 4; 25-31.

Robbins PD, Ghivizzani SC. (1998). Viral Vectors for Gene Therapy. *Pharmacology & Therapeutics*; 80; 35–47.

Schatzlein AG. (2003). Targeting of Synthetic Gene Delivery Systems. *Journal of Biomedicine and Biotechnology*: 2; 149–158.

Scheier B, Amaria R, Lewis K, Gonzalez R. (2011). Novel therapies in melanoma. *Immunotherapy*; 3;1461-1469.

Somiari S, Glasspool-Malone J, Drabick JJ, Gilbert RA, Heller R, Jaroszeski MJ, Malone RW. (2000). Theory and *in vivo* Application of Electroporative Gene Delivery. *Molecular Therapy*: 2; 178-187.

Suda T, Liu D. (2007). Hydrodynamic Gene Delivery: Its Principles and Applications. *Molecular Therapy*; 15: 2063–2069.

Sullivan SM. (2003). In Sullivan SM, Rolland A (ed). Introduction to Gene Therapy and Guidelines to Pharmaceutical Development. *Pharmaceutical Gene Delivery Systems.* Eastern Hemisphere Distribution, USA; pp. 17-31.

Tunçay M, Çalış S. (1999) İlaç taşıyıcı sistemlerde kullanılan biyoparçalanabilir sentetik ve doğal polimerler. *FABAD J. Pharm. Sci*; 24: 109-123.

Uyechi-O'Brien LS, Szoka FC (2003). In Rolland A, Sullivan SM (ed). Mechanisms for Cationic Lipids in Gene Transfer. *Pharmaceutical Gene Delivery Systems.* Eastern Hemisphere Distribution, USA. Chapter 4.

Wang X, Cao L, Wang Y, Wang X, Liu N, You Y. (2012). Regulation of let-7 and its target oncogenes (Review). *Oncology Letters*; 3; 955-960.

Ward BB, Baker Jr. JR. (2008). In Majoros IJ, Baker Jr. JR (ed). Targeted Drug Delivery in General, New Technology in Medicine. *Dendrimer Based Nanomedicine.* Pan Stanford Publishing, USA. pp: 1-16.

Willemejane J, Mir LM. (2009). Physical Methods of Nucleic Acid Transfer: General Concepts and Applications. *British Journal of Pharmacology*; 157; 207-219.

Witlox MA, Lamfers ML, Wuisman PI, Curiel DT, Siegal GP. (2007). Evolving gene therapy approaches for osteosarcoma using viral vectors: review. *Bone;* 40; *797-812.*

Wong SY, Pelet JM, Putnam D. (2007). Polymer systems for gene delivery-Past, present, and future. *Progress in Polymer Science*; 32; 799–837.

Wunderbaldinger P, Bogdanov Jr A, Weissleder R. (2000). New approaches for imaging in gene therapy. *European Journal of Radiology*; 34; 156–165.

Yaron Y, Kramer RL, Johnson MP, Evans MI. (1997). Gene therapy: Is the Future Here Yet? *Fetal Diagnosis and Therapy*; 24; 179-197.

Yi Y, Noh MJ, Lee KH. (2011). Current Advances in Retroviral Gene Therapy. *Current Gene Therapy*: 11; 218-228.

Zhang X, Edwards JP, Mosser DM. (2009). The Expression of Exogenous Genes in Macrophages: Obstacles and Opportunities. *Methods in Molecular Biology*; 531; 1-16.

Ziello JE, Huang Y, Jovin IS. (2010). Celular Endocytosis and Gene Delivery. *Molecular Medicine*; 16; 222-229.

Chapter 7

Advanced Drug Carriers Targeting Bone Marrow

Keitaro Sou

Additional information is available at the end of the chapter

1. Introduction

The progression of nanotechnology has produced engineered fine nanoparticles for use in biomedical applications. Drug delivery systems are in a particularly promising field for the use of the unique properties of nanoparticles in biomedical applications. The pharmacokinetics of nanoparticles differs considerably from that of small drug molecules. Therefore, a drug delivery system based on nanoparticles offers a novel direction of drug discovery as well as an improved delivery system for use with conventional drugs. It has been demonstrated that drug delivery systems using nanoparticles are advantageous for stable solubilization of lipophilic drugs, reduced toxicity, inhibition of enzymatic degradation of the drugs, and so on (Moghimi et al., 2001; Papahadjopoulos et al., 1991; Torchilin, 2005). Nanoparticulate drugs show longer circulation time by avoiding renal excretion compared to drugs with small molecules. Moreover, one important technology termed "PEGylation", surface modification of nanoparticles by polyethylene glycol (PEG) chains, prolonged the circulation time (Klibanov et al., 1990; Owens & Peppas, 2006). These long-circulating nanoparticles are effective to increase the passive delivery of anticancer drugs into tumor tissues having leaky blood capillaries with wide fenestrations (Matsumura & Maeda, 1986; Gabizon et al., 1994).

Practical nanotechnology and methodologies to target a specific organ or cell actively are of current interest in the development of further advanced drug delivery systems. For this purpose, the specific interaction which is typically mediated by the receptors on a cell surface must be ascertained. Furthermore, non-specific interactions must be minimized to achieve high selectivity to the target. These specific and selective mechanisms are working constantly in communication, transport, and metabolism processes in living system. Drug carriers offer a platform to target these biological mechanisms. Several results of studies have shown that the bone marrow is the principal organ for the specific uptake of bioparticles such as senescent cells, lipoproteins, and nuclei from erythroid precursor cells through the mononuclear phagocyte system (Hussain et al., 1989a; Qiu et al., 1995; Rankin, 2010). This importance suggests that the phagocytic activity of bone marrow is a potent target of nanoparticle-based drug delivery. In fact, it has been demonstrated that nanoparticles modified with a specific molecule on their surface are distributed selectively into bone marrow tissues (Harris et al. 2010; Mann et al., 2011; Moghimi, 1995; Porter et al., 1992; Schettini et al., 2006; Sou et al. 2007, 2010, 2011a). These bone marrow-specific drug carrier systems are expected to improve diagnostic and therapeutic systems to treat hematopoietic disorders. This chapter presents a review of the specific targeting of bone marrow using nanoparticles as carriers. Furthermore, future aspects of their medical applications are discussed.

2. Functions of bone marrow for blood cell turnover

Bone marrow, a soft and spongy tissue found in the hollow spaces in the interior of bones, constitutes about 4% of the total body weight of adult humans. Progenitor cell (stem cell) lines in the bone marrow produce new blood cells and stromal cells. It has been estimated that as many as 4.9×10^{11} senescent blood cells are eliminated from blood circulation per day in adult humans (Fliedner et al., 1976, 2002). Figure 1 shows that almost as many blood cells are released from bone marrow to maintain a constant number of circulating blood cells. Bone marrow possesses an efficient system that takes nutrients from blood circulation selectively for blood cell production.

Mononuclear phagocyte systems in liver and spleen have been regarded as the main pathway to eliminate senescent blood cells. However, a recent study has shown that mouse bone marrow is an important organ for eliminating white blood cells, especially neutrophils, where neutrophils are ultimately phagocytosed by bone marrow stromal macrophages (Dalli et al., 2012; Furze & Rankin, 2008; Rankin, 2010). The expression of the anti-inflammatory molecule annexin A1 by resident macrophages is necessary for clearance of senescent neutrophils, which are determined by their higher levels of CXCR4 expression and annexin V binding in the mouse bone marrow (Dalli et al., 2012). Consequently, it can be speculated that annexin A1 on bone marrow resident macrophages specifically interacts with senescent neutrophils. High uptake of white blood cells in bone marrow can also be observed in humans following administration of ^{111}In-radiolabeled white blood cells that are administered routinely to humans for the detection of occult infection which is first recognized by secondary manifestations such as increased neutrophils in the circulation or fever of unknown origin. Whole body region-of-interest analysis frequently reveals that 60–70% of the administered white blood cells localize to bone marrow, whereas 30–40% localize to liver and spleen (Sou et al., 2011a).

Chylomicrons are large lipoprotein particles that consist of triglycerides, phospholipids, cholesterol, and proteins. Hussain and co-workers reported that rabbit and marmoset bone marrow had significant uptake of chylomicrons labeled with [^{14}C] cholesterol and [^{3}H] retinol (Hussain et al., 1989b). Perisinusoidal macrophages protruding through the endothelial cells into the marrow sinuses were responsible for accumulation of the chylomicrons in the marmoset bone marrow. In contrast to marmosets, chylomicron clearance from the bone marrow of rats, guinea pigs, and dogs was much less, and the spleen in rats and guinea pigs took up a large fraction of chylomicrons. Consequently, Hussain et al. concluded that the observed differences in chylomicron metabolism result from the presence of perisinusoidal macrophages in bone marrow. It was also believed that the differences between bone marrow and spleen uptake of chylomicrons might provide insights into the role of chylomicron catabolism in these organs, both of which are involved in hematopoiesis. It was speculated that the chylomicrons play a role in the delivery of lipids to the bone marrow and spleen as a source of energy and for membrane biosynthesis or in the delivery of fat soluble vitamins. In addition, bone marrow macrophages, which are associated with erythroblasts in a hematopoietic environment, participate in erythropoiesis control, and engulfment of nuclei from erythroid precursor cells (Chasis & Mohandas, 2008; Qiu et al., 1995; Sadahira & Mori, 1999; Winkler et al., 2010; Yoshida et al., 2005). These features of bone marrow for uptake of senescent blood cells, lipoproteins, and nuclei can be original models of the specific bone marrow targeting system.

The molecular mechanism of the uptake of lipid particles such as lipoproteins and apoptotic cells plays an important role in the transport and metabolism of fats such as cholesterol, triglycerides, and phospholipids. The attractive matter on the molecular mechanism is the ligand-receptor system, which permits the specific interaction of the lipid particles with specific cells in organs. For example, low-density lipoprotein (LDL), a native lipid particles consisting with cholesterol, ApoB-100, phospholipids, and lipophilic vitamins functions to transport cholesterol and vitamins from liver to peripheral tissues. LDL receptors on cells are responsible to the binding and following endocytosis of the LDL where ApoB-100 and ApoE on the LDL act as ligands to the LDL receptors. However, once the LDL is oxidized, scavenger receptors, instead of LDL receptors, act to recognize the oxidized LDL (OxLDL) where ApoB-100 and ApoE are not ligands to the scavenger receptors. Scavenger receptors are typically expressing on the mononuclear phagocyte cells including macrophages, monocytes, and endothelial cells.

It is believed that OxLDL specifically expresses carboxyl groups on its surface and that scavenger receptors bind to the OxLDL via the carboxyl groups as ligands. Phosphatidylserine (PS), a characteristic phospholipid with a carboxyl group on its hydrophilic head group, is a known component of bilayer membrane and is asymmetrically localized in the intracellular membrane of living cells. However, PS is detected specifically on the surface of apoptotic cells that are detectable by the specific binding of annexin V to PS (Koopman et al., 1994; Martinet al., 1995). Consequently, it can be assumed that the asymmetry of the bilayer membrane disappears on the apoptosis of cells and that PS is exposed on the cell surface by the flip-flop. In addition, previous reports describe that the PS is detected on the activated platelets (Thiagarajan & Tait, 1990), senescent erythrocytes (Schroit & Zwaal, 1991), and nuclei from erythroblasts (Yoshida et al., 2005). A specific receptor to PS has been identified on the phagocytes, enabling phagocytes to recognize the biomembrane exposing PS and to eliminate it (Fadok et al., 1992, 2000).

In selective elimination of lipid particles, oxidation of the unsaturated phospholipids plays a critical role. Natural phospholipids have polyunsaturated fatty acids such as linoleic acid and arachidonic acid. These polyunsaturated fatty acids are susceptible to free radical-initiated oxidation. The general process of lipid peroxidation consists of three stages:

initiation, propagation, and termination (Catala, 2006). The initiation phase of lipid peroxidation includes hydrogen atom abstraction by which radicals such as hydroxyl (•OH) react with polyunsaturated fatty acids to produce a lipid radical (L•), which in turn reacts with molecular oxygen to form a lipid peroxyl radical (LOO•). The LOO• can abstract hydrogen from an adjacent fatty acid to produce a lipid hydroperoxide (LOOH) and a second lipid radical (Catala, 2006). The LOOH thus formed can suffer reductive cleavage by reduced metals such as Fe^{2+}, producing a lipid alkoxyl radical (LO•). Both alkoxyl and peroxyl radicals stimulate the chain reaction of lipid peroxidation by abstracting additional hydrogen atoms (Buettner, 1993). Finally, the decomposition of the alkoxyl radical produces a terminal carboxyl group. Several kinds of oxidized phospholipids having the terminal carboxyl group have been identified. These oxidized phospholipids are known as ligands or strong agonists to the scavenger receptors, especially CD36 (Gao et al., 2010; Podrez et al., 2002). Further study has indicated that the carboxyl group of oxidized phospholipid is not located in the bilayer membrane but that it extends from the cellular surface like whiskers, in the "Whisker model", to interact with the receptors (Greenberg et al., 2008; Hazen, 2008). This whisker model is expected to be important to design of surface of the drug delivery carrier, which is expected to interact with the receptors.

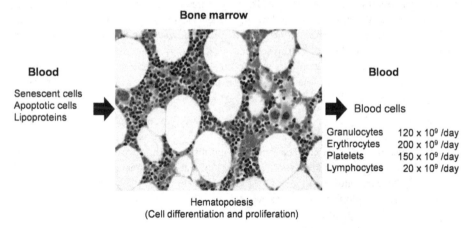

Figure 1. Bone marrow in blood cell turnover. Bone marrow can be regarded as a cell culture system in which nutrients for hematopoiesis can be supplied from circulating blood as senescent cells, apoptotic cells, lipoproteins, and so on. The blood cell turnover in an adult human is 20–200×10⁹/day which is estimated from the life time and total number of cells of each type. The image shows a hematoxylin and eosin stained rabbit bone marrow tissue section, where nuclei of hematopoietic cells are stained darkly and the circular blanks are adipocytes.

3. Engineered carriers for bone marrow targeting

Intravenous injected nano-sized materials are typically eliminated from blood circulation through a mononuclear phagocyte system (MPS). The main organs for uptake of the nanosized materials are the liver and spleen in general. Little attention has been given to the bone marrow though the bone marrow is a part of MPS because the contribution of the bone marrow for uptake of nano-sized materials is believed to be small compared with those of the liver and spleen. However, results of several studies have shown that bone marrow is the most important organ for the uptake of nanoparticles that have been modified with specific molecules on their surface as presented in Table 1.

Carrier type	Targeting	Target cells	Species	Ref
Liposome	Passive (Reduced size)	Macrophages	Dog	Schettini et al., 2006
Liposome	Active (Succinic acid-lipid) and passive (PEG-DSPE)	Macrophages	Monkey, Rabbit, Hamster	Sou et al., 2007; 2010; 2011a
Polystyrene microspheres	Active (Poloxamer 407)	Endothelial cells	Rabbit	Porter et al., 1992; Moghimi, 1995
Polymer complex	Active (Cationic peptide)	Monocytes, T-cell lineage cells	Mouse	Harris et al., 2010
Porous silicon particles	Active (E-selectin thioaptamer ligand)	Endothelium	Mouse	Mann et al., 2011
Nanoparticles of dendritic molecule	Active (Guanidinium group)	Osteoclast precursors	in vitro	Chi et al., 2010
Branched polypeptide	Active (Succinyl group)	Macrophages	in vitro	Szabó et al., 2005

Table 1. Proposed drug delivery carriers targeting bone marrow. These carriers based on surface-modified nanoparticles or polymers target bone marrow phagocytes such as macrophages and endothelial cells.

3.1. Liposomes

Liposomes are the most studied nanoparticles for drug and gene delivery to date. Great interest has been devoted to interaction between liposomes and cellular components *in vitro* and *in vivo*. Allen et al. studied the uptake of liposomes by cultured mouse bone marrow macrophages as a function of liposome composition (Allen et al., 1991). In this study, surface modification with monosialoganglioside (G_{M1}) and polyethylene glycol-lipid (PEG-PE) greatly decreased DPPC liposome uptake by bone marrow macrophages in a concentration-dependent manner. However, incorporation of PS increased liposome uptake by macrophages substantially in a concentration-dependent manner. These observations were correlated with the *in vivo* behavior of liposomes. Consequently, results of this study showed that liposome uptake by bone marrow macrophages is sensitive to the liposome composition, and that PS, which is a biological marker of apoptotic cells, accelerates the uptake of the liposomes. Several other studies have also shown the accelerated uptake of liposomes containing PS or oxidized PS by macrophages, suggesting a similar molecular mechanism on apoptotic cell clearance (Fadok et al., 1992; Greenberg et al., 2006; Ishimoto et al., 2000).

Schettini and co-workers prepared a novel liposomal formulation of meglumine antimoniate, a drug used for treating leishmaniasis, to deliver the drug to the bone marrow (Schettini et al., 2006). The liposomes were produced from distearoylphosphatidylcholine (DSPC), cholesterol, and dicetylphosphate (molar ratio of 5:4:1). The targeting of antimony to the bone marrow was improved approximately three-fold with the small liposomal formulation compared to the large liposome formulation used in dogs with visceral leishmaniasis. These liposomes had no active targeting factor to bone marrow, but the passive targeting of the liposomes to the bone marrow of dogs was improved by the reduction of vesicle size from 1200 nm to 400 nm.

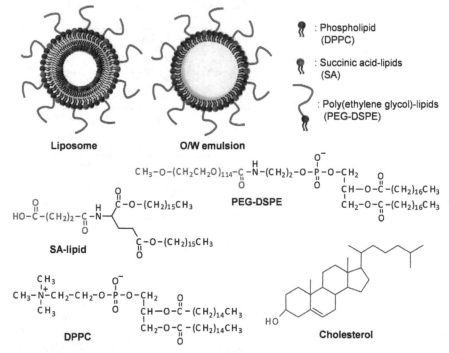

Figure 2. Lipid components of bone marrow-targeted lipid-based nanoparticles. Liposomes composed by DPPC, cholesterol and SA-lipid have high encapsulation capacity for water-soluble materials (Sou 2011b). Oil-in-water (O/W) emulsions have advantage in embedding lipophilic drugs in their oil core. The uptake of lipid-based nanoparticles by bone marrow phagocytes in rhesus monkeys, rabbits, and hamsters is induced by the incorporation of SA-lipid. PEG-DSPE enhances the uptake of the nanoparticles by bone marrow phagocytes passively by preventing the uptake by hepatic and splenic phagocytes (Sou et al. 2007; 2010; 2011a).

Sou et al. found a liposome formulation that is specifically distributed to bone marrow in rabbits and rhesus monkeys (Sou et al., 2007, 2010, 2011a). Figure 2 shows that the bone marrow-targeted liposomes comprise lipids of four kinds: 1,2-dipalmitoyl-*sn*-glycero-3- phosphocholine (DPPC), cholesterol, L-glutamic acid, *N*-(3-carboxy-1-oxopropyl)-, 1,5-dihexadecyl ester (SA-lipid), and poly(ethylene glycol) (PEG). The SA-lipid component has been identified as the active factor leading to their phagocytosis by bone marrow phagocytes, presumably macrophages in rabbits (Sou et al., 2007). Furthermore, as little as 0.6 mol% of PEG-DSPE depressed hepatic uptake but did not depress the bone marrow uptake. PEG-DSPE can be incorporated into the outer surface of preformed liposomes using the post incorporation method (Sou et al., 2000; Uster et al., 1996). Otherwise PEG-DSPE is mixed with other lipid components before preparation of liposomes. The active targeting factor of SA-lipid and passive targeting factor of PEG-DSPE appear to increase the distribution of the liposomes to bone marrow cooperatively.

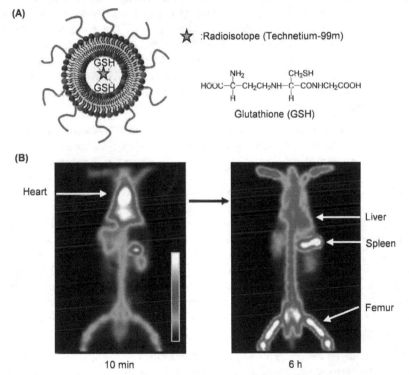

Figure 3. Imaging analysis of animal receiving technetium-99m (^{99m}Tc)-labeled bone marrow-targeted liposomes. (A) Preformed liposomes encapsulated glutathione (GSH) can be radiolabeled with ^{99m}Tc by a remote loading method (Phillips et al., 1992). (B) Gamma camera images of rabbits acquired at 10 minutes and 6 hours after injection of ^{99m}Tc-labeled bone marrow-targeted liposomes (Sou et al., 2007).

The size of the liposomes between 200–270 nm is not a significant factor for uptake by bone marrow. The liposomes were designed to have high entrapment capacity with the interfacial electrostatic interaction to form a unilamellar membrane (Sato et al., 2009; Sou et al., 2003; Sou 2011b). These characteristics are expected to facilitate the application of the bone marrow-targeted liposomes as pharmaceutical carriers to bone marrow.

To evaluate the bone marrow-targeting capability quantitatively, whole body scintigraphic imaging in living animals is a particularly powerful tool (Goins and Phillips 2001, Phillips et al., 2009, 2011). Technetium-99m (^{99m}Tc), which is a good tracer for imaging, is used widely for single photon emission computed tomography with a gamma camera. Figure 3A shows that the ^{99m}Tc labeling of the liposomes encapsulating glutathione (GSH) can be accomplished using a complex of the ^{99m}Tc and GSH in inner aqueous phase of the liposomes (Phillips et al., 1992). Stoichiometric analysis has shown a 2:1 molar ratio of GSH and ^{99m}Tc for stable complex formation (Baba et al., 1999). Images presented in Figure 3B show the distribution of ^{99m}Tc-labeled bone marrow-targeted liposomes in a rabbit at 10 min and 6 hr after intravenous injection (lipid dose: 15 mg/kg b.w.). The image at 10 min is a typical blood pool image representing large blood pool at heart and liver, where the liposomes exist in blood circulation. At 6 hr, the radioactivity at the bone including marrow is increased, although it is decreased at the heart and liver. At this point, 69.7±0.3%ID of bone marrow-targeted liposomes accumulated in bone marrow. At the same time point, the liver and spleen respectively contained much smaller amounts of 11.5±2.88 and 5.0±1.19%ID (Sou et al., 2007).

In addition to the macroscopic and quantitative observation of the distribution of the liposomes by scintigraphic imaging, histological observation by microscopic techniques enables further microscopic localization of the liposomes in bone marrow tissues. Transmission electron microscopy (TEM) is the frequent method used to observe the nanoparticle sample to determine their size and size distribution. Observations of liposomes in cells and tissues can be made using TEM (Sakai et al., 2001). Figure 4 shows that microscopic localization studies demonstrate that bone marrow macrophages are the cellular components responsible for clearance of bone marrow-targeted liposomes from circulation and that they are also responsible for their uptake by the bone marrow. The liposomes are located in the phagosomes and lysosomes of bone marrow macrophages, indicating that the bone marrow macrophages capture the liposomes through phagocytosis. Therefore, it can be speculated that bone marrow-targeted liposomes interact with a receptor on the bone marrow macrophages, which stimulates the phagocytic activity of bone marrow macrophages specifically.

Also flow cytometry analysis is a useful method to determine the targeted cell population quantitatively (Harris et al., 2010). In this method, bone marrow cells will be labeled with markers to identify specific cell subtypes. Flow cytometry analysis might be particularly useful for animal experiment in mice and rats because the markers to identify specific cell subtypes are extensive for these species. Other possible method to identify the cell type is the immunofluorescent staining. The cells type emitting fluorescence from nanoparticle carriers or cargos in tissue section could be determined from the comparative analysis with images of immunofluorescent staining (Longmuir et al., 2009).

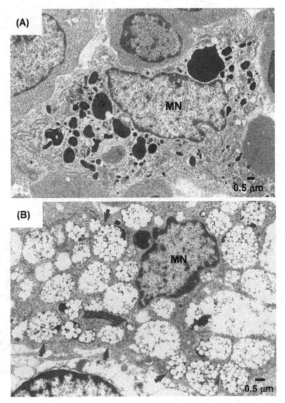

Figure 4. Transmission electron microscopic observations of bone marrow-targeted liposomes. (A) Bone marrow macrophages in a femoral bone marrow tissue section, taken from rabbit. Many phagosomes and lysosomes (electron-dense vacuoles) are visible. (B) Bone marrow macrophages in a femoral bone marrow tissue section, taken from a rabbit at 6 hr after intravenous injection of bone marrow-targeted liposomes (lipids: 15 mg/kg b.w.). Arrows indicate phagosome maturations trapping liposomes with the original diameter (average 270 nm) (Sou et al., 2007). MN: macrophage nucleus

Fluorescent techniques enable detection of the distribution of particular components labeled with fluorescent probes in live cells and tissues microscopically, with exquisite sensitivity and selectivity. For liposomes, both the lipid bilayer membrane (green fluorescent C1-BODIPY C12) and inner aqueous phase (red fluorescent Texas Red- superoxide dismutase, TR-SOD) were labeled with fluorescence probes as shown in Figure 5A. At 6 hr after injection of the dual-labeled bone marrow-targeted liposomes in rabbits (lipids: 15 mg/kg b.w.), the femoral bone marrow section was observed using confocal scanning microscopy. Figure 5B shows that the bone marrow sections have fluorescence from both the TR-SOD and C1-BODIPY C12, where the fluorescence from membrane probes and encapsulated probes are co-localized in bone marrow. This observation revealed that the bone marrow-targeted liposomes and encapsulated agents are distributed at the same locations into bone marrow tissues, clearly indicating that the encapsulated agents were delivered to bone marrow tissues by the liposomes.

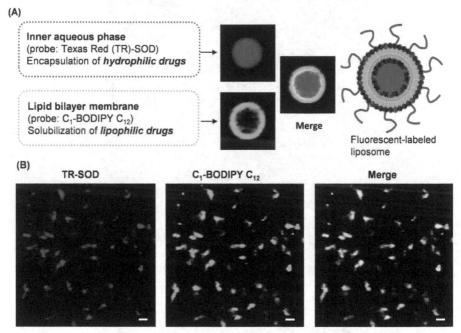

Figure 5. Histological examination of fluorescence delivered into bone marrow tissues using bone marrow-targeted liposomes as carriers. (A) Fluorescence localization in double fluorescence-labeled large multilamellar bone marrow-targeted liposomes with ca. 10 mm diameter. (B) Confocal scanning images of femoral bone marrow taken from a rabbit at 6 hr after i.v. injection of double fluorescence-labeled bone marrow-targeted liposomes (lipids: 15 mg/kg b.w.) (Sou et al., 2007). Scale bars show 20 μm.

3.2. Polymeric nanoparticles

Regarding engineered colloidal particles, Porter and co-workers observed remarkable accumulation of small colloidal particulates (150 nm and smaller diameter) that were coated by the block co-polymer poloxamer-407, a non-ionic surfactant, in the bone marrow after intravenous administration in rabbits (Porter et al., 1992). In this case, the coated colloids were sequestered by the sinusoidal endothelial cells of the bone marrow instead of macrophages. Importantly, no marked uptake was achievable with other block co-polymers having a similar structure to that of poloxamer-407, suggesting the participation of a specific interaction mechanism between the particle and the sinusoidal endothelial cell surface.

Chi and co-workers prepared dendritic amine and guanidinium group-modified nanoparticles for the delivery of model peptide drug into primary osteoclast precursor cells (bone marrow macrophages) (Chi et al., 2010). It can be speculated that positively charged guanidinium groups have favorable interactions with negatively charged functional groups in the cell membrane of osteoclast precursors (Rothbard et al., 2005). Physicochemical interaction between a positively charged drug carrier and a negatively charged cell surface can enhance the cellular uptake in cells of various kinds with a negatively charged surface. However, the selectivity to specific bone marrow cells might be low in practical applications for drug delivery carriers.

Harris and co-workers studied tissue-specific gene delivery via nanoparticle coating (Harris et al., 2010). They prepared cationic nanoparticles with plasmid DNA and then coated their cationic surface with poly anionic poly(glutamic acid)-based peptides with and without cationic insert. Particles coated with a low 2.5:1 peptide:DNA weight ratio (w/w) form two large micro-sized particles that can facilitate specific gene delivery to the liver in mice. However, the same particles coated at a higher 20:1 peptide with cationic insert:DNA (w/w) form small 200 nm particles that can facilitate specific gene delivery to the spleen and bone marrow. They have confirmed that the terminal sequence insert, cationic amino acid sequence G-dP-dL-G-dV-dR-G, to the poly(glutamic acid)-based peptides is a critical factor enhancing bone marrow and spleen-specificity of gene delivery *in vivo*. Regions of luminescence selected around the femur bones showed nearly 40-fold enhancement, and regions around the spleen showed nearly 30-fold enhancement by the cationic insert. Flow cytometry analysis of bone marrow cells from a mouse tail-vein injected with green fluorescent protein-encoding nanoparticles coated with 20:1 w/w peptide with a cationic insert revealed that green fluorescent protein expression relative to the whole population of bone marrow cells is enriched in monocyte and T-cell lineage cells. This system might be available for bone marrow-specific drug delivery and for gene delivery. The molecular mechanism at work in this system is not obvious.

E-selectin is an attractive molecular target for active targeting of a drug carrier to bone marrow because E-selectin is expressed selectively on endothelial cells of adult and fetal hematopoietic organs (Schweitzer et al., 1996). It has been suggested that the E-selectin plays a role in the homing of hematopoietic progenitor cells and that its constitutive expression on endothelial cells of hematopoietic organs is necessary in the initial step of the homing process. Mann and co-workers identified a thiophosphate-modified aptamer (thioaptamer) against E-selectin (Mann et al., 2010). They confirmed that the thioaptamer ligand selectively binds to E-selectin with nanomolar binding affinity (K_D=47 nM) while exhibiting minimal cross reactivity to P-selectin and L-selectin. Recently, they developed porous silicon particles modified with E-selectin thioaptamer ligands to target bone marrow endothelium (Mann et al., 2011). A mice study demonstrated that the accumulation of the porous silicon particles modified with E-selectin thioaptamer ligands in the bone marrow was eight times higher than control porous silicon particles, which were accumulated primarily in the liver and spleen instead of bone marrow. Histological analysis supported the presence of porous silicon particles modified with E-selectin thioaptamer ligands on the endothelial wall of the bone marrow tissue. The molecular target of this ligand-receptor reaction might be readily apparent in this system and be promising for delivering drugs to bone marrow endothelial cells specifically.

Moghimi reviewed the clearance mechanism of particulate materials from the circulation by bone marrow (Moghimi, 1995). The endothelium of bone marrow sinusoids can remove particles from circulation by both transcellular and intercellular routes. The intercellular route occurs through the fenestrate in the endothelial wall. Therefore this mechanism is strongly dependent on the particle size. The intercellular distance is less than 2 nm for the tight junctions in capillaries and less than 6 nm for post-capillary venules under normal conditions (Simionescu et al., 1978; Bundgaard, 1980). In contrast, the size of the fenestrate in the endothelial wall is reportedly 85–150 nm (Huang, 1971). These fenestrated capillaries exist in bone marrow as well as in the liver and spleen. Therefore, the intercellular route is a possible pathway to target bone marrow through circulation. Liposomes consisting of DSPC, cholesterol, PEG(5000)-DSPE, and α-tocopherol prepared in various sizes (136–318 nm diameter) have been tested for organ distribution in rabbits. None of these liposomes show a significant accumulation in bone marrow (Awasthi et al., 2003). Therefore, the passive diffusion of nanoparticles from blood circulation to extravascular space through an intercellular route is not an important factor in bone marrow targeting when no active targeting factor exists. Indeed, based on the proposed drug delivery carrier described above, the surface modification of nanoparticles with specific molecules is a critical factor to achieve bone marrow targeting with nanoparticles, although further study is necessary to ascertain details of its molecular mechanism. Consequently, discovery of receptors specifically expressing in bone marrow tissues facilitates the development of drug carriers targeting bone marrow.

4. Future prospects for bone-marrow-targeted drug carrier systems

The balance between blood cell production and removal in blood cells of each type is important to maintain the number of circulating blood cells. When blood cell production is suppressed, erythrocytopenia, leukopenia, and thrombocytopenia are induced. The blood cell production suppression results from the direct bone marrow dysfunction or indirect factor such as deficiency of the hematopoietic growth factors such as erythropoietin (EPO), granulocyte colony-stimulation factor (G-CSF), and thrombopoietin (TPO). These hematopoietic growth factors, EPO and G-CSF, have been established as recombinant products. Recombinant EPO products are used clinically for the renal anemia patients or autologous blood. These growth factors function with hematopoietic cells in bone marrow, so that a drug delivery system to target bone marrow can be expected to offer an improved therapeutic system.

Recently, Winkler and co-workers reported that the bone marrow macrophages are pivotal to maintain an endosteal hematopoietic stem cell niche and that the loss of such macrophages engenders the egress of hematopoietic stem cells into the blood (Winkler et al., 2010). They administered clodronate-loaded liposomes intravenously to deplete the bone marrow macrophages. After the macrophage depletion, hematopoietic stem cells were found in the blood. These findings provide evidence supporting the critical role that macrophages play in the support of hematopoietic cells in bone marrow. Such specific biology of bone marrow macrophages can present a therapeutic target for the treatment of hematopoietic disorders.

Leishmaniasis is an infectious disease caused by a protozoan parasite that is parasitic on resident macrophages. Promastigotes, which are injected into the skin by a sandfly, are phagocytized by macrophages. Thereafter, promastigotes transform into amastigotes inside macrophages. The amastigotes multiply in cells, including in macrophages, at various tissues. The typical symptoms in leishmaniasis are damage to the spleen and liver, and anemia by damage to bone marrow. Therefore, macrophages in bone marrow as well as in the liver and spleen are target cells in leishmaniasis treatment. Thus several nanoparticles loaded with therapeutic agents such as nanoparticles loaded with amphotericin B (Gupta & Vyas 2007; Nahar et al., 2010), PLGA nanoparticles loaded with saponin (Van de Ven et al., 2012), lipid nanoparticles loaded with oryzalin (Lopes et al., 2012), PLGA nanoparticles loaded with kinetoplastid membrane protein-11 (Santos et al., 2012) have been developed to deliver the drugs in leishmania-infected macrophages. Drug carriers targeting bone marrow, especially bone marrow macrophages, would have a great potential to deliver these therapeutic agents in leishmania-infected macrophages.

The abnormal increase of cancerous cells such as leukemia cells, which are immature white blood cells in bone marrow, suppress normal hematopoiesis. Different from a solid cancer, surgical resection is ineffective as a treatment for leukemia. Most cases of leukemia are treated using chemotherapy. Therapies are typically combined into multi-drug chemotherapy. Drug delivery systems targeting bone marrow can increase the efficacy of such methods. Moreover, bone marrow is sensitive to chemotherapy and radiation therapy. Several pharmaceuticals are available to protect soft tissues from chemotherapy and irradiation. Drug carriers targeting bone marrow offer a promising platform to deliver such pharmaceuticals to bone marrow effectively.

5. Conclusion

Conventional drug delivery to bone marrow is uncontrolled passive diffusion of drugs into bone marrow through blood circulation. The fraction of drugs reaching the target site through such passive diffusion is negligibly small. Bone marrow-targeted drug delivery carriers provide a platform to develop more efficient and safer diagnostic and therapeutic systems. These therapeutic systems can target bone and bone marrow diseases such as rheumatoid arthritis, bone regeneration and repair, bone metastases, osteoporosis, infectious diseases, multiple myeloma, and hematopoietic dysfunction.

Author details

Keitaro Sou
Waseda University, Center for Advanced Biomedical Sciences, TWIns, Tokyo, Japan
Waseda University, Faculty of Science and Engineering, Tokyo, Japan

Acknowledgement

The author thanks Dr. William T. Phillips and Dr. Beth Goins (University of Texas Health Science Center at San Antonio) for collaboration in bone marrow targeting research.

6. References

Allen, T.M.; Austin, G.A.; Chonn, A.; Lin, L. & Lee, K.C. (1991). Uptake of liposomes by cultured mouse bone marrow macrophages: influence of liposome composition and size. *Biochim Biophys Acta*, Vol. 1061, No. 1, pp. 56-64, ISSN 0005-2736

Awasthi, V.D.; Garcia, D.; Goins, B.A. & Phillips, W.T. (2003). Circulation and biodistribution profiles of long-circulating PEG-liposomes of various sizes in rabbits. *Int J Pharm*, Vol. 253, No. 1-2, pp. 121–132, ISSN 0378-5173

Baba, K.; Moretti, J.L.; Weinmann, P.; Senekowitsch-Schmidtke, R. & Ercan, M.T. (1999). Tc-glutathione complex (Tc-GSH): labelling, chemical characterization and biodistribution in rats. *Met Based Drugs* Vol. 6, No. 6, pp. 329–336, ISSN 0793-0291

Buettner, G.R. (1993). The pecking order of free radicals and antioxidants: Lipid peroxidation, α-tocopherol, and ascorbate. *Archives of Biochemistry and Biophysics*, Vol. 300, No. 2, pp. 535-543, ISSN 0003-9861

Bundgaard, M. (1980). Transport pathways in capillaries-in search of pores. *Annu Rev Physiol* Vol. 42, No., pp. 325-336, ISSN 0066-4278

Catalá A. (2006). An overview of lipid peroxidation with emphasis in outer segments of photoreceptors and the chemiluminescence assay. *Int J Biochem Cell Biol*, Vol. 38, No. 9, pp. 1482-1495, ISSN 1357-2725

Chasis, J.A. & Mohandas, N. (2008). Erythroblastic islands: niches for erythropoiesis. *Blood*, Vol. 112, No., pp. 470–478, ISSN 1528-0020

Chi, B.; Park, S.J.; Park, M.H.; Lee, S.Y. & Jeong, B. (2010). Oligopeptide delivery carrier for osteoclast precursors. Bioconjug Chem, Vol. 21, No. 8, pp. 1473-1478, ISSN 1043-1802

Dalli, J.; Jones, C.P.; Cavalcanti, D.M.; Farsky, S.H.; Perretti, M. & Rankin, S.M. (2012). Annexin A1 regulates neutrophil clearance by macrophages in the mouse bone marrow. *FASEB J*, Vol. 26, No. 1, pp. 387-396, ISSN 1530-6860

Fadok, V.A.; Voelker, D.R.; Campbell, P.A.; Cohen, J.J.; Bratton, D.L. & Henson, P.M. (1992). Exposure of phosphatidylserine on the surface of apoptotic lymphocytes triggers specific recognition and removal by macrophages. *J Immunol*, Vol. 148, No. 7, pp. 2207-2216, ISSN 0022-1767

Fadok, V.A.; Bratton, D.L.; Rose, D.M.; Pearson, A.; Ezekewitz, R.A. & Henson, P.M. (2000). A receptor for phosphatidylserine-specific clearance of apoptotic cells. *Nature*, Vol. 405, No. 6782, pp. 85-90, ISSN 0028-0836

Fliedner, T.M.; Steinbach, K.H. & Hoelzer, D. (1976). Adaptation to environmental change: The role of cell-renewal systems. In: Finckh ES, editor. *The Effects of Environment on Cells and Tissues. Excerpta Medica*, ISBN 9021903164, Amsterdam

Fliedner, T.M.; Graessle, D.; Paulsen, C. & Reimers, K. (2002). Structure and function of bone marrow hemopoiesis: mechanisms of response to ionizing radiation exposure. *Cancer Biother Radiopharm*, Vol. 17, No. 4, pp. 405-426, ISSN 1557-8852

Furze, R.C. & Rankin, S.M. (2008) The role of the bone marrow in neutrophil clearance under homeostatic conditions in the mouse. *FASEB J*, Vol. 22, No. 9, pp. 3111–3119, ISSN 1530-6860

Gabizon, A.; Catane, R.; Uziely, B.; Kaufman, B.; Safra, T.; Cohen, R.; Martin, F.; Huang, A. & Barenholz, Y. (1994). Prolonged circulation time and enhanced accumulation in malignant exudates of doxorubicin encapsulated in polyethylene-glycol coated liposomes. *Cancer Res*, Vol. 54, No. 4, pp. 987-992, ISSN 1538-7445

Gao, D.; Ashraf, M.Z.; Kar, N.S.; Lin, D.; Sayre, L.M. & Podrez, E.A. (2010). Structural basis for the recognition of oxidized phospholipids in oxidized low density lipoproteins by class B scavenger receptors CD36 and SR-BI. *J Biol Chem*, Vol. 285, No. 7, pp. 4447-4454, ISSN 1083-351X

Goins, B. & Phillips, W.T. (2001) The use of scintigraphic imaging as a tool in the development of liposome formulations. *Prog Lipid Res* Vol. 40, No. 1-2, pp. 95–123, ISSN 0163-7827

Greenberg, M.E.; Sun, M.; Zhang, R.; Febbraio, M.; Silverstein, R. & Hazen, S.L. (2006). Oxidized phosphatidylserine-CD36 interactions play an essential role in macrophage-dependent phagocytosis of apoptotic cells. *J Exp Med*, Vol. 203, No. 12, pp. 2613-2625, ISSN 1540-9538

Greenberg, M.E.; Li, X.M.; Gugiu, B.G.; Gu, X.; Qin, J.; Salomon, R.G. & Hazen, S.L. (2008). The lipid whisker model of the structure of oxidized cell membranes. *J Biol Chem*, Vol. 283, No. 4, pp. 2385-2396, ISSN 1083-351X

Gupta, S. & Vyas, S.P. (2007). Development and characterization of amphotericin B bearing emulsomes for passive and active macrophage targeting. *J Drug Target*, Vol. 15, No. 3, pp. 206-217, ISSN 1029-2330

Harris, T.J.; Green, J.J.; Fung, P.W.; Langer, R.; Anderson, D.G. & Bhatia, S.N. (2010). Tissue-specific gene delivery via nanoparticle coating. *Biomaterials*, Vol. 31, No. 5, pp. 998-1006, ISSN 0142-9612

Hazen, S.L. (2008). Oxidized phospholipids as endogenous pattern recognition ligands in innate immunity. *J Biol Chem*, Vol. 283, No. 23, pp. 15527-15531, ISSN 1083-351X

Huang, T.S. (1971). Passage of foreign particles through the sinusoidal wall of the rabbit bone marrow – an electron microscopic study. *Acta Pathol Jpn*, Vol. 21, No. 3, pp. 349-367, ISSN 0001-6632

Hussain, M.M.; Mahley, R.W.; Boyles, J.K.; Fainaru, M.; Brecht, W.J. & Lindquist, P.A. (1989a). Chylomicron–chylomicron remnant clearance by liver and bone marrow in rabbits. Factors that modify tissue-specific uptake. *J Biol Chem*, Vol. 264, No. 16, pp. 9571-9582, ISSN 1083-351X

Hussain, M.M.; Mahley, R.W.; Boyles, J.K.; Lindquist, P.A.; Brecht, W.J. & Innerarity, T.L. (1989b). Chylomicron metabolism. Chylomicron uptake by bone marrow in different animal species. *J Biol Chem*, Vol. 264, No. 30, pp. 17931-17938, ISSN 1083-351X

Ishimoto, Y.; Ohashi, K.; Mizuno, K. & Nakano, T. (2000). Promotion of the uptake of PS liposomes and apoptotic cells by a product of growth arrest-specific gene, gas6. *J Biochem*, Vol. 127, No. 3, pp. 411-417, ISSN 0021-9258

Klibanov, A.L; Maruyama, K.; Torchilin, V.P. & Huang, L. (1990). Amphipathic polyethyleneglycols effectively prolong the circulation time of liposomes. *FEBS Lett* Vol. 268, No. 1, pp. 235–237, ISSN 0014-5793

Koopman, G.; Reutelingsperger, C.P.; Kuijten, G.A.; Keehnen, R.M.; Pals, S.T & van Oers, M.H. (1994). Annexin V for flow cytometric detection of phosphatidylserine expression on B cells undergoing apoptosis. *Blood*, Vol. 84, No. 5, pp. 1415-1420, ISSN 1528-0020

Longmuir, K.J., Haynes, S.M., Baratta, J.L., Kasabwalla, N. & Robertson, R.T. (2009). Liposomal delivery of doxorubicin to hepatocytes in vivo by targeting heparan sulfate. *Int J Pharm*,Vol 382, No. 1-2, pp. 222-233, ISSN 0378-5173

Lopes, R., Eleutério, C.V., Gonçalves, L.M., Cruz, M.E. & Almeida, A.J. (2012). Lipid nanoparticles containing oryzalin for the treatment of leishmaniasis. *Eur J Pharm Sci*, Vol. 45, No. 4, pp. 442-450, ISSN 0928-0987

Mann, A.P.; Somasunderam, A.; Nieves-Alicea, R.; Li, X.; Hu, A.; Sood, A.K.; Ferrari, M.; Gorenstein, D.G. & Tanaka, T. (2010). Identification of thioaptamer ligand against E-selectin: potential application for inflamed vasculature targeting. *PLoS One*, Vol. 5, No. 9, pp. e13050, ISSN 1932-6203

Mann, A.P.; Tanaka, T.; Somasunderam, A.; Liu, X., Gorenstein D.G.; Ferrari M. (2011). E-selectin-targeted porous silicon particle for nanoparticle delivery to the bone marrow. *Adv Mater* Vol. 23, No. 36, pp. H278-282, ISSN 1521-4095

Martin, S.J.; Reutelingsperger, C.P.; McGahon, A.J.; Rader, J.A.; van Schie, R.C.; LaFace, D.M. & Green, D.R. (1995). Early redistribution of plasma membrane phosphatidylserine is a general feature of apoptosis regardless of the initiating stimulus: inhibition by overexpression of Bcl-2 and Abl. *J Exp Med*, Vol. 182, No. 5, pp. 1545-1556, ISSN 1540-9538

Matsumura, Y. & Maeda, H. (1986). A new concept for macromolecular therapeutics in cancer chemotherapy: mechanism of tumoritropic accumulation of proteins and the antitumor agent smancs. *Cancer Res.*, Vol. 46, No. 12 Part 1, pp. 6387-6392, ISSN 1538-7445

Moghimi, S.M. (1995). Exploiting bone marrow microvascular structure for drug delivery and future therapies. *Adv Drug Deliv Rev* Vol. 17, No. 1, pp. 61–73, ISSN 0169-409X

Moghimi, S.M.; Hunter, A.C. & Murray, J.C. (2001). Long-circulating and target-specific nanoparticles: theory to practice. *Pharmacol Rev*, Vol. 53, No. 2, pp. 283-318, ISSN 0031-6997

Nahar, M., Dubey, V., Mishra, D., Mishra, P.K., Dube, A. & Jain, N.K. (2010). In vitro evaluation of surface functionalized gelatin nanoparticles for macrophage targeting in the therapy of visceral leishmaniasis. *J Drug Target*, Vol. 18, No. 2, pp. 93-105, ISSN 1029-2330

Owens, D.E. 3rd & Peppas, N.A. (2006). Opsonization, biodistribution, and pharmacokinetics of polymeric nanoparticles. *Int J Pharm*, Vol. 307, No. 1, pp. 93-102, ISSN 0378-5173

Papahadjopoulos, D.; Allen, T.M.; Gabizon, A.; Mayhew, E.; Matthay, K.; Huang, S.K.; Lee. K.D.; Woodle, M.C.; Lasic, D.D.; Redemann, C. & Martin, F.J. (1991). Sterically stabilized liposomes: improvements in pharmacokinetics and antitumor therapeutic efficacy. *Proc Natl Acad Sci USA*, Vol. 88, No. 24, pp. 11460-11464, ISSN 0027-8424

Phillips, W.T.; Rudolph, A.S.; Goins, B.; Timmons, J.H.; Klipper, R. & Blumhardt, R. (1992). A simple method for producing a technetium-99m labeled liposome which is stable *in vivo*. *Nucl Med Biol* Vol. 19, No. 5, pp. 539–547, ISSN 0969-8051

Phillips, W.T.; Goins, B.A. & Bao, A. (2009). Radioactive liposomes. *Wiley Interdiscip. Rev. Nanomed. Nanobiotechnol.* Vol. 1, No. 1, pp. 69–83, ISSN 1939-5116

Phillips, W.T.; Goins, B.; Sou, K. & Bao, A. (2011). Radiolabeled liposomes as theranostic agents. In: *Nanoimaging*, Chapter 4, pp. 71-108, B. Goins and W.T. Phillips (Eds), Pan Stanford Publishing Pte Ltd., ISBN 978-981-4267-09-0, Singapore

Podrez, E.A.; Poliakov, E.; Shen, Z.; Zhang, R.; Deng, Y.; Sun, M.; Finton, P.J.; Shan, L.; Gugiu, B.; Fox, P.L.; Hoff, H.F.; Salomon, R.G. & Hazen, S.L. (2002). Identification of a novel family of oxidized phospholipids that serve as ligands for the macrophage scavenger receptor CD36. *J Biol Chem*, Vol. 277, No. 41, pp. 38503-38516, ISSN 1083-351X

Porter, C.J.; Moghimi, S.M. Illum, L. & Davis, S.S. (1992). The polyoxyethylene/polyoxypropylene block co-polymer poloxamer-407 selectively redirects intravenously injected microspheres to sinusoidal endothelial cells of rabbit bone marrow. *FEBS Lett*, Vol. 305, No. 1, pp. 62-66, ISSN 0014-5793

Qiu, L.B.; Dickson, H.; Hajibagheri, N. & Crocker, P.R. (1995). Extruded erythroblast nuclei are bound and phagocytosed by using a novel macrophage receptor. *Blood*, Vol. 85, No. 6, pp. 1630-1639, ISSN 1528-0020

Rankin, S.M. (2010). The bone marrow: a site of neutrophil clearance. *J Leukoc Biol*, Vol. 88, No. 2, pp. 241-251, ISSN 1938-3673

Rothbard, J.B.; Jessop, T.C. & Wender, P.A. (2005). Adaptive translocation: The role of hydrogen bonding and membrane potential in the uptake of guanidinium-rich transporters into cells. *Adv Drug Deliv Rev*, Vol. 57, No. 4, pp. 495-504, ISSN 0169-409X

Sadahira, Y. & Mori, M. (1999). Role of the macrophage in erythropoiesis. *Pathol Int*, Vol. 49, No. 10, pp. 841–848, ISSN 1440-1827

Sakai, H.; Horinouchi, H.; Tomiyama, K.; Ikeda, E.; Takeoka, S.; Kobayashi, K. & Tsuchida, E. (2001). Hemoglobin-vesicles as oxygen carriers: influence on phagocytic activity and histopathological changes in reticuloendothelial system. *Am J Pathol*, Vol. 159, No. 3, pp. 1079-1088, ISSN 0002-9440

Santos, D.M., Carneiro, M.W., de Moura, T.R., Fukutani, K., Clarencio, J., Soto, M., Espuelas, S., Brodskyn, C., Barral, A., Barral-Netto, M. & de Oliveira, C.I. (2012). Towards development of novel immunization strategies against leishmaniasis using PLGA nanoparticles loaded with kinetoplastid membrane protein-11. *Int J Nanomedicine*, Vol. 7, pp. 2115-2127, ISSN 1178-2013

Sato, T.; Sakai, H.; Sou, K.; Medebach, M.; Glatter, O. & Tsuchida E. (2009). Static structures and dynamics of hemoglobin vesicle (HBV) developed as a transfusion alternative. *J Phys Chem B*, Vol. 113, No. 24, pp. 8418-8428, ISSN 1520-5207

Schettini, D.A.; Ribeiro, R.R.; Demicheli, C.; Rocha, O.G.; Melo, M.N.; Michalick, M.S.; Frézard, F. (2006) Improved targeting of antimony to the bone marrow of dogs using liposomes of reduced size. *Int J Pharm*, Vol. 315, No 1-2, pp. 140-147, ISSN 0378-5173

Schroit, A.J. & Zwaal, R.F. (1991). Transbilayer movement of phospholipids in red cell and platelet membranes. *Biochim Biophys Acta*, Vol. 1071, No. 3, pp. 313-329, ISSN 0005-2736

Schweitzer, K.M.; Dräger, A.M.; van der Valk, P.; Thijsen, S.F.; Zevenbergen, A.; Theijsmeijer, A.P.; van der Schoot, C.E. & Langenhuijsen, M.M. (1996). Constitutive expression of E-selectin and vascular cell adhesion molecule-1 on endothelial cells of hematopoietic tissues. *Am J Pathol*, Vol. 148, No. 1, pp. 165-175, ISSN 0002-9440

Simionescu, N.; Simionescu, M. & Palade G.E. (1978). Open junctions in the endothelium of the postcapillary venules of the diaphragm. *J Cell Biol*, Vol. 79, No. 1, pp. 27-44, ISSN 0021-9525

Sou, K.; Endo, T.; Takeoka, S. & Tsuchida, E. (2000). Poly(ethylene glycol)-modification of the phospholipid vesicles by using the spontaneous incorporation of poly(ethylene glycol)-lipid into the vesicles. *Bioconjug Chem*, Vol. 11, No. 3, pp. 372–379, ISSN 1043-1802

Sou, K.; Naito, Y.; Endo, T.; Takeoka, S. & Tsuchida E. (2003). Effective encapsulation of proteins into size-controlled phospholipid vesicles using freeze-thawing and extrusion. *Biotechnol Prog*, Vol. 19, No. 5, pp. 1547-1552, ISSN 1520-6033

Sou, K.; Goins, B.; Takeoka, S; Tsuchida, E. & Phillips, W.T. (2007). Selective uptake of surface-modified phospholipid vesicles by bone marrow macrophages in vivo. *Biomaterials*, Vol. 28, No. 16, pp. 2655-2666, ISSN 0142-9612

Sou, K.; Goins, B.; Leland, M.M.; Tsuchida, E. & Phillips, W.T. (2010). Bone marrow-targeted liposomal carriers: a feasibility study in nonhuman primates. *Nanomedicine*, Vol. 5, No 1, pp. 41-49, ISSN 1743-5889

Sou, K.; Goins, B.; Oyajobi, B.O.; Travi, B.L.; Phillips, W.T. (2011a). Bone marrow-targeted liposomal carriers. *Expert Opin Drug Deliv*, Vol. 8, No. 3, pp. 317-328, ISSN 1744-7593

Sou, K. (2011b). Electrostatics of carboxylated anionic vesicles for improving entrapment capacity. *Chem Phys Lipids*, Vol. 164, No. 3, pp. 211-215, ISSN 0009-3084

Szabó, R.; Peiser, L.; Plüddemann, A.; Bösze, S.; Heinsbroek, S.; Gordon, S. & Hudecz, F. (2005). Uptake of branched polypeptides with poly[L-lys] backbone by bone-marrow culture-derived murine macrophages: The role of the class a scavenger receptor. *Bioconjug Chem*, Vol. 16, No. 6, pp. 1442-1450, ISSN 1043-1802

Thiagarajan, P. & Tait, J.F. (1990). Binding of annexin V/placental anticoagulant protein I to platelets. Evidence for phosphatidylserine exposure in the procoagulant response of activated platelets. *J Biol Chem*, Vol. 265, No. 29, pp. 17420-17403, ISSN 1083-351X

Torchilin, V.P. (2005). Recent advances with liposomes as pharmaceutical carriers. *Nat Rev Drug Discov*, Vol. 4, No. 2, pp. 145-60, ISSN 1474-1776

Uster, P.S.; Allen, T.M.; Daniel, B.E.; Mendez, C.J.; Newman, M.S. & Zhu, G.Z. (1996). Insertion of poly-(ethylene glycol) derivatized phospholipid into pre-formed liposomes results in prolonged in vivo circulation time. *FEBS Lett*, Vol. 386, No. 2-3, pp. 243-246, ISSN 0014-5793

Van de Ven, H., Vermeersch, M., Vandenbroucke, R.E., Matheeussen, A., Apers, S., Weyenberg, W., De Smedt, S.C., Cos, P., Maes, L. & Ludwig, A. (2012). Intracellular drug delivery in Leishmania-infected macrophages: Evaluation of saponin-loaded PLGA nanoparticles. *J Drug Target*, Vol. 20, No. 2, pp. 142-154, ISSN 1029-2330

Winkler, I.G.; Sims, N.A.; Pettit, A.R.; Barbier, V.; Nowlan, B.; Helwani, F.; Poulton, I.J.; van Rooijen, N.; Alexander, K.A.; Raggatt, L.J. & Lévesque, J.P. (2010). Bone marrow macrophages maintain hematopoietic stem cell (HSC) niches and their depletion mobilizes HSC. *Blood*, Vol. 116, No. 23, pp. 4815-4828, ISSN 1528-0020

Yoshida, H.; Kawane, K.; Koike, M.; Mori, Y.; Uchiyama, Y. & Nagata, S. (2005). Phosphatidylserine-dependent engulfment by macrophages of nuclei from erythroid precursor cells. *Nature*, Vol. 437, No. 7059, pp. 754-758, ISSN 0028-0836

Is Chronic Combination Therapy of HAART and α-ZAM, Herbal Preparation for HIV Infection Safe?

A. A. Onifade, B.H. Olaseinde and T. Mokowgu

Additional information is available at the end of the chapter

1. Introduction

Since discovery of acquired immunodeficiency syndrome (AIDS) and subsequent isolation of the virus (HIV) more than 30 million have been infected [1]. Sub-Saharan Africa was affected most with HIV infection with estimated 2/3rd of the World's HIV infected people. Nigeria is the largest populated country in Africa and it was estimated that about 3 million of the population is infected with human immunodeficiency virus [2]. Thus Nigeria is the second largest country after South Africa with largest HIV infected population in the World [1]. Nigerians like any other people in Africa are favourable to the use of herbal remedies for major illnesses, thus, that HIV infection has no cure medically serves as a catalyst to source for cure in herbal remedies [3].

Herbal remedies which are considered as herbs, herbal materials, herbal preparations and finished herbal products, that contain as active ingredients parts of plants, or plant materials, or combinations thereof used to treat a multitude of ailments throughout the world[1]. Because many HIV patients denied the use of herbal products when asked by medical practitioners, the safety of combination therapy of orthodox drugs and herbal remedies had been a major concern to many people especially when the chemical constituents of the latter product are not known and would be used for a long period [4, 5].

There was no doubt about the effectiveness of herbal remedies in HIV infection. There are many classes of herbal remedies used for HIV infection based on chemical constituent: alkaloids, carbohydrates, coumarins, flavonoids, lignans, phenolic, proteins, quinones, terpenes and tannins. There are many herbal remedies that have been found to inhibit one or more steps in HIV replication [6, 7]. Alkaloids derivatives herbal remedies (e.g. *Ancistrocladus korupensis)* from tropical liana plant inhibit reverse transcriptase and HIV induced cell fusion [8]. p14 (HIV tat regulatory protein that activates transcription of proviral DNA) had been documented to be inhibited by a carbohydrate derivative, pentosan poly-sulphate [9]. A coumarin herbal remedy in form of canolides from tropical forest tree (*Calophyllum lanigerum)* was rated as non-nucleoside reverse transcriptase inhibitor in potency [10]

However, every drug is a potential poison. Thus some herbal remedies are toxic especially when used over a long period. Despite alkaloid containing herbal remedies had been found to be very effective in HIV infection however some michellamines group of alkaloid were found to be cytotoxic thus limiting them for therapeutic use [11]. Quinones and xanthones derivatives herbal remedy were weakly effective against HIV infection and the proved effective medications were cytotoxic [10, 12].

Because HIV infection is a terminal illness, there is an increase in use of herbal remedy in Nigeria [13]. Many HIV patients resulted to herbal therapy at the on-set of HIV diagnosis before commencement of highly active antiretroviral therapy (HAART) while some use it as complementary therapy [14, 15]. The major concern is possible negative drug interaction of herbal therapy and HAART. It was documented that garlic and St John's wort negatively interact with HAART [16].

The fact that many consumers could not distinguish between the safe herbal drugs from potential harmful led to general acceptance or rejection of herbal therapy. A safe herbal therapy may become harmful if used for a long period. African potato (hypoxis) and *Sutherlandia frutescens* have been documented to be harmful when used for a long period with HAART [17]. Even chronic herbal derived vitamins and cannabis use were established to negatively influence hepatic metabolism of HAART components [18].

However, some herbal remedies have been documented to be beneficial when used with orthodox medicines. Coumarin derived herbal remedies decreased drug resistance resulting from HIV mutation associated with non-nucleoside analogue-nevirapine [19, 20]. Some herbal remedies have also shown to decreased toxicity associated with HAART. The hepatic toxicity associated with acetaminophen was reduced by Gentiana manshurica [21]

There are many herbal remedies that are used in Nigeria for HIV infection. Many of them are complementary to HAART. Toxicological studies have been done on many herbal products in Nigeria using animal modelels [22]. Unlike the assumptions that herbal remedies are harmless because of the natural source, many have been found to be toxic [23]. Thus, the researchers are trying to identify the safe herbal remedies and encourage its use while discouraged the harmful herbal products [24].

The beneficial effect of combination therapy of HAART and α-Zam an herbal remedy used as alternative therapy for HIV infection had been documented at acute and sub-acute phase [25]. The use of herbal remedy as alternative therapy to HAART had met a lot of criticisms especially when such medication has not passed through all the phases of drug trial. It is not uncommon that some HIV patients taking HAART are also using alternative herbal remedy simultaneously without the knowledge of both herbal therapist and medical practitioners

[26]. However, the benefits in association with potential toxicity of such complementary therapy at chronic phase needed an evaluation.

2. Materials and method

The materials and method had been described in earlier studies [5, 20, 22]

2.1. A-zam

This is herbal concoction that contained alkaloids, saponins, tannins, cardenolides and possibly anthraquinones [5]

2.2. Highly Active Anti-retroviral Therapy (HAART)

The drugs used in this study were Nevirapine (50mg/kg), Lamivudine (100mg/kg) and Zidovudine (300mg/kg) prepared by grinding the tablets into fine powder.

2.3. Drug preparation

10% of the herbal preparation was made to using tepid distilled water as recommended for use by herbal therapist. A fresh preparation was prepared daily.

2.4. Animals

90 male wistar rats (150-200g body weight) were acclimatised for 7 days before the start of the experiment. Throughout the time of the experiment, they were housed under standard environmental conditions, maintained on a natural light and dark cycle. The animals had free access to rat chow and portable water.

2.5. Drug administration

The freshly prepared herb and HAART were administered orally using oral canula to animals once in 24 hours. The herbal preparation and HAART (nevirapine, zidovudine and lamivudine) were administered concurrently to the groups (40 rats) receiving combination Therapy while another 4 groups (40 rats) received graded concentrations of herbal remedy alone. Animals were deprived of food before drug administration after which they were allowed access to food.

2.6. Experimental procedure

A pilot toxicity study was earlier carried out by a single dose administration of herbal preparation to rats. Results showed that neither mortality nor change in behaviour was observed even at 3200mg/Kg body weight (Onifade et al 2011). 90 wistar rats was randomised divided into 9 groups (10 rats per group) and were administered once daily for 84 days with Herbal concoction of 400mg/kg, 800mg/kg, 1600mg/kg, 3200mg/kg, 400mg/kg+HAART,

800mg/kg+HAART, 1600mg/kg+HAART, 3200mg/kg+HAART, 400mg/kg + HAART (Nevirapine, Zidovudine & Lamivudine), 800mg/kg+ HAART (Nevirapine, Zidovudine & Lamivudine) respectively. The 9th group served as control thus received rat chow and water only. All the animals were allowed to free access chow, water, fresh air and move freely. They were monitored daily for feeding pattern, behavioural or physical changes. 24 hours after the last dose (the 85th day), the diethyl ether anaesthetised animals were bled from the retro orbital plexus for haematological (total white blood cell count, red blood cell count, haemoglobin concentration, platelet count and lymphocyte counts), serum biochemical analysis (electrolytes, urea, creatinine, lipid profile, liver and renal functions tests), fertility profiles (follicle stimulating hormone, progesterone, leutenising hormone, Oestrogen, testosterone and prolactin) and sperm motility test. The liver, kidney, spleen, skin, heart and bone marrow were harvested for histological changes.

3. Results

The results were categorised as follows:

OBSERVATION- No physical or behavioural abnormalities were observed in all the groups of animals throughout the study.

LABORATORY- This is outlined into haematological, clinical chemistry (liver and renal function tests and lipid profile), fertility (fertility profile and sperm analysis) and histological results.

Substance administered	Leucocyte	Red blood cell (x 10⁶)	Haemoglobin (g/dl)	Platelet (x10⁵)	Lymphocyte %	Lymphocyte total
Ratchow& water	6400±334	7.55±1.2	13.4±2.1	3.81±1.9	68±6	4352±124
400mg/kg α-zam	9600±228*	8.34±0.7	15.3±1.8	7.19±2.56	84±9	8064±2365*
800mg/kg α-zam	9400±887*	7.88±0.56	14.3±1.2	9.65±2.85	85.6±8	8084±1890*
1600mg/kg α-zam	9700±934*	7.14±0.34	13.5±1.1	11.09±4.0	72±7.2	6984±459
3200mg/kg α-zam	6200±415	7.42±0.09	14.3±1.5	8.0±2.3	69±4.4	4278±234
0.4g/kg α-zam +HAART	7200±330	7.3±0.8	15.1±1.2	5.7±2.1	72±8.1	4100±350
0.8g/kg α-zam +HAART	8000±720	7.2±0.9	15±1.4	6.8±1.8	70±6.4	4000±270
1.6g/kg α-zam +HAART	6500±635	7.74±0.78	15.0±1.3	7.93±1.8	65±5.9	4225±519
3.2g/kg α-zam ⏐HAART	6600±756	7.22±0.82	14.6±1.6	5.56±1.7	70±3.7	4620±418

*- statistically significant
Rat chow and water only is the control and reference group

Table 1. Showing the Haematological parameters using α- Zam alone and in combination with HAART (mean and standard deviation)

Clinical chemistry- This is divided into 2: Electrolytes, urea and creatinine (Renal functions tests) and Liver functions tests and lipid profile

Substance Administered	Na+	K+	HCO3-	Cl-	Urea	Creatinine
Rat chow and water	142±2.0	4.5±0.31	30±2.2	103±2.4	6.7±0.54	62±2.1
400mg/kg α-zam	140±2.1	4.6±0.22	30±2.1	104±2.3	6.5±0.46	64±2.5
800mg/kg α-zam	144±2.7	4.4±0.27	30±2.0	105±1.9	6.6±0.32	66±1.9
1600mg/kg α-zam	143±1.5	4.5±0.34	28±2.7	103±2.9	6.8±0.45	65±2.3
3200mg/kg α-zam	144±2.0	4.6±0.21	31±0.9	102±2.8	6.9±0.3	63±1.8
0.4g/kg α-zam+HAART	143±1.9	4.6±0.3	27±3.1	104±2.2	6.7±0.5	66±3.2
0.8g/kg α-zam +HAART	142±2.1	4.6±0.2	29±2.9	103±3.4	6.6±0.4	65±2.2
1.6g/kg+HAART α-zam	141±2.9	4.7±0.18	30±1.1	104±2.3	6.6±0.4	64±1.7
3.2g/kg +HAART α-zam	142±1.8	4.7±0.21	31±0.7	103±2.7	6.8±0.55	65±2.1

Rat chow and water only is the control and reference group

Table 2. Showing the Electrolytes, Urea and Creatinine using α- Zam alone and in combination with HAART (mean and standard deviation)

substance administered	albumin	globulins	AST	ALT	Total protein	HDL	Trigly-ceride	LDL	Total cholesterol
Rat chow and water	31±5	52±5	51±7	11±2	83±13	1.1±0.2	0.8±0.3	0.4±0.2	1.8±0.13
400mg/kg α-zam	35±4	58±4	45±7.8	9±2.1	92±4.9	1.2±0.4	0.8±0.3	0.4±0.2	1.9±0.23
800mg/kg α-zam	34±4.4	59±4	49±6.9	12±2.3	93±2.7	1.3±0.3	0.7±0.29	0.4±0.1	1.8±0.19
1600mg/kg α-zam	32±2.3	57±4	54±4.3	14±3.2	89±4	1.1±0.35	0.8±0.36	0.3±0.1	1.8±0.17
3200mg/kg α-zam	30±3.2	61±3*	56±3	13±1.9	91±5	1.4±0.19	0.6±0.38	0.4±0.1	1.9±0.11
0.4g/kg α-zam +HAART	34±3.2	57±6	49±4	12±2.2	86±6	1.3±0.9	0.8±0.26	0.4±0.1	1.7±0.1
0.8g/kg α-zam + HAART	33±2.7	56±5	52±9	12±1.8	85±7	1.3±0.2	0.7±0.3	0.4±0.2	1.7±0.1
1.6g/kg α-zam +HAART	33±2.9	58±4	52±4	11±0.7	91±5	1.2±0.21	0.7±0.27	0.3±0.1	1.7±0.24
3.2g/kg α-zam +HAART	34±1.8	57±5	53±5	12±1.1	91±6	1.3±0.17	0.7±0.26	0.4±0.1	1.8±0.23

Rat chow and water only is the control and reference group

Table 3. Showing the LIVER FUNCTIONS TEST AND LIPID PROFILE using α Zam alone and in combination HAART (mean and standard deviation)

Substance administered	Follicle Stimulating Hormone (miu/ml)	Leutenizing Hormone (miu/ml)	Prolactin (ng/ml)	Estradiol (pg/ml)	Progesterone (ng/ml)	Testosterone (pg/ml)
Rat chow and water only	2.4±0.2	4.4±0.22	16.2±0.4	110±9	10.1±2.3	7.1±0.1
400mg/kg α-zam	2.8±0.1*	4.9±0.23*	16.9±0.3	114±8	10.2±2.1	7.8±0.2*
800mg/kg α-zam	2.7±0.11*	4.8±0.3	16.3±0.2	111±3	9.9±1.9	7.7±0.2*
1600mg/kg α-zam	2.7±0.12*	4.7±0.23	16.5±0.1	112±4	10.0±1.7	7.8±0.3*
3200mg/kg α-zam	2.9±0.2*	4.9±0.27	15.9±0.4	110±5.6	10.1±1.1	7.9±0.32*
0.4g/kg α-zam+HAART	2.7±0.2	4.5±0.3	16.5±0.3	111±6	10.3±2.2	7.5±0.3
0.8g/kg α-zam+HAART	2.6±0.2	4.5±0.1	16.3±0.1	111±9	10.2±1.8	7.5±0.3
1.6g/kg+HAART α-zam	2.6±0.2	4.6±0.21	16.1±0.3	112±1.8	10.2±2.5	7.6±0.23
3.2g/kg+HAART α-zam	2.5±0.2	4.5±0.18	16.3±0.3	112±2.7	10.3±3.1	7.5±0.21

*- statistically significant
Rat chow and water only is the control and reference group

Table 4. Showing the FERTILITY PROFILE using α-Zam alone and in combination with HAART (mean and standard deviation)

Substance administered	Motility (%)	Live/dead (%)	Volume (ml)	Count (x10⁷)
Rat chow& water	66±27	97±2	5.2±0.1	141±21
400mg/kg α-zam	54±22	95±3	5.2±0.1	100±34
800mg/kg α-zam	74±23	95±4	5.2±0.1	130±15
1600mg/kg α-zam	60±12	92±8	5.1±0.1	114±41
3200mg/kg α-zam	72±21	96±3	5.2±0.1	125±31
0.4g/kg α-zam+HAART	67±24	98±4	5.1±0.2	142±27
0.8g/kg α-zam+HAART	69±21	98±3	5.1±0.2	145±36
1.6g/kg α-zam+HAART	66±27	99±2	5.1±0.1	147±27
3.2g/kg α-zam+HAART	64±22	97±4	5.1±0.1	144±9

Rat chow and water only is the control and reference group

Table 5. Showing the **sperm count** using α-Zam alone and in combination with HAART (mean and standard deviation)

Substance administered	Histological Changes-Skin	Histological Changes-Spleen	Histological Changes-Testes	Histological Changes-Liver	Histological Changes-Kidney	Histological Changes-Bone Marrow
Rat chow and water only	No remarkable changes	No remarkable changes	No remarkable changes	No remarkable changes	No remarkable changes	No remarkable changes
400mg/kg α-zam	No remarkable changes	Mild congestion of splenic plexuses	No significant changes	Mild atrophy	Mild tubular atrophy and focal necrosis	Hyper-cellular marrow
800mg/kg α-zam	No remarkable changes	Mild congestion of splenic plexuses	No significant changes	Mild atrophy	Mild tubular atrophy and focal necrosis	Hyper-cellular marrow
1600mg/kg α-zam	No remarkable changes	Mild congestion of splenic plexuses	No significant changes	Mild atrophy	Mild tubular atrophy and focal necrosis	Hyper-cellular marrow
3200mg/kg α-zam	No remarkable changes	Mild congestion of splenic plexuses	No significant changes	Mild atrophy	Mild tubular atrophy and focal necrosis	Hyper-cellular marrow
0.4g/kg α-zam+ HAART	No histological changes	Normal splenic histology	Normal testicular tissue	Normal liver anatomy	Mild focal necrosis	Normal cellularity
0.8g/kg α-zam +HAART	No histological changes	Normal splenic tissue	Normal testicular tissue	Normal liver anatomy	Mild focal necrosis	Normal cellularity
1.6g/kg+HAART α-zam	No remarkable changes	Mild congestion of splenic plexuses	No significant changes	Mild atrophy	Mild tubular atrophy	Hyper-cellular marrow
3.2g/kg+HAART α-zam	No remarkable changes	Mild congestion of splenic plexuses	No significant changes	Mild atrophy	Mild tubular atrophy	Hyper-cellular marrow

Table 6. Showing the histological changes of A-Zam with HAART

4. Discussion

The effect of combination of drugs may manifest in acute or chronic phase. The acute or chronic manifestation of drug toxicity may be mild or lethal which may even result in death.

Although the combination of herbal medications with orthodox drugs had caused beneficial effects like reduction in side effects of the latter but the chronic toxicity is very fatal [21]. From the result above, none of the animal had physical or behavioural impairment thus only laboratory analysis could indicate the potential harmful effects of the combination therapy of HAART and the herbal concoction.

The fact that the animal is feeding or behaving normally does not guaranteed the total well-being especially when taking medication for a long period [25]. Although the physical and behavioural changes of the animal had to be compared with control group but there may be silent damage to cells, tissues or organs that has not manifested as systemic derangements. The health status of the animal taking potential harmful drugs can be confirmed by assessing the major laboratory parameters that are normally grouped into haematological, renal function, liver functions, lipid profiles, fertility profiles and histology of all the major organs [26].

Haematological profiles normally showed the erythrocyte, leucocyte and platelet but the apparent functionality of the immune system (lymphocyte and granulocyte) can also be obtained. When the herbal remedy was used alone in this study, there was leucocytosis with lymphocyte predominance as shown in Table 1. The lymphocyte predominance gradually changed to granulocytes as concentration increases and peak at 1600mg/kg. However, there was normal leucocytes differential irrespective of the dose when combined with HAART. There was also bone marrow hyper-cellularity when herbal medication alone was administered but normalised with HAART as shown by histological changes in Table 6. This confirmed that herbal induced leucocytosis was ameliorated by HAART induced leucopoenia [21, 22]. This showed that combination of this herbal remedy with HAART for HIV infection is beneficial if used for longer period.

Decrease in erythropoiesis (anaemia) that usually manifest early when potential bone marrow suppressive drug was administered for long period was absent with α-zam alone or combination therapy [25]. It was evident from table 1 above that the herbal remedy did not affect erythropoiesis negatively as evidenced by normal haemoglobin concentration and red cell blood count. However, A-Zam herbal remedy is associated with thrombocytosis. The platelet count increased gradually with increase in A-Zam concentration. The combination therapy of A-Zam with HAART caused significant decrease in platelet count. Thus bone marrow suppression effects of HAART components normalised the potential thrombocytosis as shown in Table 1. Chronic use of A-Zam alone or in combination therapy with HAART has no harmful effect on haematological parameters rather ameliorating side effects of associated traditional and orthodox medicines.

The role of kidney in drug excretion cannot be overemphasised. Any negative interaction of drug(s) may affect its clearance from the body. Thus, it is not unusual to noticed renal impairment while other organs and systems perform normally [26]. The combination of two potential harmful drugs may worsen the renal architecture. It was established that many of the antiretroviral therapy are potential nephrotoxic and becomes more pronounced when used in combination with another drug with similar deleterious effect [28]. Renal functions were not impaired when A-Zam alone or in combination with HAART as shown in Table 2 although mild histological changes that reduced with complementary therapy in Table 6 were observed. This study depicted a neither harmful nor beneficial effect of combination of 2 potential harmful drugs used for HIV infection [29].

Drug metabolism is majorly handled by liver. Any toxic drug will likely impair hepatic functions. Some drugs induce hepatic enzymes and apparatuses that accelerate metabolism [30]. This increases fast elimination of the toxic drug from the body. However, some drugs inhibit cytochrome P-450 thus delaying its hepatic clearance of such medication [31]. The danger is combination of cytochrome P-450 inhibitors or inducers. Table 3 showed that both HAART and herbal remedy (A-Zam) are not hepatotoxic alone or in combination. Although there were mild atrophic changes in the liver when A-Zam was used alone but the damage did not caused any significant increase in both cytosolic and mitochondrial hepatic enzymes. This result showed one of the silent cellular injuries that resolved favourably therefore not showing any plasma changes.

The metabolic status of individual is very important. The metabolic disorders associated with lipid derangement in adult are fatal. Some drugs have been noted to cause hyperlipidaemia (especially low density cholesterol and triglyceride) therefore potentiating Raeven's syndrome in adulthood [28]. The coronary index is better with hyperlipidaemia of high density proportion [30]. Any drug that lowers HDL will cause harmful effect and increases coronary index [28]. From the result in table 3, neither A-Zam alone nor its combination with HAART caused any significant harmful hyperlipidaemia. This confirmed that complementary therapy (A-Zam and HAART) is cardio-protective.

Average adult male is conscious of his fertility profile and sperm analysis. Infertility has been a major concern especially when the fault is associated with male. Many drugs affect fertility of male therefore complementary therapy of such medications constitute danger [28]. Spermatogenesis is influenced by hormonal changes. Table 4 showed deranged follicle stimulating hormone (FSH) and testosterone in rats with A-Zam therapy portraying a potential danger. However, combination of HAART with A-Zam ameliorated the fertility hormonal changes which was collaborated with sperm sperm analysis (total sperm count) in Table 5. Plasma and semen analysis showed derangement which did not manifested with significant testicular injury as shown in table 6.

The histology of heart and skin as shown in table in Table 4 were not affected by herbal remedy or its combination with HAART. This confirmed the earlier studies that some herbal remedy are not dermato-toxic [25, 32]. Despite there was no significant changes in liver and renal functions parameters, it was clearly evident there were mild injury to kidney and liver with chronic A-Zam administration alone. However, complementary therapy of HAART and A-Zam reduced the toxic injuries on liver, kidneys and bone marrow. This histological result in confirmed the safety of chronic complementary therapy of HAART and A-Zam as documented in earlier studies [20, 33].

5. Conclusion

This study concluded that the chronic complementary therapy of herbal remedy (A-Zam) with HAART is safe and beneficial as evidenced by side effects amelioration of both orthodox and traditional medicines in wistar rat in this study.

Author details

A. A. Onifade*, B.H. Olaseinde and T. Mokowgu
Immunology Unit, Chemical Pathology Department,
College of Medicine, University of Ibadan, Ibadan, Nigeria

6. References

[1] UNAIDS/WHO (2010) "UN Millenium Goals report 2010"

[2] Federal Ministry of Health (2010) Technical Report on the 2008 National HIV/Syphilis Sero-prevalence Sentinel Survey among pregnant women attending Antenatal Clinics in Nigeria. Department of Public Health National AIDS/STI Control Programme, Abuja: Nigeria

[3] Elujoba AA (2005): Medicinal plants and herbal medicines in the management of opportunistic infections in people living with HIV/AIDS, Our experience so far. *Being a Guest lecture presented at the National Scientific Conference organized by the Nigerian Society of Pharmacognosy (NSP) at Zaria, Nigeria* 2005:11-12

[4] WHO (2002) Traditional Medicine; Growing Needs and Potential, WHO Policy Perspectives on Medicines. *World Health Organization, Geneva;* pp. 1–6.

[5] Onifade A.A, Jewell A.P, Okesina A.B, Ojezele M, Nwanze J.C, Saka G.O, Yong K, Adejumo B. I, Igbe A.P & Egunjoobi A.O (2010) The Phytochemistry and Safety profile of α-Zam, herbal remedy used for treatment of HIV infection in Nigeria, Trop J of Health Sci.18 (1) 40-45

[6] De Clereq (2000) Current lead natural products for the chemotherapy of human immunodeficiency virus infection, Med. Res. Rev 20, 323-349

[7] Kong J M, Goh N K, Chia L S and Chia T F (2003) Recent advances in traditional plant drugs and orchids, Acta Pharmacol. Sin 24, 7-21

[8] Matthee G, Wright AD, König G (1999) HIV reverse transcriptase inhibitors of natural origin. Planta Med; 65: 493–506

[9] Watson K, Gooderham N J, Davies D S and Edwards R J (1999) Interaction of the transactivating protein HIV-1 tat with sulphated polysaccharides, Biochem Pharmacol; 57: 775–83

[10] Dharmaratne HRW, Tan GT, Marasinghe GPK, Pezzuto JM (2002). Inhibition of HIV-1 reverse transcriptase and HIV-1replicationbyCalophyllum coumarins and xanthones, PlantaMed; 68: 86–87

* Corresponding Author

[11] Bringmann G, Wenzel M, Ross Kelly T, Boyd MR, Gulakowski RJ, Kaminsky R (1999) Octadehydromichellamine, a structural analog of the anti-HIV michellamines without centrochirality, Tetrahedron; 55: 1731–40

[12] Cos P, Maes L, Vlientinck A and Pieters L (2008) Plant-derived leading compounds for chemotherapy of human immunodeficiency virus (HIV) infection- an update (1998-2007), Planta Med 74; 1323- 1337

[13] Onifade A A, Jewell AP, Okesina AB, Oyeyemi BO, Ajeigbe KO et al (2012) Attitude of medical practitioners to herbal remedy for HIV infection in Nigeria, J Medicine & Med Sci 3 (1) 30-33

[14] Onifade AA, Jewell1 AP and Okesina AB(2011) virologic and immunologic outcome of treatment to HIV infection with herbal concoction , A-Zam , among clients seeking herbal remedy in Nigeria, Afr J Tradit Complement Altern Med. 8(1):37-44

[15] Nagata JM, Jew AR, Kimeu JM, Salmen CR, Bukusi EA, Cohen CR (2011) 2011 Medical pluralism on Mfangano Island: use of medicinal plants among persons living with HIV/AIDS in Suba District, Kenya, J Ethnopharmacol 17;135(2):501-9

[16] Nyika A (2007) Ethical and regulatory issues surrounding African traditional medicine in the context of HIV/AIDS, Dev World Bioeth, 7 (1):25-34

[17] Mills E, Cooper C and Kanfer I (2005) Traditional African medicine in the treatment of HIV, Lancet Infect Dis, 5(8):465-467

[18] Dhalla S, Chan KJ, Montaner JS, Hogg RS (2006), Complementary and alternative medicine use inBritish Columbia–a survey of HIV positive people on antiretroviral therapy, Complement Ther Clin Pract, 12 (4): 242-248

[19] Yu D, Suzuki M, Xie L, Morris-Natschke S L and Lee K H (2003) Recent progress in the development of coumarin derivatives as potent anti-HIV agents, Med Res Rev; 23: 322–45

[20] Onifade AA Jewell AP, Okesina AB, Yong K, Ojezele M, et al (2011) Effect of combination of HAART and α-zam, herbal preparation for HIV infection in rats J HIV/AIDS Research 3 (2) 38-42

[21] Wang AY, Lian LH, Jiang YZ, Wu YL and Nan JX (2010) Gentiana manshurica Kitagawa prevents acetaminophen-induced acute hepatic injury in mice via inhibiting JNK/ERK MAPK pathway ,World J Gastroenterol; 16 (3):384-91

[22] Abere TA and Agoreyo FO (2006). Antimicrobial and toxicological evaluation of the leaves of Baissea axillaries Hua used in the management of HIV/AIDS, BMC Complement Alter Med.21; 6: 22

[23] Keay RNJ, Onochie CFA, Standfield DP (1964) Nigerian Trees by Federal Department of Forest Research in Nigeria. Offset Lithography of the University Press, Nigeria: 18-19; 65–67

[24] Sofowora A (2002) Plants in African traditional medicine- An overview. Trease and Evans Pharmacognosy, 15th Edition, W B Saunders London, Pages 20-45

[25] Onifade A A, Jewell AP, Okesina AB, Yong K, Ojezele M, et al (2011) chronic toxicity profiles of α-zam, herbal concoction used for HIV infection in Nigeria, Intern Res J Biochem & Bioinformatics 1 (5) 124-130

[26] Onifade AA, Jewell AP, Okesina AB (2011) Are herbal remedies effective in HIV infection? Lambert Academy Publishers (LAP) Page 110-178 ISBN 978-3-8443-2594-2 *(https: www. Lap-publishing.com)*

[27] Ladenheim D, Horn O, Werneke U, Phillpot M, Murungi A, Theobald N, Orkin C (2008)Potential health risks of complementary alternative medicines in HIV patients, HIV Med. ;9(8):653-9

[28] Burtis C A, Ashwood E R and Bruns D E (2008) Tietz fundamentals of clinical chemistry, 6th edition,(Saunders publishers) Missouri,USA page 363-696. ISBN-978-0-7216-3865-2

[29] Bepe N, Madanhi N, Mudzviti T, Gavi S, Maponga CC, Morse GD (2011)The impact of herbal remedies on adverse effects and quality of life in HIV-infected individuals on antiretroviral therapy, J Infect Dev Ctries. 1;5(1):48-53

[30] Maek-a-nantawat W, Phonrat B, Dhitavat J, Naksrisook S, Muanaum R, Ngamdee V, Pitisuttithum P (2009) Safety and efficacy of CKBM-A01, a Chinese herbal medicine, among asymptomatic HIV patients, Southeast Asian J Trop Med Public Health. 40(3):494-501.

[31] Russo R, Autore G and Severino L (2009) Pharmaco-toxicological aspects of herbal drugs used in domestic animals, Nat Prod Commun. 4(12):1777-84.

[32] Liu (2007). The use of herbal medicines in early drug development for the treatment of HIV infections and AIDS, ExpertOpinInvestigDrugs;16 (9):1355-64.

[33] Moltó, José; Miranda, Cristina; Malo, Sara; Valle, Marta; Andreu, Angels; Bonafont, Xavier; Clotet, Bonaventura (2012) Use of herbal remedies among HIV-infected patients: Patterns and correlates, Med Clin (Barc)138:93-8.

Chapter 9

Nanoparticles Toxicity and Their Routes of Exposures

Ahmet Aydın, Hande Sipahi and Mohammad Charehsaz

Additional information is available at the end of the chapter

1. Introduction

1.1. Nanotechnology and nanomaterials

Nanotechnology is a new area that presents small sized materials, structures, devices, and systems in last few decades. We hear about many materials and systems that contain nanomaterials nowadays. Most of the producers present their products as materials having excellent characteristics.

Due to their small size, nanotechnology based materials have unique characteristics such as magnetic, optical, thermal, mechanical, electrical, electron configuration density when compared with macromolecules. Nanomaterials are generally at the 1–100 nm scale and have a vast range of applications such as in medicine, electronics and energy production. Cosmetics, sunscreens, coatings, batteries, fuel additives, paints, pigments, tires and cement are the examples of consumer products that based on nanotechnology. Nanomaterials may also used for special medical purposes such as to produce novel drug delivery systems, to enhance the performance of medical devices, or to produce diagnostic-imaging materials [1].

1.2. Nanomedicine

The European Science Foundation [2] defines 'Nanomedicine' as the science and technology of diagnosing, treating and preventing disease and traumatic injury, of relieving pain, and of preserving and improving human health, using molecular tools and molecular knowledge of the human body. It is discussed under five main sub-disciplines as:

- Analytical tools
- Nanoimaging
- Nanomaterials and nanodevices
- Novel therapeutics and drug delivery systems
- Clinical, regulatory and toxicological issues.

Although most nanotechnology deal with nanoparticles (NPs) sized below 100 nm, in nanomedicine including drug delivery systems particle size is ranged from a few nanometers to 1000 nm. Nanomedicines in practice are generally sized 5–250 nm [3]. In contrast to small sized nanomaterials, this relatively big dimension in drug delivery systems is sufficient to load the drugs onto the particles [4].

1.3. Nanotechnology based novel drug delivery systems

Nanosized drug delivery systems have already entered routine clinical use and Europe has been pioneering in this field [2]. Novel drug delivery systems are improving steadily in recent years. Main goals of these improvements are to achieve targetting of drug more specifically, to reduce toxicity of drug without the interfering of efficacy, to achieve biocompatibility, and to develop safe new medicines [4]. Nanotechnology is extensively used to produce the drug carriers having such kind of advantages, for example, carbon nanotubes (CNTs) are being used in targeted anticancer drug formulations and it has been shown to greatly improve the anticancer activity in animal models. Paclitaxel is another extensively studied anticancer molecule of which NP drug delivery formulation is prepared. This formulation enhanced cytotoxicity of paclitaxel on tumor cells *in vitro* and increased therapeutic efficacy in an animal model [5]

Nanomedicines produced with nanotechnology based engineered materials include proteins, polymers, dendrimers, micelles, liposomes, emulsions, NPs and nanocapsules [3].

2. Nanotoxicology issue of novel drug delivery systems

2.1. Toxicological aspects of NPs

Although nanoscale drug delivery systems are designed to reduce toxicity of drugs and to increase biocompatibility [6], there might be some risks because of the unique characteristics of them. Due to these challenge, "nanotoxicology" term was adopted and defined as the science dealing with the effects of nanodevices and nanostructures in living organisms [7].

Nanoparticles have intrinsic toxicity profiles. Properties of nanoparticles that might increase the toxicity potential include **i)** particle size, **ii)** surface area and charge, **iii)** shape/structure, **iv)** solubility, and **v)** surface coatings [1]. Small size of NPs give rise to a high surface area per unit mass, and this surface area is often correlated with higher biological reactivity. In addition, formation of free radicals such as superoxide anion or hydroxyl radical may also be increased with high surface area. Accordingly oxidative stress may play an important role in NP toxicity especially for metal-based NPs. For example, inflammatory responses to NPs can be explained with these free radical formation [8].

Data on potential human and environmental exposure and dose-response relationship will be necessary to determine potential risks of nanomaterials following inhalation, oral or dermal routes of exposure. Significance of dose, dose rate, dose metric, and biokinetics are very useful parameters for the safety evaluation of newly engineered NPs.

One of the most common entry routes for NPs is inhalation. *In vivo* studies have demonstrated lung inflammation as a result of exposure to NPs [9]. Systemic distribution of NPs has been reported into the blood stream and lymphatic pathways [10].

Another important route for NP entry is the skin, from accidental exposure and use of cosmetics and other topical applications. Although the outer layer of the epidermis, the stratum corneum, protects against environmental insults, tittanium dioxide (TiO$_2$) has been shown to penetrate the stratum corneum and even hair follicles [11]. Penetration of nanosized TiO$_2$ (5–20 nm) into the skin and its interaction with the immune system has also been demonstrated [12].

Dey et al. [13] have demonstrated that nanosized alumina is internalized and significantly increases manganese superoxide dismutase (MnSOD) protein levels, indicating that the effect of alumina may occur, in part, via alteration of cellular redox status. It was also indicated that NP exposure can cause increased proliferation and anchorage-independent transformation in JB6 cells.

De Jong et al. [4] have summarized more striking toxicological effects of NPs in Table 1.

2.2. Proposed mechanism of NP induced toxicity

2.2.1. Oxidative stress

Through many researches, reactive oxygene species (ROS) production is increased at NP exposure. This phenomenon is called oxidative stress. Knaapen et al. [14] suggested three main factors which cause ROS release: (i) active redox cycling on the surface of NPs, particularly the metal-based NPs [15,16] (ii) oxidative groups functionalized on NPs; and (iii) particle–cell interactions, especially in the lungs where there is a rich pool of ROS producers like the inflammatory phagocytes, neutrophils and macrophages. Overproduction of ROS activates cytokines and upregulates interleukin (IL), kinases and tumor necrosis factor-α (TNF-α) as an indicators of proinflammatory signaling processes as a counter reaction to oxidative stress [17].

Miura et al. reported that the expressions of ho-1 and mt-2A, well-known oxidative stress related genes, were up-regulated by nano-silver treatment. These results indicated that apoptosis induction by silver nanoparticles (Ag NPs) may be created by ROS generation [18].

Potential role of oxidative stress as a mechanism of toxicity of AgNPs were evaluated by Hussain et al. [19]. In this study ROS generation following 6 h of exposure to Ag (15, 100 nm) at 0, 5, 10, 25, and 50 g/mL was investigated. The level of ROS in cells increased in a concentration dependent manner and was statistically increased from 10 g/mL concentration. Ag (15, 100 nm) treatment at 25 and 50 g/mL resulted in an approximately 10-fold increase in ROS generation over control levels.

Description of finding, *in vivo*	Particle type
NPs cause pulmonary inflammation in the rat.	All PSP
Later studies show that inflammation is mediated by surface area dose.	SWCNT, MWCNT
NPs cause more lung tumors than fine particles in rat chronic studies. Effect is surface area mediated.	PSP only.
NPs cause progression of plague formation (ApoE-/-mice)	SWCNT, PM2.5
NPs affect immune response to common allergens.	Polystyrene, CB, DEP
NPs can have access to systemic circulation upon inhalation and instillation.	Specific NP, dependent on surface coating.
Description of finding, *in vitro*	
NPs cause oxidative stress *in vivo* and *in vitro*, by inflammatory action and generation of surface radicals.	PSP, NP general, CNT
NPs inhibit macrophage phagocytosis, mobility and killing.	CB, TiO_2
NPs cause platelet aggregation.	PM, SWCNT, fullerenes, latex-COOH surface
NPs exposure adversely affects cardiac function and vascular homeostasis.	PM, SWCNT
NPs interfere with Ca-transport and cause increased binding of pro-inflammatory transcription factor NF-kB.	CB (<100 nm), ROFA, PM2.5
NPs can affect mitochondrial function.	Ambient NP
NPs can translocate to the brain from the nose.	MnO_2, Au, carbon
NPs do affect rolling in hepatic tissue.	CB

NP: nano particle, PSP: poorly soluble particles, DEP: diesel exhaust particles, SWCNT: single wall carbon nanotube, MWCNT: multi walled carbon nanotube, CB: carbon black, titanium dioxide:TiO_2, PM: particulate matter, ROFA: residual oil fly ash, manganese dioxide: MnO_2, PM2.5: particle mass fraction in ambient air with a mean diameter of 2.5 μm.

Table 1. Toxicological effects of engineered and combustion NPs [4].

In another study intractions of AgNPs with human fibrosarcoma (HT-1080) and human skin/carcinoma (A431) cells was undertaken. When the cells was challenged with AgNPs (6.25 μg/mL), signs of oxidative stress such as decrease in oxyradical scavengers including reduced glutathione (GSH) and superoxide dismutase (SOD) as well as increase in lipid peroxidation were seen. Authors mentioned that observed SOD inactivation might be due to generation of peroxy radicals after AgNPs exposure [20].

Induction of oxidative stress and apoptosis by AgNPs in the liver of adult zebrafish was studied by Choi et.al. The results indicated that the levels of malondialdehyde (MDA), a product of cellular lipid peroxidation, and total GSH were increased in the tissues after treatment with AgNPs. The mRNA levels of the oxyradical scavenging enzymes catalase (CAT) and glutathione peroxidase 1a (GPx 1a) were reduced in the tissues. Authors concluded that the increased level of hepatic MDA indicates that AgNPs induced oxyradicals in the liver. In addition, the induction of an endogenous antioxidant, GSH, suggests that the liver tissues respond defensively to the increased level of oxyradicals. Also the reduction of the levels of CAT and GPx may thus result in the accumulation of hydrogen peroxide (H_2O_2) and other oxyradicals [21]. The elevated oxidative stress can damage lipids, carbohydrates, proteins and DNA.

Some investigations reported that TiO_2 increased intracellular ROS generation and MDA concentration in a dose-dependent manner [22,23]. The mechanism by which TiO_2 NPs can generate free radicals is through decreasing the activities of antioxidant enzymes such as SOD, CAT, GPx and glutathione reductase (GR) or intracellular levels of antioxidants such as GSH and ascorbic acid [24-27].

Ramkumar et al. reported that the ratio of GSH/GSSG, a good indicator of the levels of cellular oxidative stress, was found to be decreased dose dependently in the TiO_2 treated cells [22] and thus preserving the GSH-mediated antioxidant defense that is critical for cell survival. It is possible that the loss of GSH may compromise cellular antioxidant defenses and led to the accumulation of ROS and free radicals that are generated in response to exposure to NPs or as by products of normal cellular function.

In line with these findings, Sun et al. investigated the generating of superoxide (O_2^-) and H_2O_2 after long-term exposure to TiO_2 NPs in mice [28]. Results showed that the production rates of O_2^- and H_2O_2 in TiO_2 treated group were significantly higher than those of control. It is also reported that exposure to TiO_2 NPs elicits lipid peroxidation levels in the mouse lung. Since ROS act as second messengers in intracellular signaling cascades [29], the increase in ROS by TiO_2 NPs exposure may play an important role in the modulation of gene expression and resultant inflammation or apoptosis.

Li et al. investigated the oxidative stress associated with gold NPs (Au NPs) in human lung fibroblast cells [30]. It was observed that the Au NPs treated cells generated significantly more lipid hydroperoxides, a positive indicator of lipid peroxidation, than the control cells. In addition, MDA modified protein adducts were evaluated by western blotting as a further verification of the presence of lipid peroxidation. MDA reacts readily with protein or DNA forming adducts which are considered to be highly genotoxic. The results obtained from this study clearly showed that the amount of proteins alkylated by MDA was significantly more in the AuNPs treated samples than that in control samples.

Jia et al. [31] reported that Au NPs can catalyze nitric oxide (NO), a reactive nitrogen species, generation from endogenous S-nitroso adducts with thiol group (RSNOs) whenever they come into contact with fresh blood serum. RSNOs, such as S-nitrosoalbumin, S-nitrosocystein and S-nitrosoglutathione, is a more abundant and stable form of NO in blood since NO has a relative short lifetime in blood because of its reactivity with various blood components. One notable reaction of RSNO dissociation to yield NO is catalyzed by metal ions including Au NPs. NO reacts rapidly with O_2^- and produces a harmful peroxynitrite (ONOO⁻) species. ONOO- can disrupt lipids, DNA, and proteins.

Another study, conducted by Tedesco et al. [32], investigated the oxidative stress and toxicity of AuNPs in *Mytilus edulis* (blue mussel). In this study *M. edulis* was exposed to 750 ppb AuNP (average diameter 5.3 ± 1 nm) for 24 hours to investigate in vivo biological effects of nanoparticles. Traditional biomarkers and an affinity procedure selective for thiol-containing proteins were used to study toxic and oxidative stress responses. Protein thiols can play a role in antioxidant defense and absorption of ROS. *M. edulis* that was exposed to Au NP were displayed a decreased amount of thiol containing proteins in comparison both to controls and those treated with cadmium chloride ($CdCl_2$) (a well known pro-oxidant). This result was consistent with direct oxidation of thiols by ROS induced by AuNP. Also this was supported by more traditional independent measures of biological and oxidative stress such as lysosomal membrane stability and lipid peroxidation. Lysosomal membrane stability measured as neutral red retention time showed a decrease for both Au NP and $CdCl_2$ treatments confirming significant biological stress. The effect was stronger in the case of Au NP than $CdCl_2$. This study also showed that Au NP caused significant lipid peroxidation in digestive gland of *M. edulis*. This study suggested that *M. edulis* is a suitable model animal for environmental toxicology studies of nanoparticles.

Due to the interesting magnetic and electrical properties with good chemical and thermal stabilities, spinal ferrite nanoparticles such as nickel ferrite are used in bioapplications including magnetic resonance imaging, drug delivery and hyperthermia [33-37]. However, little is known about the toxicity of spinal ferrite nanoparticles at the cellular and molecular levels. Ahamed et al. investigated oxidative stress mediated apoptosis induced by nickel ferrite nanoparticles in human lung epithelial (A549) cells [38]. In this study the potential of nickel ferrite nanoparticles to induce oxidative stress was assessed by measuring the ROS and GSH levels in A549 cells. Results showed that the nickel ferrite nanoparticles significantly induced the production of ROS and reduced the level of intracellular GSH in these cells. Further, co-treatment with the antioxidant L-ascorbic acid migrated the ROS generation and GSH depletion due to nickel ferrite nanoparticles exposure. These results indicated that nickel ferrite nanoparticles induced oxidative stress in A549 cells by induction of ROS and depletion of GSH.

2.2.2. Phagocytosis of NPs and inflammation

In respiratory tract, mucociliary clearance removes particulate matter (PM) in <6 μm diameter. Alveolar macrophages engulf and process particles that are not cleared by mucociliary action and coughing. Upon phagocytosis macrophages are activated to release substantial amounts of oxygen radicals, proteolytic enzymes, proinflammatory mediators and growth-regulating proteins. These mediators may lead to both acute and chronic lung inflammation [17].

As other NPs, the toxicity of Ag NPs appears to be driven by their oxidative and inflammatory nature, which then drives genotoxic and cytotoxic outcomes [39].

Carlson et al. [40], investigated the size-dependent cellular interactions of Ag NPs in rat alveolar macrophages (NR8383) cell culture. In this study cells were exposed to 0, 5, 10 and

25 µg/mL Ag NPs (15 nm, 30 nm and 55 nm) for 24 hours and levels of characteristic markers of macrophage activation such as TNF-α, macrophage inhibitory protein-2 (Mip-2), IL-1β and IL-6. The results demonstrated significant levels of TNF-α, Mip-2, IL-1β at 5, 10 and 25 µg/mL for all sizes of Ag NPs comparing to the control group. However, there was no detectable level of IL-6 upon exposure to Ag NPs. Also the cytotoxicity of Ag NPs were evaluated by MTT metabolic activity assay (3-(4,5-Dimethylthiazol-2-yl)-2,5-diphenyltetrazolium bromide) and membrane integrity (lactic dehydrogenase (LDH)) assays. The results of the MTT viability assay showed a significant decrease in mitochondrial function of alveolar macrophages exposed to Ag NPs at 15 nm, 30 nm, or 55 nm for 24 h at concentrations ranging from 10 to 75 µg/mL. It was noted that compared to the smaller nanoparticles (15 and 30 nm), 55 nm did not exhibit significant toxicity until 50-75 µg/mL. Similarly to the MTT data, the results of LDH assay showed a dose-dependent decrease in cell viability compared to control cells after 24 h of exposure to Ag NPs. Ag NPs at 15 and 30 nm exhibited significant cytotoxicity at 10-75 µg/mL, whereas 55 nm required a concentration of 75 µg/mL to markedly decrease cell viability according to LDH assay results.

In another study, Park et al. [41] measured secreted NO levels, as a second messenger in inflammatory signaling, to investigate the correlation of nitrosative-oxidative stress and cytotoxicity induced by Ag NPs. The mouse peritoneal macrophage (RAW264.7) cell line were exposed to 0.2, 0.4, 0.8 and 1.6 µg/mL Ag NPs (68.9 nm) for 24, 48, 72 and 96 hours. Results showed that NO secretion was increased 2-fold over the control group by Ag NPs at 1.6 µg/mL. Also TNF-α level was increased almost 2.8-fold and GSH level was decreased by the same concentration comparing to control group. Ultimately, the phagocytosis of Ag NPs stimulated inflammatory signaling through the ROS generation in macrophages followed by the induced secretion of TNF-α. The increase of TNF-α can cause damage of cell membrane and apoptosis. Authors concluded that ionization of Ag NPs can be a major factor for all these results in cells.

Park et al. [42] also conducted a 28-day oral administration study in mice to investigate toxicity and inflammatory responses of 0.25, 0.5 and 1 mg/kg Ag NPs (42 nm). Evaluation of inflammatory responses by repeated administration of AgNPs were conducted by measurement of pro-inflammatory cytokines (IL-1, TNF-α and IL-6), Th1-type cytokines (IL-12 and interferon-gamma), Th2-type cytokines (IL-4, IL-5, IL-10) and transforming growth factor beta (TGF-β) concentrations in serum. The results showed that IL-1 was significantly increased by Ag NPs. TNF-α and IL-6 were increased almost 2.8-fold and 9.5-fold of the control group, respectively. Also both Th1-type cytokines and Th2-type cytokines showed a significant increase. TGF-β which is known as tissue damage-related cytokines, was also increased in a dose-dependent manner.

Also some studies reported that exposure to TiO$_2$NPs results in pulmonary inflammation, pulmonary edema, macrophages accumulation and pneumonocyte apoptosis [28, 43-45].

Jacobsen et al. [46] studied inflammatory potential after intratracheal instillation of 5 different types of nanoparticles (CB, gold clusters, fullerense C60, SWCNT and quantum dots) for pulmonary effects in apolipoprotein E knockout mice. Results indicated significant increases in mRNA levels of Mip-2, IL-6 and macrophages/monocyte chemoattractant protein-1 (Mcp-1) in lung tissue following 3h and 24h instillation of SWCNT, CB and quantum dots. Also gold and fullerense C60 were found less potent at the three end points when compared to others.

Gosens et al. [47] administered a single dose of 1.6 mg/kg bw of single (50 nm) and agglomerated (250 nm) gold particles in the rat lung by intratracheal instillation. Findings showed that both single and agglomerated particles were taken up by macrophages. Both particles increased inflammatory cells and pro-inflammatory cytokine production. The effects were the least for 50 nm Au NPs.

In line with these findings, Cho et al. [48] reported that Au NPs sized at 13 nm induced acute inflammation and apoptosis in the liver of BALB/c mice after intravenous administration.

Downs et al. [49] measured TNF-α and IL-6 in plasma samples of the rats intraperitoneally treated with silica NPs (15 nm and 55 nm) and crystalline silica (quartz) particles (400 nm). The largest increases in the plasma levels of cytokines were found in the animals exposed to 125 mg/kg (the highest dose) of both the 15 nm and 55 nm silica NPs and the quartz particles. A remarkable increase in the levels of both TNF-α and IL-6 was found in the rats treated with the 15 nm silica NPs at 50 mg/kg dose (middle dose), but not at the 25 mg/kg dose (low dose). Treatment with the 55 nm silica NPs resulted in a 1.5-fold and a 2.3-fold increase in TNF-α and IL-6 levels at 125 mg/kg, respectively, but no change was observed in IL-6 levels at the 25 mg/kg doses. Quartz particles showed a 2.3-fold and 2.1-fold induction of TNF-α and IL-6 production, respectively, at the 100 mg/kg dose.

2.2.3. Genotoxicity

NanoGenotoxicology is yet another new term that was coined to represent the growing trend of research into NP-induced genotoxicity and carcinogenesis [17]. Although there is still no exact correlation between NP-induced genotoxicity and lung cancer from epidemiological studies and *in vivo* rodent experiments, it is pointed out in literature that long-term inflammation and oxidative stress present in tissue can eventually induces DNA damage in cells and tissues. Continuous ROS production in the cell can cause gene mutations/deletions leading to mutagenesis, carcinogenicity, and subsequently development of tumors and cancer. Particularly the metal based NPs like Ag NPs [19], Au NPs [30] and TiO2 NPs [22] are important for that kind of ROS production and genetic damage. As a result of DNA damage induced by NPs, single-strand DNA breaks, double-strand breaks, DNA deletions and genomic instability in the form of increase in 8-hydroxy-2-deoxyguanosine levels are formed [50]. According to Mroz et al.[51] long-term exposure of cells to NPs displayed genome instability under comet assay analysis, altered cell cycle kinetics in flow cytometry and induced protein expression of p53, having a critical role in responding to various stresses that cause DNA damage, and DNA repair-related proteins.

Li et al. [52] studied the genotoxicity of 5 nm Ag NPs using two standard genotoxicity assays, the Salmonella reverse mutation assay (Ames test) and the *in vitro* micronucleus assay. Results demonstrate that 5 nm AgNPs did not induce mutations in five different *S. typhimurium* strains (TA102, TA100, TA1537, TA98 and TA1535). However, Ag NPs displayed concentration-dependent genotoxicity in the human lymphoblast TK6 cell micronucleus assay. Ag NPs produced statistically significant increases in micronucleus frequency in the assay. The data suggest that the *in vitro* micronucleus assay may be more appropriate than the Ames test for evaluating the genotoxicity of the AgNPs.

Ahamed et al. [53] investigated the ability of uncoated or polysaccharide-coated Ag NPs (25 nm) to elicit DNA damage within two types of mammalian cells; mouse embryonic stem cells (mES) and mouse embryonic fibroblasts (MEF). mES and MEF cell lines were exposed to AgNPs at a concentration of 50 μg/mL for a duration of up to 72 hours. Results showed that the proteins p53 and Rad51, responsible for DNA double-strand repair, were up-regulated in two types of mammalian cells. Also in this study DNA double strand breakage induced by AgNPs was confirmed by both immunofluorescent and immunoblot analysis of phospho-H2AX which is ordinarily induced by DNA double-strand breakage. Results indicated that phosphorylation of the histone H2AX were induced by AgNPs. Also this study suggested that the polysaccharide coated AgNPs are more individually distributed and exhibited more severe damage than uncoated AgNPs. This finding may be related with the agglomeration of the uncoated particles and restriction of their cellular distribution.

In an *in vivo* study, Kim et al. [54] conducted a 90-day whole-body inhalation study (6 hours day/5 days a week) to AgNPs (18 nm) in rats at low (0.7×106 particles/cm^3), middle (1.4×106 particles/cm^3) and high (2.9×106 particles/cm^3) doses. After sacrificing of rats, micronucleus induction was measured in the bone marrow according to the test guideline 474 issued by OECD. Authors found out that AgNPs did not affect either the frequency of micronucleated polychromatic erythrocytes (PCE) as an indicator of DNA damage or the PCE / (PCE+NCE) ratio as an indicator of toxicity to bone marrow cells (NCE: normochromatic erythrocytes) in male and female rats. The authors concluded that exposure to AgNPs by inhalation for 90 days does not induce genetic toxicity in male and female rat bone marrow *in vivo*.

Also the same authors conducted an *in vivo* micronucleus assay after 28-day oral administration of Ag NPs. The results were similar to those of inhalation study [55].

A number of studies have shown that TiO2 NPs exhibited genotoxicity in cultured cell lines [56-58]. Kang et al. [59], studied the genotoxic effects of TiO2 NPs (20-100 μg/ml) in human peripheral blood lymphocyte cells using alkaline single cell gel electrophoresis (Comet) and cytokinesis block micronucleus (CBMN) assays. The CBMN assay results showed that the micronuclei frequency increased in a dose-dependent manner. Also cells had a significant olive tail moment which indicates unrepaired DNA strand breaks in comet assay.

Similarly, Wang et al. [60] investigated the toxicity of ultrafine TiO2 particles in cultured human B-cell lymphoblastoid cell line (WIL2-NS). Significant increases in the micronuclei frequency were detected by the CBMN assay in a dose-dependent manner. In the comet assay, 3-fold increase in %Tail DNA were found when the cells were treated with ultrafine TiO_2 at a dose of 65 µg/mL for 24 hours exposure. In the olive tail moment a 5-fold elevation was found at the same dose and exposure duration. Also a linear relationship was determined between the mutation frequency and concentration in the clonal selection assay for the hypoxanthine-guanine phosphoribosyl transferase (HPRT) gene.

Toyooka et al. [61] examined the genotoxicity of TiO_2 NPs (5 nm) and microparticles (<5000 nm) in the lung adenocarcinoma epithelial cell line (A549) based on the phosphorylation of histone H2AX (γ-H2AX) as a new sensitive biomarker for DNA damage. Results showed that TiO_2 particles have the ability to generate γ-H2AX and this was more remarkable with nanoparticles than microparticles.

Contrary to above studies, a number of investigations showed that TiO_2 NPs didn't induce DNA damage and mutation using the Ames test, micronucleus assay, comet assay, and etc. [62-68].

Au NPs are also recognized in their ability to contribute in genotoxicity. Schulz et al. [69] investigated two genotoxic endpoints, alkaline comet assay in lung tissue and micronucleation in PCE of the bone marrow, 72 hours after a single instillation of 18 µg uncoated Au NPs in different sizes (2, 20 and 200 nm) into the trachea of male adult Wistar rats. Results indicated that AuNPs in the different sizes were non-genotoxic and showed no systemic and local adverse effects at the given dose.

Also the genotoxicity of zinc oxide nanoparticles (ZnO NPs), widely used in cosmetics and sunscreens, was evaluated in some studies. Sharma et al. [70] investigated the genotoxicity of these nanoparticles in primary human epidermal karatinocytes using comet assay. Results showed a significant induction in DNA damage in cells exposed to 8 and 14 µg/mL ZnO NPs for 6 hours comparing to control group. Finding demonstrated that ZnO NPs are assimilated by the human epidermal karatinocytes and induce cytotoxic and genotoxic responses.

Also in another study Sharma et al. [71] highlighted the *in vitro* genotoxicity of ZnO NPs in human liver cells (HepG2). Similarly significant increase in DNA damage was observed in cells in the comet assay.

Fen Song et al. [50] analyzed the induction of reticulocyte micronuclei and oxidative DNA damage in ICR female mice after intraperitoneal injection of metal oxides (CuO, Fe_2O_3, Fe_3O_4, TiO_2) and Ag NPs at various doses (0, 1, 3 mg/mouse). The results of the micronucleus assay demonstrated significant increases in micronucleated reticulocyte formation after the intraperitoneal administration of CuO, Fe_2O_3, Fe_3O_4, TiO_2 and Ag NPs. Also the levels of 8-hydroxydeoxyguanosine (8-OH-dG) which is one of the most well studied biomarkers to measure the oxidative damage in DNA was evaluated in liver and bone marrow DNA and urine after the administration of metal oxide and Ag NPs. The urinary level of 8-OH-dG was significantly increased by the CuO at each time point of the urine analysis. Although the increases in the urinary levels of 8-OH-dG for the other nanoparticle treatments were not significant, all of the other metal compounds showed higher levels of urinary 8-OH-dG than the control. The 8-OH-dG levels in the bone marrow immediately increased after the injection of CuO, and continued to increase up to 24 h after administration. Also the 8-OH-dG levels in the liver DNA of the mice treated with 3 mg CuO were significantly higher than those in the non-treated control. The increase of 8-OH-dG levels in the liver DNA continued for 72 h after the administration of 1 and 3 mg doses of CuO. The other nanoparticles did not cause an increase in the liver 8-OH-dG level at 24 h after administration. Authors concluded that metal oxide nanoparticles can cause genotoxic effects *in vivo*. Among them, the CuO NPs were the most potent, iron oxide NPs also showed relatively high toxicity and TiO_2 and Ag NPs showed low toxicity.

3. Toxicity assessment of novel drug delivery systems

Lack of full toxicological knowledge about nanomaterials including novel drug delivery systems lead to the misperception regarding all nanomaterials pose a significant health risk. Under such realistic conditions, many engineered NPs are unlikely to induce adverse effects although effects of chronic and low level exposures are still largely unknown. Owing to extensive toxicological studies it will be possible to do exact risk assessment related with NPs.

Identification of potential health risks is a prerequisite for assessing the safety of the new products that are being developed. That is why, nanotoxicology area is gaining increasing importance with the growth of nanotechnological applications. Safety evaluation of nanomaterials through toxicological research will also provide information about their undesirable properties. These information will also help to avoid their possible adverse effects [7].

Toxicity studies on nanoparticles are generally conducted at very high doses. With high doses, any NP can be identified as toxic in living systems. A more realistic approach will be to discriminate high doses tested and tests under real exposure conditions. Therefore non *in vivo* assays for the purpose of extrapolating the responses to *in vivo* results may reduce and avoid a lot of laboratory animals. Beside occupational exposure to NP where they are produced and intentional use of consumer goods containing NP should be evaluated. With respect to nanomedicine, *in vivo* tests will always be mandatory for nanotechnology-based therapeutics and diagnostics [72].

As mentioned by Oberdorster [72], a tiered testing system to assess NP toxicity was suggested by a working group of the International Life Sciences Institute (ILSI) [73]. Table 2 lists the tiered testing strategy including **physico-chemical characterization prior to and during testing in cell-free, cellular** and *in vivo* **assays**. Studies designed to determine whether *in vitro* assays are predictive for *in vivo* effects have come to opposite conclusions.

4. Dose concepts in NP toxicology

Classical mass dose trend applied in conventional toxicological research may not be sufficient in nanotoxicological testing due to the extensively large surface area compairing with large particles. Oberdorster [74] studied the toxicity of ultrafine and fine TiO_2 measuring polymorphonuclear neutrophils in lung lavage fluid as an index of inflammation and they found ultrafine TiO_2 as more toxic than fine TiO_2 considering mass unit dose. When considered surface area, the toxicity was equivalent.

• **Physico-chemical characterization**
• **Cell-free assays** (solubility; ROS generating potential; chemreactivity; agglomeration/aggregation; zeta potential; other)
• **Cellular assays** [primary cells; cell-lines; (primary and secondary organs); co-cultures]
• **In vivo assays** [generally rodents; diverse methodologies (resp. tract; skin; GI-tract)]
• **Question**   Can any of the in vitro tests be used to predict in vivo toxicity?

Table 2. Tiered testing system to assess NP toxicity (ILSI Report) [73]

In vivo and *in vitro* test correlation is critical point in safety evaluations. The dose unit considered in the evaluations may affect the correlations between *in vitro* and *in vivo* tests directly. Say et al. studied fine and nanoparticle toxicity assessing in alveolar macrophages and a pulmonary epithelial cell line and then comparing them with the in vivo pulmonary inflammation induced by the same particles in rats [75]. They could not find a significant *in vitro – in vivo* correlation and suggested more sophisticated in vitro cell culture systems to gauge the relative toxicity of nanoparticles *in vivo*. When these results were analyzed according to the new approach suggested by Rushton et al. [76] who used NP surface area as a dose unit, the *in vitro* and *in vivo* results of Say et al. were correlated significantly.

5. Conclusion

As said by Oberdorster [72], nanotechnology, nanomedicine and nanotoxicology are closely related disciplines aimed at the improvement of human life. As a result of introducing of nanotechnology based nanomaterial into nanomedicine, novel and superior diagnostic, therapeutic and preventive systems have emerged. The safety assessment of these new materials is mandatory to recognize risks and avoid potential hazards. This assessment also provide useful information to avoid disinformation about the toxicity potential of nanosized systems. At this point nanotoxicology will have a crucial role. Material scientists, physicians, pharmacists and toxicologists should be included in nanotechnological developments as a team aproach.

As a result, it is important that safety assessments and health risks of novel drug delivery systems including nanomaterials should be made with the available and produced data. Nanomaterials should be evaluated on case-by-case basis in place of general evaluations for NPs.

Author details

Ahmet Aydın*, Hande Sipahi and Mohammad Charehsaz

Yeditepe University, Faculty of Pharmacy, Department of Toxicology, Istanbul, Turkey

6. References

[1] Society of Toxicology. SOT: Developing Safe Products Using Nanotechnology. http://www.toxicology.org (accessed 20 April 2012).

[2] European Science Foundation. ESF: Nanomedicine. http://www.esf.org (accessed 20 April 2012).

[3]] Garnett MC and Kallinteri P. Nanomedicines and Nanotoxicology: Some Physiological Principles. Occupational Medicine 2006;56:307–311.

[4] De Jong WH and Borm PJA. Drug Delivery and Nanopartciles. Applications and Hazards. International Journal of Nanomedicine 2008;3(2):133-149.

[5] Win KY, and Feng SS. *In Vitro* and *In Vivo* Studies on Vitamin E TPGS-emulsified Poly(D,L-lactic-co glycolic acid) Nanoparticles for Paclitaxel Formulation. Biomaterials 2006; 27:2285-91.

[6] Rangasamy M and Parthiban KG. Recent Advances in Novel Drug Delivery Systems. International Journal of Research in Ayurveda & Pharmacy 2012;1(2):316-326.

[7] Oberdörster G, Oberdörster E, and Oberdörster J. Nanotoxicology: An Emerging Discipline Evolving from Studies of Ultrafine Particles. Environmental Health Perspectives 2005; 113:823–839.

[8] Donaldson K, Aitken R, Tran L, Stone V, Duffin R, Forrest G, and Alexander A. Carbon Nanotubes: A Review of Their Properties in Relation to Pulmonary Toxicology and Workplace Safety. Toxicological Sciences 2006;92(1):5–22

[9] Dailey LA, Jekel N, Fink L, Gessler T, Schmehl T, Wittmar M, Kissel T, Seeger W. Investigation of The Proinflammatory Potential of Biodegradable Nanoparticle Drug Delivery Systems in The Lung. Toxicology and Applied Pharmacology 2006;215:100–108.

[10] Medina C, Santos-Martinez MJ, Radomski A, Corrigan OI and Radomski MW. Nanoparticles: pharmacological and toxicological significance. British Journal of Pharmacology 2007;150:552–558.

[11] Lademann J, Weigmann H, Rickmeyer C, Barthelmes H, Schaefer H, Mueller G, Sterry W. Penetration of Titanium Dioxide Microparticles in a Sunscreen Formulation Into The Horny Layer and The Follicular Orifice. Skin Pharmacology and Applied Skin Physiology 1999;12(5):247-56.

[12] Kreilgaard M. Influence of Microemulsions on Cutaneous Drug Delivery. Advanced Drug Delivery Reviews 2002;54 Suppl.1 S77–S98.

[13] Dey S, Bakthavatchalu V, Tseng MT, Wu P, Florence RL, Grulke EA, Yokel RA, Dhar SK, Yang H, Chen Y, and Clair DK. Interactions Between SIRT1 and AP-1 Reveal a

---

* Corresponding Author

Mechanistic Insight Into the Growth Promoting Properties of Alumina (Al2O3) Nanoparticles in Mouse Skin Eepithelial Cells. Carcinogenesis 2008;29(10):1920–1929.

[14] Knaapen AM, Borm PJA, Albrecht C, Schins RPF. Inhaled Particles and Lung Cancer. Part A: Mechanisms. International Journal of Cancer 2004;109:799–809.

[15] Fahmy B, Cormier SA. Copper Oxide Nanoparticles Induce Oxidative Stress and Cytotoxicity in Airway Epithelial Cells. Toxicology In Vitro 2009;23:1365–71.

[16] Lopez N, Norskov JK. Catalytic CO Oxidation by a Gold Nanoparticle: A Density Functional Study. Journal of American Chemical Society 2002;124:11262–3.

[17]] Jia'en Li J, Muralikrishnan S, Ng CT, Yung LYL and Bay BH. Nanoparticle-Induced Pulmonary Toxicity. Experimental Biology and Medicine 2010;235:1025-1033.

[18] Miura N, Shinohara Y. Cytotoxic Effect and Apoptosis Induction by Silver Nanoparticles in Hela Cells. Biochemical and Biophysical Research Communinations 2009;390:733-737.

[19] Hussain SM, Hess KL, Gearhart JM, Geiss KT, Schlager JJ. In Vitro Toxicity of Nanoparticles in BRL 3A Rat Liver Cells. Toxicology in Vitro 2005;19:975-983.

[20] Arora S, Jain J, Rajwade JM, Paknikar KM. Cellular Responses Induced by Silver Nanoparticles: in Vitro Studies. Toxicology Letters 2008;179:93-100.

[21] Choi JE, Kim S, Ahn JH, Youn P, Kang JS, Park K, Yi J, Ryu DY. Induction of Oxidative Stress and Apoptosis by Silver Nanoparticles in the Liver of Adult Zebrafish. Aquatic Toxicology 2010;100:151-159.

[22] Ramkumar KM, Manjula C, Gnanakumar G, Kanjwal MA, Sekar TV, Paulmurugan R, Rajaguru P. Oxidative Stress-Mediated Cytotoxicity and Apoptosis Induction by TiO2 Nanofibers in Hela Cells. European Journal of Pharmaceutics and Biopharmaceutics 2012;81:324-333.

[23] Gurr JR, Wang AS, Chen CH, Jan KY. Ultrafine Titanium Dioxide Particles in the Absence of Photoactivation Can Induce Oxidative Damage to Human Bronchial Epithelial Cells. Toxicology 2005;213:66–73.

[24] Hu RP, Zheng L, Zhang T, Cui YL, Gao GD, Cheng Z, Chen J, Tang M, Hong FS. Molecular Mechanism of Hippocampal Apoptosis of Mice Following Exposure to Titanium Dioxide Nanoparticles. Journal of Hazardous Materials 2011;191:32-40.

[25] Ma LL, Liu J, Li N, Wang J, Duan YM, Yan JY, Liu HT, Wang H, Hong FS. Oxidative Stress in the Brain of Mice Caused by Translocated Nanoparticulate TiO2 Delivered to the Abdominal Cavity. Biomaterials 2010;31:99-105.

[26] Liu HT, Ma LL, Liu J, Zhao JF, Yan JY, Hong FS. Toxicity of Nanoanatase TiO2 to Mice: Liver Injury, Oxidative Stress. Toxicological and Environmental Chemistry 2010;92:175-186.

[27] Long TC, Tajuba J, Sama P, Saleh N, Swartz C, Parker J, Hester S, Lowry GV, Veronesi B. Nanosized Titanium Dioxide Stimulates Reactive Oxygen Species in Brain Microglia and Damages Neurons in Vitro. Environmental Health Perspectives 2007;115:1631-1637.

[28] Sun Q, Tan D, Zhou Q, Liu X, Cheng Z, Liu G, Zhu M, Sang X, Gui S, Cheng J, Hu R, Tang M, Hong F. Oxidative Damage of Lung and its Protective Mechanisim in Mice Caused by Long-Term Exposure to Titanium Dioxide Nanoparticles. Journal of Biomedical Materials Research Part A 2012; DOI: 10.1002/jbm.a.34190.

[29] Valko M, Rhodes CJ, Moncol J, Izakovic M, Mazur M. Free Radicals, Metals and Antioxidants in Oxidative Stress-Induced Cancer. Chemico-Biological Interactions 2006;160:1-40.

[30] Li JJ, Hartono D, Ong CN, Bay BH, Yung LYL. Autophagy and Oxidative Stress Associated with Gold Nanoparticles. Biomaterials 2010;31:5996-6003.

[31] Jia HY, Liu Y, Zhang XJ, Han L, Du LB, Tian Q, Xu YC. Potential Oxidative Stress of Gold Nanoparticles by Induced-No Raleasing in Serum. Journal of the American Chemical Society 2009;131:40-41.

[32] Tedesco S, Doyle H, Blasco J, Redmond G, Sheehan D. Oxidative Stress and Toxicity of Gold Nanoparticles in Mytilus edulis. Aquatic Toxicology 2010;100:178-186.

[33] Willard MA, Kurihara LK, Carpenter EE, Calvin S, Harris VG. Chemically Prepared Magnetic Nanoparticles. International Materials Reviews 2004;49:125-170.

[34] Lee JH, Huh YM, Jun YW, Seo JW, Jang JT, Song HT, Kim S, Cho EJ, Yoon HG, Suh JS, Cheon J. Artificially Engineered Magnetic Nanoparticles for Ultra-Sensitive Molecular Imaging. Nature Medicine 2007;13:95-99.

[35] Rana S, Gallo A, Srivastava RS. Misra RK. On the Suitability of Nanocrystalline Ferrites as a Magnetic Carrier for Drug Delivery: Functionalization, Conjugation and Drug Release Kinetics. Acta Biomaterialia 2007;3:233-242.

[36] Sun C, Lee JH, Zhang M. Magnetic Nanoparticles in MR Imaging and Drug Delivery. Advanced Drug Delivery Reviews 2008;60:1252-1265.

[37] Chertok B, Moffat BA, David AE, Yu F, Bergemann C, Ross BD, Yang VC. Iron Oxide Nanoparticles as a Drug Delivery Vehicle for MRI Monitored Magnetic Targeting of Brain Tumors. Biomaterials 2008;29:487-496.

[38] Ahamed M, Akhtar MJ, Siddiqui MA, Ahmad J, Musarrat J, Al Khedhairy AA, AlSalhi MS, Alrokayan SA. Oxidative Stress Mediated Apoptosis Induced by Nickel Ferrite Nanoparticles in Cultured A549 Cells. Toxicology 2011;283:101-108.

[39] Johnston HJ, Hutchison, G, Christensen, FM, Peters, S, Hankin, S, Stone V. A Review of the in Vivo and in Vitro Toxicity of Silver and Gold Particulates: Particle Attributes and Biological Mechanisims Responsible for the Observed Toxicity. Critical Reviews in Toxicology 2010;40(4):328-346.

[40] Carlson C, Hussain SM, Schrand AM, Braydich-Stolle LK, Hess KL, Jones RL, Schlager JJ. Unique Cellular Interaction of Silver Nanoparticles: Size-Dependent Generation of Reactive Oxygen Species. Journal of Physical Chemistry B 2008;112:13608-13619.

[41] Park EJ, Yi J, Kim Y, Choi K, Park K. Silver Nanoparticles Induce Cytotoxicity by a Torjan-Horse Type Mechanism. Toxicology in Vitro 2010;24:872-878.

[42] Park EJ, Bae E, Yi J, Kim Y, Choi K, Lee SH, Yoon J, Lee BC, Park K. Repeated-Dose Toxicity and Inflammatory Responses in Mice by Oral Administration of Silver Nanoparticles. Environmental Toxicology and Pharmacology 2010;30:162-168.

[43] Warheit DB, Webb TR, Sayes CM, Colvin VL, Reed KL. Pulmonary Instillation Studies with Nanoscale TiO2 Rods and Dots in Rats: Toxicity is Not Dependent Upon Particle Size and Surface Area. Toxicological Sciences 2006;91:227–236.

[44] Warheit DB, Webb TR, Reed KL, Frerichs S, Sayes CM. Pulmonary Toxicity Study in Rats with Three Forms of Ultrafine-TiO2 Particles: Differential Responses Related to Surface Properties. Toxicology 2007;230:90–104.

[45] Chen HW, Su SF, Chien CT, Lin WH, Yu SL, Chou CC, Chen JJW, Yang PC. Titanium Dioxide Nanoparticles Induce Emphysema-Like Lung Injury in Mice. The Journal of the Federation of American Societies for Experimental Biology 2006;20:1732–1741.

[46] Jacobsen NR, Moller P, Jensen KA, Vogel U, Ladefoged O, Loft S, Wallin H. Lung Inflammation and Genotoxicity Following Pulmonary Exposure to Nanoparticles in ApoE-/- Mice. Particle and Fibre Toxicology 2009;6(2):1-17.

[47] Gosens I, Post JA, Fonteyne LJJ, Jansen EHJM, Geus JW, Cassee FR, Jong WH. Impact of Agglomeration State of Nano and Submicron Sized Gold Particles on Pulmonary Inflammation. Particle and Fibre Toxicology 2010;7(37):1-11.

[48] Cho WS, Cho M, Jeong J, Choi M, Cho HY, Han BS, Kim SH, Kim HO, Lim YT, Chung BH, Jeong J. Acute Toxicity and Pharmacokinetics of 13 nm-Sized PEG-Coated Gold Nanoparticles. Toxicology and Applied Pharmacology 2009;236:16-24.

[49] Downs TR, Crosby ME, Hu T, Kumar S, Sullivan A, Sarlo K, Reeder B, Lynch M, Wagner M, Mills T, Pfuhler S. Silica Nanoparticles Administered at the Maximum Tolerated Dose Induce Genotoxic Effects through an Inflammatory Reaction wile Gold Nanoparticles Do Not. Mutation Researh 2012;745:38-50.

[50] Song MF, Li YS, Kasai H, Kawai K. Metal Nanoparticle-Induced Micronuclei and Oxidative DNA Damage in Mice. Journal of Clinical Biochemistry and Nutrition 2012;50(3):211-216.

[51] Mroz RM, Schins RP, Li H, Jimenez LA, Drost EM, Holownia A, MacNee W, Donaldson K. Nanoparticle-driven DNA Damage Mimics Irradiation-related Carcinogenesis Pathways. European Respiratory Journal 2008;31:241–51.

[52] Li Y, Chen DH, Yan J, Chen Y, Mittelstaedt RA, Zhang Y, Biris AS, Heflich RH, Chen T. Genotoxicity of Silver Nanoparticles Evaluated Using the Ames Test and in Vitro Micronucleus Assay. Mutation Research 2012;745:4-10.

[53] Ahamed M, Karns M, Goodson M, Rowe J, Hussain SM, Schlager JJ, Hong Y. DNA Damage Response to Different Surface Chemistry of Silver Nanoparticles in Mammalian Cells. Toxicology and Applied Pharmacology 2008;233:404-410.

[54] Kim JS, Sung JH, Ji JH, Song KS, Lee JH, Kang CS, Yu IJ. In Vivo Genotoxicity of Silver Nanoparticles after 90-Day Silver Nanoparticles Inhalation Exposure. Safety and Health at Work 2011;2:34-38.

[55] Kim YS, Kim JS, Cho HS, Rha DS, Kim JM, Park JD, Choi BS, Lim R, Chang HK, Chang YH, Kwon IH, Jeong J, Han BS, Yu IJ. Twenty-Eight-Day Oral Toxicity, Genotoxicity and Gender-Related Tissue Distribution of Silver Nanoparticles in Sprague-Dawley Rats. Inhalation Toxicology 2008;20:575-583.

[56] Falck GC, Lindberg HK, Suhonen S, Vippola M, Vanhala E, Catalan J, Savolainen K, Norppa H. Genotoxic Effects of Nanosized and Fine TiO2. Human & Experimental Toxicology 2009;28:339-352.

[57] Rahman Q, Lohani M, Dopp E, Pemsel H, Jonas L, Weiss DG, Schiffmann D. Evidence that Ultrafine Titanium Dioxide Induces Micronuclei and Apoptosis in Syrian Hamster Embryo Fibroblasts. Environmental Health Perspectives 2002;110:797-800

[58] Türkez H, Geyikoglu F. An in Vitro Blood Culture for Evaluating the Genotoxicity of Titanium Dioxide: the Responses of Antioxidant Enzymes. Toxicology and Industrial Health 2007;23:19-23.

[59] Kang SJ, Kim BM, Lee YJ, Chung HW. Titanium Dioxide Nanoparticles Trigger p53-Mediated Damage Response in Peripheral Blood Lymphocytes. Environmental and Molecular Mutagenesis 2008;49:399-405.

[60] Wang JJ, Sanderson BJ, Wang H. Cyto- and Genotoxicity of Ultrafine TiO2 Particles in Cultured Human Lymphoblastoid Cells. Mutation Research 2007;28:99-106.

[61] Toyooka T, Amano T, Ibuki Y. Titanium Dioxide Particles Phosphorylate Histone H2AX Independent of ROS Production. Mutation Research 2012;742:84-91.

[62] Hackenberg S, Frichs G, Froelich K, Ginzkey C, Koehler C, Scherzed A, Burghartz M, Hagen R, Kleinsasser N. Intracellular Distribution, Geno- and Cytotoxic Effects of Nanosized Titanium Dioxide Particles in the Anatase Crystal Phase on Human Nasal Mucosa Cells. Toxicology Letters 2010;195:9-14.

[63] Hackenberg S, Friehs G, Kessler M, Froelich K, Ginzkey C, Koehler C, Scherzed A, Burghartz M, Kleinsasser N. Nanosized Titanium Dioxide Particles Do Not Induce DNA Damage in Human Peripheral Blood Lymphocytes. Environmental and Molecular Mutagenesis 2010,52:264-268.

[64] Landsiedel R, Ma-Hock L, Van Ravenzwaay B, Schulz M, Wiench K, Champ S, Schulte S, Wohlleben W, Oesch F. Gene Toxicity Studies on Titanium Dioxide and Zinc Oxide Nanomaterials Used for UV-Protection in Cosmetic Formulations. Nanotoxicology 2010;4:364-381.

[65] Kocbek P, Teskac K, Kreft ME, Kristl J. Toxicological Aspects of Long-Term Treatment of Keratinocytes with ZnO and TiO2 Nanoparticles. Small 2010,6:1908-1917.

[66] Warheit DB, Hoke RA, Finlay C, Donner EM, Reed KL, Sayes CM. Development of a Base Set of Toxicity Tests Using Ultrafine TiO2 Particles as a Component of Nanoparticle Risk Management. Toxicology Letters 2007;171:99-110.

[67] Theogaraj E, Riley S, Hughes L, Maier M, Kirkland D. An Investigation of the Photo-Clastogenic Potential of Ultrafine Titanium Dioxide Particles. Mutation Research 2007;634:205-219.

[68] Naya M, Kobayashi N, Ema M, Kasamoto S, Fukumuro M, Takami S, Nakajima M, Hayashi M, Nakanishi J. In Vivo Genotoxicity Study of Titanium Dioxide Nanoparticles Using Comet Assay Following Intratracheal Instillation in Rats. Regulatory Toxicology and Pharmacology 2012;62:1-6.

[69] Schulz M, Hock LM, Brill S, Strauss V, Treumann S, Groters S, Ravenzwaay BV, Landsiedel R. Investigation on the Genotoxicity of Different Sizes of Gold Nanoparticles Administered to the Lungs of Rats. Mutation Research 2012;745:51-57.

[70] Sharma V, Singh SK, Anderson D, Tobin DJ, Dhawan A. Zinc Oxide Nanoparticle Induced Genotoxicity in Primary Human Epidermal Keratinocytes. Journal of Nanoscience and Nanotechnology 2011;11(5):3782-3788.

[71] Sharma V, Anderson D, Dhawan A. Zinc Oxide Nanoparticles Induce Oxidative Stress and Genotoxicity in Human Liver Cells (HepG2). Journal of Biomedical Nanotechnology 2011;7(1):98-99.

[72] Oberdorster G. Safety Assessment for Nanotechnology and Nanomedicine: Concepts of Nanotoxicology. Journal of Internal Medicine 2010;267:89–105.

[73] Oberdorster G, Maynard A, Donaldson K, Castranova V, Fitzpatrick J, Ausman K, Carter J, Karn B, Kreyling W, Lai1 D, Olin S, Monteiro-Riviere N, Warheit D, Yang and A Report From the ILSI Research Foundation / Risk Science Institute Nanomaterial Toxicity Screening Working Group. Principles for characterizing the potential human health effects from exposure to nanomaterials: elements of a screening strategy. Particle and Fibre Toxicology 2005;2:8.

[74] Oberdorster G: Pulmonary Effects of Inhaled Uultrafine Particles. International Archives of Occupational and Environmental Health 2001;74:1-8.

[75] Sayes CM, Reed KL, Warheit DB. Assessing Toxicity of Fine and Nanoparticles: Comparing In Vitro Measurements to In Vivo Pulmonary Toxicity Profiles. Toxicological Sciences 2007; 97:163–80.

[76] Rushton EK, Jiang J, Leonard SS et al. Concept of assessing nanoparticle hazards considering nanoparticle dosemetric and chemical / biological response-mixes. Journal of Toxicology and Environmental Health, Part A 2010;73:445–461.

Permissions

The contributors of this book come from diverse backgrounds, making this book a truly international effort. This book will bring forth new frontiers with its revolutionizing research information and detailed analysis of the nascent developments around the world.

We would like to thank Ali Demir Sezer, for lending his expertise to make the book truly unique. He has played a crucial role in the development of this book. Without his invaluable contribution this book wouldn't have been possible. He has made vital efforts to compile up to date information on the varied aspects of this subject to make this book a valuable addition to the collection of many professionals and students.

This book was conceptualized with the vision of imparting up-to-date information and advanced data in this field. To ensure the same, a matchless editorial board was set up. Every individual on the board went through rigorous rounds of assessment to prove their worth. After which they invested a large part of their time researching and compiling the most relevant data for our readers. Conferences and sessions were held from time to time between the editorial board and the contributing authors to present the data in the most comprehensible form. The editorial team has worked tirelessly to provide valuable and valid information to help people across the globe.

Every chapter published in this book has been scrutinized by our experts. Their significance has been extensively debated. The topics covered herein carry significant findings which will fuel the growth of the discipline. They may even be implemented as practical applications or may be referred to as a beginning point for another development. Chapters in this book were first published by InTech; hereby published with permission under the Creative Commons Attribution License or equivalent.

The editorial board has been involved in producing this book since its inception. They have spent rigorous hours researching and exploring the diverse topics which have resulted in the successful publishing of this book. They have passed on their knowledge of decades through this book. To expedite this challenging task, the publisher supported the team at every step. A small team of assistant editors was also appointed to further simplify the editing procedure and attain best results for the readers.

Our editorial team has been hand-picked from every corner of the world. Their multi-ethnicity adds dynamic inputs to the discussions which result in innovative outcomes. These outcomes are then further discussed with the researchers and contributors who give their valuable feedback and opinion regarding the same. The feedback is then collaborated with the researches and they are edited in a comprehensive manner to aid the understanding of the subject.

Apart from the editorial board, the designing team has also invested a significant amount of their time in understanding the subject and creating the most relevant covers. They scrutinized every image to scout for the most suitable representation of the subject and create an appropriate cover for the book.

The publishing team has been involved in this book since its early stages. They were actively engaged in every process, be it collecting the data, connecting with the contributors or procuring relevant information. The team has been an ardent support to the editorial, designing and production team. Their endless efforts to recruit the best for this project, has resulted in the accomplishment of this book. They are a veteran in the field of academics and their pool of knowledge is as vast as their experience in printing. Their expertise and guidance has proved useful at every step. Their uncompromising quality standards have made this book an exceptional effort. Their encouragement from time to time has been an inspiration for everyone.

The publisher and the editorial board hope that this book will prove to be a valuable piece of knowledge for researchers, students, practitioners and scholars across the globe.

List of Contributors

Hamid Sadeghian
Department of Laboratory Sciences, School of Paramedical Sciences, Mashhad University of Medical Sciences, Mashhad, Iran

Atena Jabbari
Department of Chemistry, School of Sciences, Ferdowsi University, Mashhad, Iran

Amani M. Elsayed
Department of Pharmaceutics, Faculty of Pharmacy, Taif University, Taif, Saudi Arabia

Utkarshini Anand, Tiam Feridooni and Remigius U. Agu
Biopharmaceutics and Drug Delivery Laboratory, College of Pharmacy, Faculty of Health Professions, Dalhousie University, Halifax, NS, Canada

Yousef Javadzadeh and Sanaz Hamedeyazdan
Biotechnology Research Center and Faculty of Pharmacy, Tabriz University of Medical Sciences, Iran

Viness Pillay, Pradeep Kumar, Yahya E. Choonara and Lisa C. du Toit
University of the Witwatersrand, Faculty of Health Sciences, Department of Pharmacy and Pharmacology, Parktown, Johannesburg, South Africa

Girish Modi
University of the Witwatersrand, Faculty of Health Sciences, Division of Neurosciences, Department of Neurology, Parktown, Johannesburg, South Africa

Dinesh Naidoo
University of the Witwatersrand, Faculty of Health Sciences, Division of Neurosciences, Department of Neurosurgery, Parktown, Johannesburg, South Africa

Erdal Cevher and Emre Şefik Çağlar
Department of Pharmaceutical Technology, Faculty of Pharmacy, Istanbul University, Beyazıt, Istanbul, Turkey

Ali Demir Sezer
Department of Pharmaceutical Biotechnology, Faculty of Pharmacy, Marmara University, Haydarpaşa, Istanbul, Turkey

Keitaro Sou
Waseda University, Center for Advanced Biomedical Sciences, TWIns, Tokyo, Japan
Waseda University, Faculty of Science and Engineering, Tokyo, Japan

A. A. Onifade, B.H. Olaseinde and T. Mokowgu
Immunology Unit, Chemical Pathology Department, College of Medicine, University of Ibadan, Ibadan, Nigeria

Ahmet Aydın, Hande Sipahi and Mohammad Charehsaz
Yeditepe University, Faculty of Pharmacy, Department of Toxicology, Istanbul, Turkey

Printed in the USA
CPSIA information can be obtained
at www.ICGtesting.com
JSHW011420221024
72173JS00004B/605

9 781632 421197